OXFORD MEDICAL PUBLICATIONS

Young People
and
Physical Activity

Young People
and
Physical Activity

Neil Armstrong and Joanne Welsman

Children's Health and Exercise Research Centre
University of Exeter, UK

Oxford   New York   Melbourne   Toronto
OXFORD UNIVERSITY PRESS
1997

Oxford University Press, Great Clarendon Street, Oxford OX2 6DP

Oxford   New York

Athens   Auckland   Bangkok   Bogota   Bombay   Buenos Aires
Calcutta   Cape Town   Dar es Salaam   Delhi
Florence   Hong Kong   Istanbul   Karachi
Kuala Lumpur   Madras   Madrid   Melbourne
Mexico City   Nairobi   Paris   Singapore
Taipei   Tokyo   Toronto

and associated companies in
Berlin   Ibadan

Oxford is a trade mark of Oxford University Press

Published in the United States
by Oxford University Press Inc., New York

A catalogue record for this book is available from the British Library

Library of Congress Cataloging-in-Publication Data

Armstrong, Neil.
Young people and physical activity / Neil Armstrong and Joanne Welsman
p.   cm. — (Oxford medical publications)
Includes bibliographical references and index.
ISBN 0 19 262660 4 (Hbk)—ISBN 0 19 262659 0 (Pbk)
1. Exercise—Physiological effect.   2. Exercise for children.
3. Physical fitness for children.   I. Welsman, Joanne.   II. Title.   III. Series.
RJ133.A75   1997
613.7'042—dc20   96–26617 CIP

Typeset by
Advance Typesetting Ltd, Oxfordshire

Printed in Great Britain by Biddles Ltd, Guildford and King's Lynn

Preface

This book has been written for scientists, physicians, paramedics, teachers, lecturers, coaches, and students interested in the study of paediatric exercise science. An understanding of the basic principles of exercise physiology is assumed and the principal objective of the book is to provide a comprehensive, state of the art overview of the physiological responses to physical activity in young people. The dramatic increase in published research over the last decade precludes complete coverage of the topic but the book is extensively referenced to allow the reader to pursue areas of interest in more depth.

Children and adolescents are not mini-adults. They are growing and maturing at their own rate and their physiological responses to physical activity vary as they progress through childhood and adolescence into adult life. Part I provides a foundation and a framework for subsequent sections of the book by reviewing somatic growth and sexual maturation. Individual variation is emphasized and the effects of physical activity on aspects of growth and maturation are examined.

In Part II two chapters are devoted to discussion of the ethical, methodological, and conceptual problems of assessing and interpreting children's and adolescents' responses to exercise. In the light of these issues young people's aerobic and anaerobic performance is analysed in relation to chronological age, maturation, and sex.

Part III discusses the effects of physical activity on aspects of young people's health and well-being. The techniques available for the study of physical activity are critically examined and the current physical activity patterns of children and adolescents are reviewed. Subsequent chapters focus on physical activity in relation to aerobic fitness, muscular strength, coronary artery disease, body fatness, diabetes, skeletal health, and mental health. The final chapter in Part III describes problems which may arise through intensive participation in sport and exercise during childhood and adolescence.

The final section of the book addresses the issue of promoting physical activity. Biological, psychological, sociological, and environmental correlates of physical activity are examined, key role models are identified, and strategies for the promotion of active lifestyles are presented.

Throughout the text emphasis is placed upon critical analysis of the research literature and potential areas for further research are identified.

Much remains to be learned about young people's responses to physical activity, and if this book stimulates interest in paediatric exercise science and encourages other scientists to initiate research programmes devoted to the promotion of young people's health and well-being it will have served its purpose.

Exeter   N.A.
July 1996   J.W.

Acknowledgements

The origins of this book lie with the formation of the Coronary Prevention in Children Research Group of Neil Armstrong, John Balding, Peter Gentle, and Brian Kirby at Exeter University in 1985. Joanne Welsman joined the group as a research assistant in 1987. The Research Group developed into a Research Centre and many of the data reported here were generated by a Centre team of outstanding research students and technical staff. David Childs, Jenny Frost, and Sue Vooght merit special mention. Much of our research has been funded by the British Heart Foundation, the Northcott Devon Medical Foundation, the Darlington Trust, the Healthy Heart Research Trust, and the University of Exeter, and we gratefully acknowledge their support.

The staff of Oxford University Press advised and gently encouraged us to keep the book moving to completion. Alison Husband made it possible through her devoted and tireless secretarial efforts. Dr Alan Nevill and Dr Martin Lee commented eruditely on drafts of Chapters 3 and 13, respectively. We have enjoyed the intellectual stimulation provided by our friends in the European Pediatric Work Physiology Group and we have been particularly fortunate to have Dr Brian Kirby as mentor as he has provided us with unwavering support and inspiration for over a decade.

Finally, without the 2500 young people who have visited the Research Centre and willingly given their time, blood, and energy we could not have indulged ourselves in the exciting study of the exercising child and adolescent. To them we dedicate this book with the hope that it will make a contribution to promoting young people's health and well-being.

Acknowledgements

The origins of this book lie with the formation of the Collingian Division in...

Contents

PART I
Physical activity: growth and maturation

'Physical activity', 'exercise', and 'physical fitness' are terms which are often used interchangeably, but this can be confusing as they are not synonymous. Physical activity is a complex set of behaviours which encompasses any bodily movement, produced by skeletal muscles, that results in energy expenditure above the resting level.[317] Physical activity is therefore a component of total energy expenditure, which also includes resting metabolism, the thermic effect of food, and growth.[131]

Exercise is a subcategory of physical activity that is planned, structured, repetitive, and often results in the improvement or maintenance of one or more of the components of physical fitness.[316] Exercise training is the systematic use of exercise of specific intensities, durations, and frequencies to attain a desired effect. The principles of exercise training are described in Table III.1, p. 100.

Physical fitness is a concept which refers to a set of attributes that relate to the ability to perform physical activity.[316] It is extremely difficult to define and we have some empathy with Professor Karpovich who once commented that, 'physical fitness is the ability to pass physical fitness tests'. However, physical fitness may be usefully conceived as ten separate components grouped into two broad categories.[363, 364] In this taxonomy agility, balance, reaction time, speed and co-ordination are the skill-related aspects of physical fitness. Aerobic fitness, muscular strength, muscular endurance, flexibility, and body fatness are the health-related concepts. We define the components of health-related fitness in Table III.2, p. 101.

As young people grow they also mature but although the concepts are related they are probably under separate genetic regulation.[1503] Maturation refers to the tempo and timing of progress towards the mature biological state.[967] For example, sexual maturity is reproductive capability and skeletal maturity is a fully ossified skeleton. Maturation differs from growth in that although biological systems mature at different rates all individuals reach the same endpoint and become fully mature.[5] Growth refers to an increase in the size of the body or any of its parts and there may be wide variations in endpoints such as stature. Growth does not cease when maturity is attained but continues throughout life as in almost all tissues and organs there is a recurring cycle of growth, death, and replacement. Individual parts of the body do not necessarily grow at the same rate and therefore the relative size and mass of tissues and organs change through the life cycle. Variations in growth and maturation have profound effects upon aspects of physical activity, physical fitness, and physical performance.

The term 'development' is commonly used in association with growth and maturation but it often refers to a broader concept which includes the behavioural as well as the biological domain. Growth, maturation, and development interact with one another but may operate on different time-scales. A young person's social or emotional development may be well advanced, although their biological growth and/or maturation are delayed, or vice versa. This book focuses on the biological domain but reference is made to behavioural processes where appropriate. The role of physical activity in promoting mental health and well-being is discussed in Chapter 13 and some behavioural issues are addressed in Part IV where we discuss the promotion of physical activity.

The first year of life is called 'infancy' with 'childhood' being defined as the period from the first birthday to the onset of puberty.[967] For a myriad of reasons which will emerge throughout the text few secure data are available on the responses of young children to physical activity and, with some notable exceptions, the extant literature focuses on children of eight years of age and above.

'Puberty' refers to the somatic and physiological changes that occur in young people as the gonads change from the infantile to the adult state. It is not complete until the individual becomes functionally capable of producing a child.[979] Puberty is triggered by the neuro-endocrine system and produces a number of changes not directly related to sexual function. These include the adolescent growth spurt, the appearance of secondary sexual characteristics, and alterations in body composition. Adolescence is sometimes used to refer to the psychological changes associated with puberty[1504] but as the literature still refers to the 'adolescent growth spurt' in this text we will adopt the convention of using 'adolescence' synonymously with 'puberty'.

In England, puberty is recognized in law as having been reached by the age of 12 years for girls and 14 years for boys[1403] but in biological terms it is extremely difficult to categorize puberty in relation to chronological age because of the wide individual variations in onset, progress through puberty, and completion. Chronological age is often used as a point of reference for growth and maturation but the fact that individual biological clocks do not run in accord with the calendar cannot be ignored, especially when trying to interpret the influence of physical activity on physical performance, physical fitness, or health.

Having clarified key terms and concepts which will be used throughout the text, Part I will focus on somatic growth and sexual maturation to provide a framework for subsequent chapters.

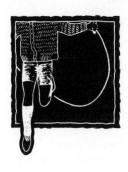

1

Physical activity: somatic growth and sexual maturation

Somatic growth

Somatic growth is characterized by individual variation both between and within sexes. It is under neuroendocrine and genetic control but influenced by environmental factors. The complex interaction of hormones involved in the regulation of somatic growth during childhood and adolescence has been debated at length[221, 1178, 1229, 1230, 1565] but may be summarized as follows.

Growth hormone (GH) from the anterior pituitary and somatomedins, which are produced primarily in the liver, play a central role in maintaining normal growth during childhood. GH is released in a pulsatile manner throughout the day although the largest pulses occur during sleep. The amount of GH in circulation increases from childhood through adolescence, reaching its maximum coincident with peak rate of growth in stature (standing height). GH plays an important metabolic role in mobilizing lipids from adipose tissue and therefore sparing carbohydrates, but its effects on linear growth are mediated by somatomedins. The release of somatomedins is stimulated by GH and they in turn stimulate the linear growth of long bones and therefore increases in stature.

The actions of GH and somatomedins do not occur in isolation and thyroid hormones and insulin from the pancreas are necessary for the full effects of GH to be expressed. Calcitonin and parathyroid hormone regulate circulating calcium which is essential for normal skeletal growth and maturation (see Chapter 12 for a discussion). Adrenocorticosteroids are also necessary for optimal growth and maturation but excess secretion of adrenocortical hormones during childhood causes a stunting of growth in stature.

During adolescence both androgens and oestrogens promote skeletal growth and maturation (see later in this chapter for a discussion of their effects on sexual maturation). Androgens (e.g. testosterone) have a much more potent effect than oestrogens on linear growth of bones and this is related to the greater skeletal growth of boys. Testosterone underpins the male adolescent spurt in muscle mass (see Chapter 8) whereas oestrogens have a less marked effect on protein anabolism and the blunted female increase in muscle mass is primarily due to adrenal androgens.

In boys, but apparently not in girls, increased secretion of gonadal and adrenal sex steroids causes an increase in GH secretion and inevitably an enhanced stimulation of somatomedins.[967, 1226] This effect helps to explain some of the sex differences in growth described in this chapter.

Table 1.1. Overview of hormones involved in somatic growth and sexual maturation

Hormone	Origin	Principal effects
Growth hormone (GH)	Anterior pituitary	Stimulates somatic growth mediated by somatomedins. Mobilizes lipids, spares carbohydrates
Follicle-stimulating hormone (FSH)	Anterior pituitary	Stimulates oestrogen production in girls and sperm production in boys
Luteinizing hormone (LH)	Anterior pituitary	Stimulates oestrogen production and triggers ovulation in girls. Promotes testosterone production in boys
Adrenocorticotrophic hormone	Anterior pituitary	Promotes secretion of androgens and glucocorticoids from adrenal cortex. Mobilizes lipids, spares carbohydrates
Thyroxine and triiodothyronine	Thyroid	Augments the effects of GH. Stimulates metabolic rate
Calcitonin	Thyroid	Decreases circulating calcium, important in skeletal growth and maturation
Parathyroid hormone	Parathyroids	Increases circulating calcium, important in skeletal growth and maturation
Glucocorticoids	Adrenal cortex	Mobilize lipids, increase blood glucose concentration. Depress inflammatory and immune responses
Mineralocorticoids	Adrenal cortex	Regulate sodium and potassium homeostasis
Androgens	Adrenal cortex	Promote growth and maturation

cont'd

Hormone	Origin	Principal effects
Insulin	Pancreas	Augments the effects of GH. Decreases the concentration of blood glucose
Glucagon	Pancreas	Increases the concentration of blood glucose
Somatomedins	Liver	Stimulate the linear growth of long bones
Testosterone	Testes (also adrenal cortex)	In boys, promotes sexual and skeletal maturation, bone growth, adolescent spurt in muscle mass
Oestrogens	Ovaries (also adrenal cortex)	In girls, promotes sexual and skeletal maturation and accumulation of body fat

Stature

The most obvious change from birth to adulthood occurs in stature and because of the relative ease of its measurement stature is the most widely used indicator of growth. The difficulties in accurately measuring stature and related anthropometric variables should not, however, be underestimated.[921, 1247, 1611] In addition, stature varies during the course of the day being greatest in the morning and decreasing throughout the day. 'Shrinkage' occurs as a result of the force of gravity compressing the fibrous discs of cartilage that separate the vertebrae. The diurnal variation may be as much as 1–2 cm, even in children.[967, 1403] Nevertheless, all young people follow the same pattern of growth from infancy through adolescence but there are significant individual differences in both timing and magnitude of change in stature. Figure 1.1 describes a typical rate of gain (or velocity of growth) in stature.

During infancy body length increases by about 25 cm and in the second year another 12–13 cm or so are added so that by the age of two years the child has attained about 50% of adult stature. Thereafter there is a steady deceleration of growth down to a rate of about 5–6 cm per annum before the initiation of the adolescent growth spurt. The adolescent growth spurt has been described by fitting curves to a series of measurements taken on the same young people at different ages.[e.g. 185, 191, 1397] Despite the methodological nuances of using different curve-fitting techniques[183] valuable information on the time of onset of the spurt and the peak rate of growth (peak height velocity, PHV) has emerged.[183, 968, 979] In longitudinal studies PHV

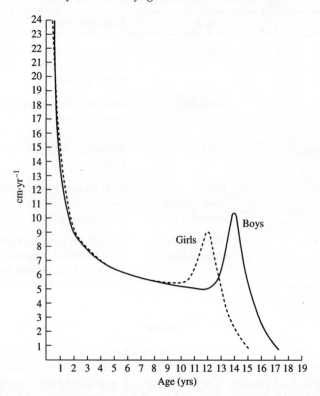

Fig. 1.1. Typical individual curves for stature in boys and girls. From Tanner, J.M., Whitehouse, R.J. and Takaishi, M. (1966). Standards from birth to maturity for height, weight, height velocity and weight velocity: British children, 1965–1. *Archives of Disease in Childhood*, **41**, 454–71. Reprinted with permission.

has often been used as a marker of somatic maturity and other variables of interest (e.g. peak oxygen uptake) have been examined in relation to PHV.[808, 1041, 1280] Beunen and Malina[183] have provided a comprehensive critique of the extant literature.

In the Western world girls are, on average, in advance of boys by about 2 years with the onset of their spurt occurring between about 8.5 and 10.3 years of age and PHV being reached between 11.4 and 12.2 years. Corresponding ages for boys are 10.3–12.1 years and 13.4–14.4 years.[968] There is, however, considerable variation among individual children in both the timing of the initiation of the spurt and the timing and magnitude of PHV. Very early maturing boys may reach PHV at 12.0 years having initiated their spurt at about 10.5 years, while very late maturers may begin their spurt at 14.5 years, and reach PHV at about 16 years. Corresponding variation occurs in girls and there is therefore some overlap between boys and girls.[1504]

The average boy increases in stature by about 7 cm in the first year of his adolescent growth spurt, by about 9 cm in the second year, and by about 7 cm in the final year. After this, the rate of growth rapidly decreases to about 3 cm in the year following the spurt and to around 2 cm in subsequent years until adult stature is attained at about 18 years of age. In girls, the velocity of growth is somewhat lower, perhaps 6, 8, and 6 cm per year during the three year period of the spurt. Girls attain their adult stature at about 16 years of age.

Up to the initiation of the adolescent growth spurt there is little difference between the average stature of boys and girls. Because their spurt normally begins earlier girls are often taller than boys by the age of 11 years although the balance is usually redressed by 14 years of age. The sex difference in adult stature is, on average, 13 cm but this is primarily due to the boys experiencing two extra years of preadolescent growth at 5 cm per year. The difference in magnitude of the growth spurt being only about 3 cm.

Correlations between the size of the individual as a child and as an adult (autocorrelations) provide some insight into the genetics of growth. During infancy there is little relationship between current and adult stature and correlations between the child's length and his/her parents' stature are generally low. From the age of 2–3 years until the onset of puberty growth tracks quite well and autocorrelations between current stature and adult stature may be as high as $r = 0.8$. Correlations between stature measured during adolescence and adult stature decline relative to those during childhood. This is due to individual variation in the timing, duration, and magnitude of the adolescent growth spurt which appears to be under different genetic regulation. The overall genetic effects on stature are not fully understood but it has been estimated that the contribution of the genotype to adult stature is about 60%.[967] Tall children do not always have tall parents but they have a tendency to do so.

Body mass

Body mass triples during infancy and by the end of the second year it has quadrupled. From about the age of 2 years there is a slight, but constantly accelerating, rate of increase in mass prior to the adolescent growth spurt. The spurt in mass is similar to that in stature but normally occurs from 0.2–0.4 year later in boys and 0.3–0.9 year later in girls (Fig. 1.2). The difference is related, in part, to sex differences in body composition.[183] The spurt in boys' body mass is primarily due to gains in skeletal tissue and muscle mass with fat mass remaining relatively stable. Girls experience less dramatic rises in skeletal tissue and muscle mass but a continuous rise in fat mass. Boys gain, on average, 43.8 kg between the ages of 7 and 18 years while girls experience an increase in mass of about 33.5 kg over the same time period.[371, 1370]

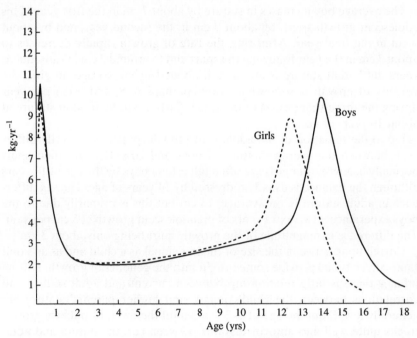

Fig. 1.2. Typical individual curves for body mass in boys and girls. From Tanner, J.M., Whitehouse, R.J. and Takaishi, M. (1966). Standards from birth to maturity for height, weight, height velocity and weight velocity: British children, 1965–1. *Archives of Disease in Childhood*, **41**, 454–71. Reprinted with permission.

Muscle mass comprises about 25% of body mass at birth. It increases with chronological age and marked sexual differences become apparent during and after the adolescent growth spurt. Peak muscle growth velocity occurs later than PHV and is often coincidental with the peak velocity of shoulder width. Girls also experience an adolescent spurt in muscle mass but it is much less dramatic than that of boys. Relative muscle mass increases from 42–54% of body mass in boys between 5 and 17 years. In girls, it increases from 40–45% of body mass between 5 and 13 years and then, in relative terms, declines after 13 years of age due to the increase in fat accumulation during adolescence.[967] We return to the growth of muscle mass in relation to strength in Chapter 8.

At birth, 10–12% of total body mass is fat. During childhood girls have only slightly more body fat than boys, perhaps 18% and 16% of body mass, respectively, at the age of 8 years.[559] During the adolescent growth spurt, girls' body fat increases to about 25% of body mass while boys decline to about 12–14% body fat.[664, 968] This extra fat may be advantageous to girls in some situations. It aids buoyancy, it helps to maintain body temperature and provides a significant energy store. However, in activities which require moving body mass on land girls are generally penalized for carrying excess fat mass. The increase in body fat during puberty contributes to the changing shape of the female adolescent and subsequent alterations in centre of gravity. These adaptations may adversely affect performance in activities such as gymnastics which may have been taken up several years earlier with a very different body shape and strength to mass ratio. In Chapter 10 we address physical activity and body fatness.

Young children have a relatively large body surface area in relation to their mass, and the ratio between the two diminishes with increasing age. The implications of changes in body size and the relationship between body mass and surface area are discussed in detail in Chapter 3 and developed in relation to aerobic function, anaerobic function, and muscular strength in Chapters 4, 5, and 8, respectively.

Other dimensions

Most body dimensions follow a growth curve similar to that of stature but there is wide variation in timing of growth spurts. During infancy, trunk length is the fastest growing component of stature but from then until puberty the legs account for 66% of the total increase in stature. Growth in leg length ceases earlier than growth in trunk length and trunk growth, therefore, makes a greater contribution to increase in stature during the adolescent growth spurt. During early adolescence, young people have relatively long legs but the appearance of long-leggedness disappears with the subsequent increase in trunk length. For a short period in early adolescence, the leg length of girls tends to be slightly longer than that of boys. By the age of 12 years boys have normally surpassed girls in leg length but they do not catch up with girls in trunk length until about 14 years of age. The longer period of preadolescent growth in boys is largely responsible for the fact that men's legs are longer than women's in relation to trunk length.[967, 979, 1504]

The hands and feet accelerate their growth first, then the calf and forearm, followed by the hips and chest, and then the shoulders. There is, therefore, a transient stage where some youngsters have relatively large hands and feet, but by the time the adolescent spurt has ended, hands and feet are a little smaller in proportion to arms, legs, and stature. The timing and speed of these changes may have dramatic effects on several aspects of physical performance.

At puberty, differences in body shape become apparent between the sexes and perhaps the most obvious concerns the shoulders and hips. Girls have greater hip (bicristal) breadths than boys from middle childhood but the difference becomes more marked during adolescence. The differential growth of the female pelvis, which causes it to become wider, shallower, and roomier than the male pelvis is one of the reasons why older girls tend to throw out their heels when they run, as their thighs have to create a greater angle to bring their knees together. Boys catch up to girls in bicristal breadth in late adolescence and the sex difference in young adulthood is negligible compared to that of biacromial (shoulder) breadth. With the possible exception of the ages 10–12 years, boys have greater shoulder breadth than girls at all ages, but the difference becomes readily apparent following boys' marked adolescent spurt in biacromial breadth. Boys gain about twice as much in shoulder breadth compared to hip breadth during the spurt, whereas there is only a small difference in the amount gained in the two breadth dimensions in girls.[967, 1504]

As even small differences in shoulder breadth can result in large differences in upper trunk muscle, this partially explains why strength differences between older boys and girls are much greater in the upper body than in the legs. When greater upper body muscle mass is combined with the greater leverage of longer arms, one of the reasons for boys' generally better performances in throwing, rowing, and racquet sports becomes readily apparent. The relative broadening of the hips in girls lowers their centre of gravity. This provides greater stability and may be the primary reason why girls normally have better balance than boys.

Sexual maturation

The detailed endocrinology of sexual maturation has been well documented[1503, 1504, 1613] but it can be summarized as follows.

During childhood serum concentrations of the gonadotrophic hormones follicle-stimulating hormone (FSH) and luteinizing hormone (LH) are low and stable, with much overlap between girls and boys. Late in childhood, the hypothalamus stimulates the anterior pituitary gland to release FSH and LH and circulating concentrations begin to rise first in girls, reflecting their earlier onset of puberty, and then in boys. The first sign of the onset of puberty is an increase in LH secretion during sleep, which gradually extends into the waking part of the day as puberty progresses. In girls, just before menarche, FSH and LH develop a cyclic pattern related to the menstrual cycle but their production remains fairly constant in boys with the attainment of sexual maturity.

In boys, LH stimulates the production and secretion of testosterone by the testes and FSH stimulates sperm production. In girls, FSH and LH are responsible for ovulation and stimulation of oestrogen by the ovaries. Testosterone and dihydrotestosterone, an androgen which is derived from testosterone, are responsible for the enlargement of the testes, penis, scrotum, seminal vesicles and prostate, voice changes, and the growth and coarseness of pubic, axillary, and facial hair during male sexual maturation. Oestrogens—oestradiol is the most potent—stimulate the growth and maturation of females' primary and secondary sexual characteristics including ovaries, uterus, vagina, fallopian tubes, external features of the female genitalia, breasts, and pubic and axillary hair.

Androgens and oestrogens also have effects on muscle growth, fat accumulation, and skeletal maturation and these are discussed in Chapters 8, 10, and 12, respectively.

Secondary sex characteristics

Tanner[1503] described a five-point scale with which to assess the development of breasts in girls, genitalia in boys, and pubic hair in both sexes (Table 1.2). The scale is normally used in conjunction with a series of appropriate photographs which are available in several texts.[e.g. 967, 1503] There is some lack of precision in the technique as an individual in say, the early phase of stage 3 breast development is rated the same as an individual in the late phase of this stage and there is no consistent relationship between rate of progress through the stages. Nevertheless, Tanner staging provides a useful method of estimating maturity in cross-sectional studies and a valuable framework upon which to hang our discussion of sexual maturation.

The sequence of events through which adolescents pass is not exactly the same for each individual but it is much less variable than the time at which events occur. For example, some adolescents will complete their genital development in less than 2 years, while others may take five or more years to complete the process.[979]

The first sign of puberty in boys is usually the enlargement of the testes accompanied by changes in the texture and colour of the scrotal skin. The penis then begins to enlarge and pubic hair to appear. Data reported in Malina and Bouchard's[967] comprehensive text suggests that boys normally enter genitalia stage two (G2) within the age range 11.0–12.4 years and pubic hair stage two (PH2) within the age range 12.2–13.4 years. G5 is reached in the range 14.6–17.3 years and PH5 in the range 14.9–16.1 years. In comparison, PHV normally occurs within the age range 13.8–14.1 years when most boys are in G4 and PH4. At about the same time the voice change (breaking of the voice) begins and is completed about 1 year later. The first ejaculation of semen during wakefulness has been reported to occur between the ages of 12.5 and 16.5 years. Axillary hair normally appears about 1.5–2 years after pubic hair and facial hair occurs about 1 year later. Occasionally, however, axillary hair may appear before the onset of pubic hair and the relationship between facial hair and axillary hair is also variable.[979] The development of both pubic hair and genitalia is normally complete before hair grows on the chin.[1503] These data clearly

Table 1.2. Secondary sex characteristics

Stage	Pubic hair development (boys and girls)	Genital development (boys)	Breast development (girls)
1	No true pubic hair	Testes, scrotum, and penis same size and proportion as early childhood	Elevation of papilla only
2	Sparse growth of long slightly pigmented downy hair, straight or only slightly curled	Enlargement of scrotum and testes and reddening and change in texture of scrotal skin. Little or no enlargement of penis	Elevation of breast and papilla as a small mound. Enlargement of areolar diameter
3	Considerably darker, coarser, and more curly hair spreading over the pubic symphysis	Increase in penis length, smaller increase in breadth. Further growth of scrotum	Further enlargement and elevation of breast and areola
4	Adult-type hair but covering smaller area with no spread to medial surface of thighs	Further increase in both length and breadth of penis, development of glans. Further enlargement of testes and scrotum with darkening of scrotal skin	Areola and papilla further enlarged forming a secondary mound above level of the breast
5	Adult in quantity and type distributed in an inverse triangle. It has spread to the medial surface of thighs but not up the linea alba or elsewhere above the base of the triangle*	Adult in size and shape. No further enlargement of penis takes place	Adult stage with projection of papilla but recession of areola to breast contour. Secondary mound present in stage 4 no longer present

* Stage 5 is the endpoint of adolescent growth in pubic hair but in about 80% of men and 10% of women pubic hair spreads beyond the triangular pattern. This point is rarely reached before the mid twenties and may be rated as stage 6.

Adapted from Tanner, J.M. (1962). *Growth at Adolescence*. Oxford, Blackwell, pp. 32–7, and Marshall, W.A. and Tanner, J.M. (1986). Puberty. In F. Falkner and J.M. Tanner (Eds.), *Human Growth, volume 2*. London, Plenum Press, pp. 180–8.

illustrate the individual variation in entering, progressing through and completing male adolescence.

Similar variability is seen in the onset, progression, and completion of female adolescence. The first event is normally the appearance of the breast bud (breast stage two, B2). Pubic hair usually appears a little later but in about one-third of girls pubic hair appears before the breast bud. The sequences of pubic hair and breast development show considerable independence so, of girls in B3, 25% may be in PH1 and 10% in PH5.[1503] The range of ages reported by Malina and Bouchard[967] for the onset of B2 is 10.6–11.4 years and for the onset of PH2, 10.4–12.1 years. B5 is reached in the range 13.7–15.6 years and PH5 in the range 13.9–15.2 years. PHV normally occurs within the age range 11.5–12.1 years. Menarche occurs relatively late in puberty, on average between 12.8 and 13.5 years.[967] It is independent of other pubertal characteristics and although most girls are in B4 and either PH3 or PH4 some may still be in B2 and/or PH1. Menarche is, however, closely associated with PHV although the hormonal significance of this is unknown. Almost all girls experience menarche when velocity in stature is falling and menarche tends to occur at the time of maximum deceleration of growth and stature.[1504]

Maturity indicators

In the exercise sciences maturity is usually assessed using one or more of the indicators of somatic (PHV), sexual (e.g. Tanner staging), or skeletal (see Chapter 12) maturity. There is a variation among these indicators and no single measure gives a complete description of the tempo of growth and maturation through childhood and adolescence. Nevertheless, they seem to be sufficiently associated with one another for each to indicate a general maturity factor during adolescence.[182, 958]

The technique of choice probably varies with the study design and all methods have their limitations. The determination of skeletal age is relatively expensive and the ethics of exposing children to repeated radiation must be considered very carefully[143] (and see Chapter 2). The use of PHV as a maturational marker is limited to longitudinal studies and requires frequent measurements if meaningful results are to be obtained.[183] Tanner staging is probably the method of choice in cross-sectional studies but it lacks precision and although there are no potential side-effects it may be personally embarrassing to young people. In order to prevent embarrassment some investigators have asked the subject to assess his/her own sexual maturity using Tanner staging photographs[466, 1090] but the validity of this approach remains to be proven. Correlations between adolescents' self-assessment and physicians' assessments have ranged from $r = 0.63$–0.93 for girls and $r = 0.59$–0.88 for boys.[1226] In our laboratory we have found the self-report maturity assessment of 11–13-year-olds to have little relationship with the assessment of an experienced nurse.

Serum or salivary levels of adrenal (e.g. dehydroepiandrosterone sulphate, DHEA-S) and gonadal (e.g. testosterone) androgens have been related to pubertal status,[285, 1322] including Tanner staging.[3] Their use as indicators of sexual maturity in the exercise sciences is appealing[758, 1623] but large diurnal fluctuations and inter-individual variation limit the precision in estimating pubertal status. Androgen levels may, however, be useful in confirming the prepubescent state of children.[758, 871] Similarly, age at menarche is a convenient marker of sexual maturity but it is only capable of dividing girls into pre- and post-menarcheal state. [e.g. 205]

Physical activity and somatic growth

Malina[952, 953, 955, 959, 960, 963, 964] has published a series of excellent papers which comprehensively review and periodically update the data relating physical activity and exercise training to growth. We will sample selectively from these reviews and readers requiring more detail are referred to the original papers.

Early studies of the effects of physical activity on somatic growth suggested an increase in stature with exercise training.[186, 1350] The observed changes were, however, quite small and subject selection and maturity status were not controlled. A later study[1251] offered a conflicting view and noted that participants in an interscholastic touch football programme, though taller, gained less in stature over a 2 year period, between the ages of 14 and 16 years, than non-participants. Several subsequent reports[925, 1130, 1196] concluded on the basis of these data that exercise training may slow down growth in stature. However, as the original author reported,

since the athletic group is composed of boys who have matured earlier, age considered, than the group of non-athletic boys, the athletic boy is not going to grow as much as the non-athletic boy over the period studied.[1251, p. 115]

it is likely that the observed differences in growth rates simply reflected maturity status.

More recent longitudinal studies from Belgium[184, 185] and Canada[1041, 1042] provide some insights into the association of physical activity with growth. The Belgian study followed 32 active and 32 inactive boys from 12–18 years of age. Active boys were those who participated in sport activities for more than 5 h·wk^{-1} during the first 3 years of the study in addition to compulsory school physical education classes of between 1 and 3 h·wk^{-1}. Inactive boys participated in less than 1.5 h·wk^{-1} of sport activities in addition to compulsory physical education. In the Canadian study 14 active boys were compared with 11 inactive boys from 10–16 years of age. The boys were classified active or inactive on the basis of activity questionnaires, teacher assessment of activity level, and a sport participation inventory. Active and inactive Canadian and Belgian boys did not differ in stature, in ages at PHV, or in PHV, which suggests that growth is not influenced by level of physical activity either positively or negatively.

Data on young athletes need to be considered in the context of the often extremely selective criteria applied to the sport, including selection according to characteristics associated with early maturity in some sports[245] and late maturity in others.[689] When this is taken into account both longitudinal[962, 965, 1356, 1446] and cross-sectional[291, 335] data indicate that the size attained by young athletes in a whole range of sports does not appear to be affected by intensive training. We can therefore endorse Malina's[964] conclusion that,

allowing for population variability, sample size, and variations in descriptions of habitual physical activity and training for sport, the data suggest that regular physical activity, sport participation, and training for sport has no effect on attained stature, timing of PHV, and rate of growth in stature.[964, p. 765]

Physical activity and sexual maturation

Successful young female athletes tend to be delayed in menarche and the possibility that exercise training may delay sexual maturation has been comprehensively debated.[1171, 1228, 1619, 1711] In contrast, boys who are successful in youth sports tend to be advanced in maturation.[154, 245, 552] The explanation may lie in preselection for specific sports. Boys participate more in team games and sports which depend upon strength and power, the boy with delayed pubertal development is therefore at a distinct disadvantage. Conversely, the characteristics associated with delayed adolescent maturation in females may be more suitable for performance in activities popular with girls, such as gymnastics and dance.[154, 953, 964] Late maturing girls tend to be more linear in shape, longer-legged, narrower hipped, and less fat than their early maturing peers. It has been suggested that early maturing girls may be socialized away from sports competition whereas late maturing girls may not experience these pressures and may even have increased motivation to compete based on early success in their sport.[1228]

The literature describing menarcheal age in selected groups of female athletes is extensive.[954, 978, 1450, 1593] Many of the studies, however, rely on small sample sizes and retrospective, questionnaire-based data. Factors such as dietary restriction, sleep patterns, family size, training load, and sport-specific selection criteria are rarely considered.[150, 1171] The association between menstrual dysfunction and intensive participation in competitive sport is developed further in Chapter 14 but we will explore possible explanations for a relationship between sexual maturation and physical activity in both boys and girls in the following sections.

Physical activity and the critical mass—critical fat hypothesis

This often cited hypothesis, proposed by Frisch and her associates,[584-587] postulated that a certain level of body mass (about 48 kg) or body fatness (about 17%) is necessary for menarche, and because exercise training, especially if combined with dietary restriction, causes a reduction in body mass or body fat it may delay menarche. Although still widely quoted in the popular press Frisch's work has been severely criticized on both methodological and statistical grounds.[1619] In brief, her method of estimating body fatness was indirect and lacked the necessary precision to define a critical fat level and her interpretation of associational data as causative cannot be sustained. Furthermore, subsequent studies have been unable to verify the hypothesis and the available evidence does not support the view that menarche is triggered by a set weight or body composition.[191, 295, 372, 494]

Physical activity and hormonal mechanisms

Malina[958, 950, 960] has suggested that the association between exercise training and delayed menarche may be hormonal. He has proposed that intensive training, and perhaps an associated energy drain, alter circulating levels of gonadotrophic and ovarian hormones, and in turn, delay menarche. Although the theory is plausible hormonal data on prepubertal and pubertal athletes are sparse. Furthermore, observations are usually based upon single assessments of hormone levels in plasma or serum. This raises several methodological problems as hormones are normally episodically secreted and it is unlikely that single samples are representative of 24 h levels of circulating hormones. The presence of a hormone does not necessarily imply that it is biochemically active and there is variation in tissue responsiveness in maturing children. The target cells must be capable of responding for a hormone to have any effect.[958]

Low resting levels of LH and FSH but normal levels of prolactin and thyroid-stimulating hormone have been observed in 12–15-year-old ballet dancers who were delayed in menarche and breast development but not in pubic hair. Progression in sexual maturation occurred during times of decreased activity.[1593] Lower plasma levels of oestrone, testosterone, and androstenedione have been reported in 11-year-old gymnasts compared with swimmers of the same age and prepubertal status but the two groups did not differ in concentrations of gonadotrophins or DHEA-S.[1154] The fact that prepubertal gymnasts and swimmers had similar levels of DHEA-S although the gymnasts had been training longer than the swimmers does not support the suggestion that training prolongs the prepubertal stage.[247]

In small samples of 13–18-year-old swimmers basal oestradiol levels were shown to differ between pre- and post-menarcheal groups at the start of a 24 week training programme. Levels in both groups decreased during the first 12 weeks, and were followed by a rise after 24 weeks. Overall, the oestradiol levels of the premenarcheal swimmers after 24 weeks were not different from at the start of the programme but a lower basal level than pre-training was noted in post-menarcheal girls following the 24 week training programme. Both groups had similar basal plasma levels of adrenocorticotrophic hormone (ACTH), cortisol, prolactin, and testosterone throughout the programme.[304] On the basis of these results it is difficult to implicate exercise training as a causative factor of delayed sexual maturity in girls.

Endurance running is associated with reduced testosterone levels in adult males[1642] but this may not be the case in adolescent boys[1267] and it has been suggested that testosterone metabolism in adolescents may not be comparable with that in adults.[108] Basal levels of testosterone and ACTH were monitored over two competitive seasons in male swimmers, aged 12–16 years, reported changes were variable and within the normal physiological range.[305] In a group of non-athletes, classified according to Tanner's stages, no differences in postmaximal exercise concentrations of serum GH or testosterone were detached.[530] These results suggest that, in males at least, no critical pubertal stage with enhanced hormonal response to exercise exists.

Physical activity and sleep

Sleep apparently plays a role in the maturation process. The pulsatile release of LH is associated with the number of sleep cycles in late prepubertal or early pubertal children and deep sleep affects the release of GH. Exercise training during the day presumably encourages longer sleep and more slow-wave sleep but anxiety related to competition may adversely affect sleep patterns.[960, 1124] In the waking state competition-related stress has been associated with both increased and decreased LH concentrations.[1368] The effects of any interaction between exercise training and sleep on hormonal responses remain unclear and require further study before firm conclusions can be drawn.

There is no convincing evidence for permanent alterations in reproductive function following intensive exercise training[1520] and, on the basis of the available data, we must conclude that the case for physical activity as a causative factor in altering the rate of sexual maturity remains to be proven. We revisit these issues in Chapter 14.

Summary

All young people follow the same pattern of somatic growth from infancy through adolescence but it is characterized by individual variation, both between and within sexes, in the timing and magnitude of changes. Girls tend to experience the onset of puberty about two years in advance of boys and for a short period are often taller and heavier than boys. At puberty differences in body shape become readily apparent between the sexes and boys experience marked increases in muscle mass. These changes can have dramatic effects on physical performance.

The sequence of events through which all adolescents pass during sexual maturation is similar but the timing at which events occur and the rate of progression through stages have wide individual variations. Some young people may be sexually mature whilst others of the same chronological age are still waiting for the onset of puberty.

A number of maturity indicators have been identified and they have been used extensively in the exercise sciences. No single measure gives a complete description of the tempo of growth and maturation but skeletal, somatic, and sexual maturity indicators appear to be sufficiently associated with one another for each to provide an indication of maturity during adolescence.

Physical activity, specifically exercise training, has been associated with both somatic growth and sexual maturity. The data are, however, not extensive and any influence of physical activity or exercise training on the rates or endpoints of somatic growth or sexual maturation remains to be proven.

PART II
Aerobic and anaerobic exercise

All forms of physical activity involve muscular contraction and for this to occur energy generated during the breakdown of high-energy phosphates is required. The intramuscular stores of the principal high-energy phosphate, adenosine triphosphate (ATP), are limited and for muscular contraction to be sustained for more than a few seconds ATP must be resynthesized. There are three energy systems through which ATP may be generated. Two of these do not require oxygen and are therefore termed 'anaerobic energy systems' the third system is dependent upon the presence of oxygen and is termed the 'aerobic system'.

At the onset of maximal exercise ATP is resynthesized from an intramuscular reservoir of another high-energy phosphate, creatine phosphate. If maximal exercise continues for longer than a few seconds, energy provision from the second anaerobic system (glycolysis) increases. Here, glucose or glycogen is degraded to pyruvate via a complex series of enzymatic reactions which result in the production of ATP.[1101] Near the beginning of exercise, when oxygen consumption is low, and during intensive exercise when pyruvate production exceeds the capacity of the aerobic energy system to oxidize it, excess pyruvate is reduced to lactate. Intramuscular lactate production causes lactate to accumulate in the blood where it can be measured relatively easily and used in the assessment of both aerobic and anaerobic performance (see Chapters 2, 4, and 5).

The oxygen transport system is relatively slow to adapt to the demands of exercise and the rate at which ATP can be generated anaerobically greatly exceeds that of the aerobic energy system. The aerobic system is, however, the most efficient system in terms of ATP production and, because of its ability to use pyruvate, free fatty acids (FFA), and amino acids as substrates, it has a much greater capacity for energy generation than the anaerobic systems.[1101] Prolonged exercise therefore depends upon the ability to deliver oxygen to the muscles. However, during physical activity no single energy system operates in isolation and the relative intensity and duration of the activity dictates which system is the predominant provider of ATP.

Data quantifying stores of energy substrates in children and adolescents are scarce and data from girls are almost non-existent. Concentrations of muscle ATP and creatine phosphate similar to those of adults have been reported in boys aged 11–13 years although a progressive increase in high-energy phosphate (phosphagen) stores from 11–16 years of age has also been indicated.[512, 518] During exercise of the same relative intensity the rate of phosphagen depletion appears similar in children compared to adults,[513, 514] suggesting that children are as capable as adults of high-intensity, short duration exercise where energy requirements are fuelled almost exclusively by the high-energy phosphates.

Data from muscle biopsy studies indicate that children and adolescents are less able than adults to generate energy from glycolysis. Muscle glycogen stores (mmol·kg^{-1} wet weight) in 11–12-year-old boys are less than 70% of those in adults and increase progressively to adult levels throughout adolescence.[514] The rate of glycogen utilization during exercise at near maximal exercise is also lower in boys than in adults and is reflected by lower intramuscular lactate levels.[518, 521, 525] As discussed in Chapter 2, the use of invasive techniques to investigate the intramuscular environment in healthy children is now generally considered unethical. This has imposed limitations upon the expansion of our understanding of energy metabolism in the growing child although recent advances in [^{31}P]-magnetic resonance spectroscopy[1323, 1707] may help to clarify the development of these characteristics.

The physiological and metabolic responses of the adult to exercise have been well documented and appropriate protocols for the assessment of aerobic and anaerobic exercise performance are well established.[675, 936] Comparatively less is known about the exercising child although there are sufficient data to confirm that the young person cannot be considered a 'mini-adult'. Apparatus, techniques, and protocols designed to assess the aerobic and anaerobic performance of adults are rarely directly applicable to children and adolescents. In Chapter 2 we discuss the many methodological problems associated with the measurement of young people's aerobic and anaerobic performance and suggest appropriate protocols which accommodate the physical, physiological, and metabolic differences between children, adolescents, and adults.

In order to understand the growth and maturation of aerobic and anaerobic performance differences in body size must be accounted for. It is conventional to express performance measures in simple ratio with body mass. In Chapter 3 we highlight the theoretical limitations of this convention and explore the validity of alternative statistical methods of removing the influence of body size and mass from measures of physiological performance.

In the light of the ethical, methodological, and conceptual issues surrounding the interpretation of children's and adolescents' aerobic and anaerobic responses to exercise, these performance characteristics are examined in Chapters 4 and 5 respectively with reference to sex, age, and maturation. Chapter 5 also explores the trainability of anaerobic performance in children and adolescents and the relationships between aerobic and anaerobic performance during this period. The response of aerobic fitness to training is discussed in Chapter 7.

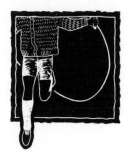

2
Measurement of aerobic and anaerobic exercise

Ethical considerations

The involvement of children and adolescents in experimental research within the exercise sciences raises clear ethical issues: in essence, the researcher must consider whether the experimental procedures they wish to use are ethical in young subjects, and whether the value of the knowledge gained outweighs the risks, either physiological or psychological, to the young subject.[1255] Such issues have been debated at length and the consensus view is that there is no general legal or ethical bar to the participation of children and adolescents in non-therapeutic research (i.e. research which is of no direct benefit to the young person).[1683, 1684] Notwithstanding this position, children should only be involved when the information required is unobtainable from similar investigations with adults. Issues regarding the provision of 'informed consent' to participate in a research project are somewhat less clear as, in some countries, there are no legal guidelines regulating the age at which children and adolescents can consent for themselves, or the parent on their behalf. Therefore, both the parent and the young person should provide written consent, and the researcher must consider carefully the maturity and independence of the child or adolescent and the likely expectations of their parents. It is, of course, essential that the young person is a willing participant in any project and coercion from any party must be guarded against. It has been recommended that experimental procedures should place the young person at no more than negligible risk of harm (i.e. no greater than the risks of harm ordinarily encountered in daily life). Procedures suggested to represent 'negligible risk'[1684] are summarized in Table 2.1.

Measurement of peak aerobic performance

Maximal or peak oxygen uptake?

The rate at which muscles can generate energy from aerobic metabolism depends upon the ability of the pulmonary, cardiovascular, haematological, and cellular mechanisms to transport oxygen from the atmosphere to the contracting muscles and the ability of the tissues to use oxygen to catabolize

Table 2.1. Experimental procedures representing 'negligible risk' to young people

---

- Observation of behaviour

- Physical examinations

- Changes in diet

- Non-invasive physiological monitoring

- Obtaining blood and urine samples

---

fuels.[1523] Maximal oxygen uptake ($\dot{V}O_{2\,max}$), the highest rate at which an individual can consume oxygen during exercise, limits the capacity to perform aerobic exercise and is therefore widely accepted as the best single index of aerobic fitness.[98]

$\dot{V}O_2$ plateau criterion

The increase in oxygen uptake with increasing exercise intensity was originally demonstrated in a series of experiments carried out by Hill and co-workers.[720, 721] They reported a linear relationship between $\dot{V}O_2$ and running speed up to a critical velocity beyond which further increases in running speed were not matched by a corresponding increase in $\dot{V}O_2$. As the subject was able to continue exercising at intensities beyond the plateau in $\dot{V}O_2$, it was assumed that the additional energy requirements were being satisfied by anaerobic metabolism with consequent lactate accumulation and eventual exhaustion. Although investigators have questioned the theoretical[1108] and methodological[1080] validity of the $\dot{V}O_2$ plateau concept, its demonstration during a progressive exercise test to exhaustion continues to be the criterion most frequently used to establish $\dot{V}O_{2\,max}$.[102, 1080, 1523]

During an incremental exercise test to exhaustion, it is rare for an absolute levelling in $\dot{V}O_2$ to be observed, therefore, several less rigorous definitions of a plateau have been proposed (Table 2.2). The most commonly applied criterion with children is the requirement for an increase in $\dot{V}O_2$ of ≤ 2.0 mL·kg^{-1}·min^{-1} for a 5–10% increase in exercise intensity.[1377]

Clearly, some plateau definitions are more stringent than others and there is the added complication that criteria based upon a per body mass ratio may not represent a consistent relative $\dot{V}O_2$ increase in individuals of differing body size (see Chapter 3). Many children complete a laboratory exercise test to exhaustion without demonstrating a $\dot{V}O_2$ plateau regardless of the definition applied. In those studies which have tested large numbers

Table 2.2. Criteria for defining a $\dot{V}O_{2\,max}$ plateau

---

- An increase in $\dot{V}O_2$ less than 150 mL·min⁻¹ or 2.1 mL·kg⁻¹·min⁻¹ with a 2.5% increase in treadmill speed[1510]

- A rise in $\dot{V}O_2$ of less than 2 standard deviations below that of the mean of changes between previous exercise intensities[1045]

- An increase in $\dot{V}O_2$ of less than 5% over the final stages of the exercise test[485, 1212]

- An increase in $\dot{V}O_2$ of ≤2.0 mL·kg⁻¹·min⁻¹ for a 5–10% increase in exercise intensity[1377]

---

of untrained subjects, around 30–50% of children achieve a plateau during cycle ergometer or treadmill testing.[85, 98, 804, 1212]

The absence of the classical $\dot{V}O_2$ plateau in the majority of children at maximal exercise raises questions as to whether the values elicited are truly maximal. Several studies have failed to identify significant differences in the maximal values for $\dot{V}O_2$ obtained from subjects demonstrating a plateau compared with those who do not.[359, 383, 1216] Others have actually noted significantly higher values for $\dot{V}O_2$ in the non-plateau group.[77, 804] As a result of these studies it has become more usual, and arguably more appropriate, to define the highest oxygen uptake achieved during a test to voluntary exhaustion as *peak* $\dot{V}O_2$ rather than $\dot{V}O_2$ *max* which implies that a plateau in $\dot{V}O_2$ has been demonstrated.[69, 81] Recent studies have confirmed this view by measuring children's $\dot{V}O_2$ during exhaustive exercise at intensities beyond those completed during an initial peak $\dot{V}O_2$ test.[84, 1263] We exercised 10-year-old boys and girls to exhaustion, on two separate occasions, at the same treadmill speed but at 2.5% and 5% higher gradients than achieved during a previously completed peak $\dot{V}O_2$ test. These 'supramaximal' bouts failed to elicit significant increases in $\dot{V}O_2$ confirming that a plateau is not a necessary prerequisite for maximal aerobic performance in young people.[84]

Several investigators have sought explanations for children's failure to demonstrate $\dot{V}O_2$ plateaux during exercise to exhaustion. Rowland[1256] has suggested that metabolic differences between adults and children prevent young people from generating the required additional energy from anaerobic metabolism. This is supported by indications of increased anaerobic metabolism, such as a higher respiratory exchange ratio (RER) (the ratio of carbon dioxide expired to oxygen consumed; $\dot{V}CO_2/\dot{V}O_2$), and blood lactate, in children and adolescents who consistently demonstrate a $\dot{V}O_2$ plateau in repeated testing compared to those who do not.[383] Considerable evidence exists to refute this with several studies failing to observe significant differences in post-exercise blood lactates between plateau and non-plateau groups.[77, 84, 98]

Others have investigated the theory that the demonstration of a plateau is related to leg muscle mass. In subjects studied longitudinally,[804] a $\dot{V}O_2$ plateau was associated with both lower peak $\dot{V}O_2$ and smaller leg muscle mass as determined from anthropometric measures. It was suggested that subjects with higher leg muscle mass were less likely to reach a plateau as a result of reduced vasoconstriction during uphill treadmill running thus permitting a continued upward drift in $\dot{V}O_2$. However, these conclusions are confounded by the application in this study of a 150 mL·min^{-1} plateau criterion which would not be equally stringent across the age range studied (12–21.5 years) considering the range of body size this represents. Recent data from our laboratory, using magnetic resonance imaging (MRI) to assess thigh muscle volume, indicate no effect of muscle volume on the demonstration of a plateau in 10-year-old girls[1671] and boys (unpublished data).

Although it has been suggested that better test to test reliability is achieved when a $\dot{V}O_2$ plateau is observed[383] the weight of evidence indicates that peak $\dot{V}O_2$ measured using a jogging or running protocol is as reliable in young people as $\dot{V}O_{2\,max}$ is in adult groups.[213, 1146, 1216]

Secondary criteria

Increasingly, investigators are questioning the validity of the $\dot{V}O_2$ plateau as the principal criterion of maximal aerobic exercise. Although it has been suggested that a plateau criterion for defining $\dot{V}O_{2\,max}$ can be used in very active children[174] others have argued that alternative termination criteria may be more applicable.[72, 1214] The termination of maximal exercise tests with young people is usually dictated by the point of voluntary exhaustion (i.e. when the individual is unwilling or unable to continue exercising despite strong verbal encouragement).[81] Signs of intense effort include, unsteady gait, hyperpnoea, sweating, facial flushing, and grimacing. With well-habituated subjects and experienced laboratory staff, such subjective signs of exhaustion provide valuable confirmation of maximal effort in young subjects.[72]

Secondary criteria for establishing maximal effort based upon heart rate, RER, and blood lactate are frequently applied in the absence of a $\dot{V}O_2$ plateau.[81, 851, 1262] A problem arises in recommending target values for these parameters which are applicable throughout childhood and adolescence. The formula, 220 minus age, provides a reasonably accurate prediction of maximal heart rate for adults but is of limited use with young subjects as maximal values remain fairly stable throughout childhood and adolescence. In our laboratory we have recorded heart rates at peak $\dot{V}O_2$ ranging from 185–225 beats per minute (bpm) in prepubertal children and adolescents.[84, 85] Mean maximal heart rates close to 200 bpm are frequently reported during treadmill running[85, 98, 1332] hence the recommendation that a target heart rate of 200 bpm be set to confirm maximal effort in children.[81, 1262] In view of the variability of maximal heart rate during childhood, the pitfalls of such a recommendation for the evaluation of individual test results are obvious. Here, the additional proviso that heart rate should level off over the final exercise stages[81] may be a useful guideline.

The RER provides an indication of exercise effort. During the initial stages of a progressive exercise test, values approximating 0.8 are typical, rising to exceed 1.0 in adults at $\dot{V}O_{2\,max}$. It has been recommended that, in children and adolescents, a value of 0.99^{1262} or 1.0^{81} should be observed at peak $\dot{V}O_2$. Examination of published literature indicates a considerable range in the RER achieved by young people at peak $\dot{V}O_2$, signalling caution with the application of a single, specific criterion. Values ranging from 0.99^{1146}–1.1^{1214} have been reported. As is the case with adults, cycle ergometry typically elicits higher RER in young people, with typical values ranging from 1.06–1.11.[213, 1271]

In addition to the influence of the exercise modality, both RER and heart rate may be affected by the test protocol[379, 1215] further confounding the issue. The proposal that age-specific criteria of peak $\dot{V}O_2$ be developed[1214] appears untenable in the light of both the methodological influences upon and the considerable individual differences observed in peak exercise responses. The recommendation for individual laboratories to develop their own norms for defining maximal effort[1262] may be more practicable than the rigid adoption of published criteria but it is essential that authors clearly report the termination criteria used to enable others to interpret the data. In the presence of clear subjective indications that a child has performed maximally, heart rate and RER do provide the investigator with valuable confirmatory markers.[72]

High post-exercise blood lactate levels are often used with adults as a subsidiary criterion of peak $\dot{V}O_2$, with values of 8–10 mmol·L^{-1} reported as indicative of maximal effort.[102] A similar criterion has been suggested for use with children although a lower target value of 6 mmol·L^{-1} [378, 851, 1494] has been set in order to accommodate children's typically lower blood lactate responses to exercise (see Chapter 4). Post-exercise blood lactate in children and adolescents is, however, probably the least reliable marker of maximal effort during a single test as large inter-individual differences are evident. Levels at peak $\dot{V}O_2$ may range from less than 4.0 mmol·L^{-1} to in excess of 13 mmol·L^{-1}. [72, 378, 1658] Many methodological factors influence the level of post-exercise blood lactate, including the mode of exercise and protocol employed, the timing of post-exercise sampling relative to the cessation of exercise, and the lactate sampling and assay procedures employed.[1622, 1659] These issues are discussed later in this chapter.

Estimation of peak oxygen uptake from submaximal and performance tests

Tests which enable peak $\dot{V}O_2$ to be predicted from submaximal responses are particularly attractive with young subjects as the individual is not required to exercise to exhaustion. The most frequently used procedure is the prediction of peak $\dot{V}O_2$ from a single submaximal heart rate and the corresponding $\dot{V}O_2$ or power output using the Astrand nomogram.[102] Unfortunately, this nomogram was derived from adult responses to exercise and its applicability to children and adolescents is limited. Cardiopulmonary responses to exercise in young people differ from those in adults and the use of the Astrand nomogram with young subjects generally results in large errors[193, 276] and may underestimate directly measured peak $\dot{V}O_2$ by as much as 26%.[1689]

The limitations of using maximal performance tests such as the 12 min run and the more recently popularized 20 m progressive shuttle run are well documented.[40, 43] Such tests are more a reflection of factors such as the environment, the individual's pace judgement, running economy, and motivation to perform maximally than peak $\dot{V}O_2$. Other authors have remarked that the prediction of peak $\dot{V}O_2$ from an endurance run is little better than a prediction based upon measures of stature, mass, and skinfolds,[376] or is a complicated way of identifying tall or fat children.[1377] The laboratory determination of peak $\dot{V}O_2$ appears to be the only valid measure of children's and adolescents' peak aerobic fitness.[81]

Laboratory determination of peak oxygen uptake

Ergometers

The majority of published data on the peak $\dot{V}O_2$ of children and adolescents are derived from either cycle ergometer or treadmill exercise. Both modes of exercise have advantages and disadvantages and the choice ultimately depends upon considerations of cost and the nature of any ancillary measures investigators wish to make.[1379]

Although previously popular, particularly for the prediction of peak $\dot{V}O_2$ from submaximal data, the step bench is now rarely used to determine peak $\dot{V}O_2$, except in remote areas,[324] and its limitations for maximal testing are readily apparent. Exercise intensity depends upon step frequency, step height, and the subject's body mass. Children's relative lack of body mass combined with the local muscle fatigue experienced during stepping means that the test is rarely terminated by cardiopulmonary insufficiency. Furthermore, to be effective, subjects must step up and down in time with a consistent rhythm which many children find difficult. Consequently, peak $\dot{V}O_2$ may be 25–30% lower than that elicited during treadmill exercise.[81]

Cycle ergometry has the advantages of being a portable, relatively cheap, and less noisy mode of exercise than treadmill ergometry and it may induce less anxiety in young subjects.[1262] Care must be taken to ensure that the ergometer is suitably modified to accommodate children's smaller body size,[739] for example, by altering the length of the pedal cranks and saddle pillar. There is considerably less upper body movement during cycling which greatly facilitates the measurement of heart rate, blood pressure, and blood lactate during exercise. Children may, however, experience difficulty in maintaining the required pedal rhythm[739] and it is easy to voluntarily slacken pace in the latter stages of a test making it difficult to elicit peak $\dot{V}O_2$. Peak $\dot{V}O_2$ determined during cycle ergometry is typically 8–10% lower than treadmill determined values.[67, 85, 213] Treadmill running engages a larger muscle mass than cycling with the result that the peak $\dot{V}O_2$ obtained is more likely to be limited by central rather than peripheral factors.[1375, 1379] In cycling there is greater specific involvement of the quadriceps muscle[799] and the effort required to push the pedals is high in relation to muscle strength,[727] resulting in increased anaerobic metabolism as blood flow through the quadriceps is restricted.[792] Muscle lactate accumulation eventually terminates the exercise test before the limits of the cardiovascular system are reached.

As a result of these limitations, the treadmill is the most appropriate mode of exercise for most paediatric testing but in situations where a mobile[803] or temporary laboratory is established by necessity, for example in a school[85, 450] cycle ergometry may well provide the only practical mode of exercise.

Protocols

Several standardized exercise protocols, such as Balke, Bruce, James, or MacMaster protocols, are widely used for paediatric exercise testing in clinical settings with published norms available for various subject groups regarding the expected number of stages completed. see [1262] The majority of research laboratories have developed their own protocols which are suited to the specific aims of their investigations and are appropriate for required ancillary measures. Progressive exercise tests to exhaustion may be either continuous or discontinuous as the measurement of peak $\dot{V}O_2$ has been shown to be protocol-independent.[379, 1414] Continuous tests with exercise stages of 1 or 2 min reduce the total duration of the test, an important factor when considering the shorter attention span of young children. Discontinuous tests may be more practical when repeated submaximal measures such as blood lactate or cardiac output are required. The duration of each incremental stage may vary according to whether or not near steady-state measures of $\dot{V}O_2$ and blood lactate are required. Although children characteristically increase $\dot{V}O_2$ rapidly at the onset of exercise (see Chapter 4) and reach a near steady-state within 2 min, it may take up to 3 min for blood lactate to appropriately reflect the exercise intensity.[1656]

The majority of studies with healthy children and adolescents employ a running protocol whilst in clinical situations a walking protocol may be preferable. It is well documented that walking protocols may elicit significantly lower peak $\dot{V}O_2$ than running protocols.[1146, 1374]

Diurnal and seasonal variation in peak oxygen uptake

Few studies have attempted to quantify diurnal or seasonal variation in young people's peak $\dot{V}O_2$. A study of twelve 13–16-year-olds[375] reported no significant differences in peak $\dot{V}O_2$ determined six times in the morning and six times in the afternoon. A subsequent study by the same author[376] failed to identify any significant seasonal effect upon peak $\dot{V}O_2$ in Canadian youngsters. In contrast, Astrand[99] recorded improvements in young Swedes' 'working capacity' over the school year with a deterioration during the summer vacation. Data from a study reporting high springtime values of peak $\dot{V}O_2$ in boys[383] are difficult to interpret due to the subjects' involvement in training and competition. Other studies have both supported[1387] and refuted[803, 1381] seasonal variation but in view of the consistency of peak $\dot{V}O_2$ values observed in the world literature, the influence of seasonal or diurnal variation may be considered minimal.

Measurement of anaerobic performance

Documentation of the development of anaerobic performance in young people is scarce compared with the abundant literature describing the development of aerobic power. Data describing the anaerobic characteristics of girls are notably lacking. This may, in part, be attributed to the lack of standardized, valid, and reliable testing protocols with which to assess young people's anaerobic performance.[144] Whilst protocols for anaerobic performance assessment are well established and validated for adults[231] their application to children and adolescents is less secure.

The *power* of an energy system refers to the maximal amount of energy which may be generated from that system during maximal exercise per unit time. The *capacity* of a given system refers to the total amount of energy available within the system to perform maximal exercise.[231] Tests of anaerobic performance fall broadly into two categories: (1) those that attempt to measure power, for example, the Margaria Step and Force–Velocity Tests;[975, 1084] and (2) those that assess the total capacity of a system such as the Cunningham and Faulkner Treadmill Test[382] and the estimation of the maximal accumulated oxygen deficit (MAOD).[1020] Some tests, such as the Wingate Anaerobic Test (WAnT),[110] attempt to assess both peak and mean power. The main advantages and limitations of anaerobic performance tests are summarized in Table 2.3.

Table 2.3.   Tests for anaerobic performance: advantages and limitations

Test	Characteristic measured	Advantages	Limitations
Wingate Anaerobic Test (WAnT)	Peak power and mean power	Can be adapted to measure arm or leg performance	Resistance does not allow optimization of both peak and mean power
		Safe and easy to administer with young people	Considerable aerobic component
		Moderate to good correlations with field performance	Not specific to many sporting activities
			Heavily reliant upon subject motivation
Margaria Step Test (MST)	Peak power	Does not require expensive equipment	Requires good co-ordination to perform optimally
Force–Velocity Test	Peak power	Optimized power output derived from a series of values	Not well validated with children and adolescents
Cunningham and Faulkner Treadmill Test	Maximal anaerobic capacity	Mode of exercise reflects many sports activities	Duration of test indicates a high aerobic contribution
			Heavily reliant upon subject motivation
Maximal Accumulated Oxygen Deficit (MAOD)	Maximal anaerobic capacity	Less sensitive to motivational factors than other tests of anaerobic capacity	Questionable assumption of linearity between $\dot{V}O_2$ and exercise intensity at supramaximal intensities

Test protocols for the measurement of anaerobic performance

The Wingate Anaerobic Test (WAnT)

The WAnT was developed at the Wingate Institute in Israel in the mid 1970s[110] based upon a prototype introduced by Cumming.[377] The test consists of a 30 sec maximal effort on a cycle ergometer against a constant mechanical force. Although predominantly used to determine the anaerobic performance of the legs, the test is easily modified for upper body assessment using arm-cranking.[141, 231] The majority of information regarding children's anaerobic performance to date is derived from this test or a modification of it.

Variables typically measured during the test include: peak power, the highest power output recorded in any 5 sec period, the mean power sustained over 30 sec, and the rate of fatigue (percentage drop in power output from the highest to lowest value). Peak power was previously assumed to reflect the maximal rate of energy generation from the phosphagen system but the demonstration of the rapid involvement of glycolysis with consequent lactate accumulation in the very early stages of the test[756] suggests that it may be preferable to consider peak power as a reflection of the ability of the leg muscles to produce high mechanical power in a short time period.[141] Similarly, mean power is no longer presumed to reflect the capacity of the glycolytic system, as the duration of the test may be insufficient to truly exhaust the mechanisms for glycolytic energy generation.[1315, 1566] Mean power is thus considered a measure of the ability to sustain high power output (i.e. muscular endurance).[141]

The optimal braking force (resistance) should elicit the highest values possible for both peak and mean power[141] but since the introduction of the WAnT it has proved difficult to establish definitive guidelines for appropriate resistances for athletic and non-athletic adults and even more problematic for young subjects. Originally set as 75 g·kg^{-1} (0.74 N·kg^{-1})[1] for a lower limb assessment on a Monark ergometer[110] this resistance has been shown to be too low to optimize adults' performance. Several studies have identified mean resistances ranging from 85–98 g·kg^{-1} to elicit the highest mean power in adults[455, 528, 1148] with a higher resistance required to maximize peak power.[455, 1148]

The limitations of setting a mass-related resistance when performance on the test is better related to muscle mass or fat-free mass[141] are readily apparent. Identification of an appropriate resistance is a particular problem during growth and maturation due to the changes in body composition that occur during this time (see Chapter 1). Few studies have investigated the optimal resistance required for children but, on a Monark ergometer,

---

[1] Although the correct SI unit for force is the newton (N), within this text we have continued with the convention of reporting WAnT resistances in g·kg^{-1} to avoid confusion with the extant literature.

values for active but non-athletic 13–14-year-old boys of 70 g·kg⁻¹ and 67 g·kg⁻¹ for girls have been reported.[455]

In an attempt to circumvent some of the problems associated with the application of a standardized resistance for all subjects, several studies have determined the optimal resistance to elicit peak power for individual subjects from a force–velocity test (described below) completed prior to the WAnT.[534, 1560, 1562] The mean optimal resistance (Fopt) of 68 g·kg⁻¹ identified for 12–13-year-old girls[1562] corresponds almost exactly to that observed by previous authors.[455] However, a much higher value of 85 g·kg⁻¹ has been reported for similar aged boys.[1562] The need to adjust resistances for young people at different stages of maturation is highlighted by the finding of a mean Fopt of 64 g·kg⁻¹ in 7-year-old boys[1561] compared with mean Fopt of 93 and 98 g·kg⁻¹ in 13-year-old boys and girls, respectively.[1622]

Obviously, this procedure requires additional testing time and may not always be feasible. Furthermore, the load derived is optimal for peak power and may therefore be inappropriate to maximize mean power. Other investigators continue to apply a standardized force of 75 g·kg⁻¹ [535, 1519] which is in accordance with current published guidelines recommending forces between 67 and 77 g·kg⁻¹ according to sex and mass.[144] A recent study[308] indicated that resistances of 65, 75, and 80 g·kg⁻¹ elicit similar values for peak (5 sec) and mean (30 sec) power in 6–12-year-old boys and girls, suggesting that a wide range of resistances may be equally applicable.

To become accepted, a laboratory test of exercise performance must be valid (i.e. it must measure the performance variable it is designed to measure) and the results produced must be consistent and reproducible.[935] With children and adolescents, the validity and reliability of a test should ideally be demonstrated across the full maturational range, as the changes in body size, composition, and metabolic responses to exercise which occur during this period may influence the ability to perform the test correctly.

Studies with healthy, athletic adults have yielded test-retest correlation coefficients for the WAnT ranging from $r = 0.91$ to $r = 0.97$[147, 528, 1148] suggesting good reproducibility. Documentation of the WAnT's reliability with healthy young people is scarce. It would appear that the test is somewhat less reproducible than in adults with coefficients ranging from $r = 0.89$ to $r = 0.93$ reported for 10–12-year-old children.[455] An unpublished study in our laboratory found the test-retest correlation coefficient for WAnT peak power to be higher than that for mean power ($r = 0.97$ vs. $r = 0.75$) in 14 well-habituated 10-year-old girls tested on two consecutive weeks. Despite the high correlation, peak power (W) scores were significantly higher ($P < 0.05$) on the second test (334.3 vs. 304.5 W) indicative of a significant learning effect with young children. Further confirmation of the reliability of the WAnT, using more appropriate methods than calculation of a correlation coefficient,[196] is required in groups of normal children and adolescents.

Whereas a laboratory measured peak $\dot{V}O_2$ is the established criterion against which other aerobic performance tests are assessed, there is no similar 'gold-standard' anaerobic test. This has confounded attempts to establish the validity of the WAnT and other anaerobic tests. Indirect validation has thus been attempted by examining the relationships between WAnT performance, and performance during other activities or athletic events demanding high-intensity, short-duration efforts.

Strong relationships have been observed between WAnT indices and field measures of anaerobic performance. In 10–15-year-old boys WAnT, peak power and mean power correlated with a 40 m dash ($r = 0.84$) and a 300 m run ($r = 0.85$) speed, respectively.[149] Similarly, mean power was highly related to 25 m swimming time in a mixed-sex group of 8–12-year-old competitive ($r = -0.87$) and recreational swimmers ($r = -0.90$).[748] Other studies have yielded somewhat weaker relationships with correlation coefficients ranging from 0.53–0.71 recorded between WAnT indices and sprint running performance in 7–13-year-old subjects.[1519, 1561, 1562] In some populations no significant relationship has been identified.[1562] The WAnT, and field tests of anaerobic performance appear to reflect similar performance characteristics but the magnitude of the correlation coefficients suggests that WAnT performance is not highly predictive of field performance. Nevertheless, WAnT performance has been improved following appropriate anaerobic training[660, 1248] (and see Chapter 5).

The intensity and duration of an exercise bout will dictate the relative contribution to ATP production from each of the three energy systems with the rate of ATP utilization precisely matched to resynthesis. As a result, it is almost impossible to design a performance test which completely isolates a given energy system. Nevertheless, the acceptance of a particular laboratory or field test as a valid indicator of anaerobic performance depends upon demonstration of the test's ability to stress predominantly anaerobic metabolic pathways.

With adults, studies have established the high anaerobic component of the WAnT through laboratory-measured indices of anaerobic metabolism. Correlation coefficients ranging from $r = 0.60$ to $r = 0.84$ between fast twitch muscle fibre area or percentage and performance on the WAnT have been observed.[148, 751, 773] The results of muscle biopsy studies further testify to significant glycolytic contribution. Muscle lactate levels have been shown to reach 46.1 mmol·kg^{-1} dry weight just 10 sec into the test, increasing to 73.9 mmol·kg^{-1} by the end of the test.[756]

The invasive techniques used to determine biochemical evidence of anaerobic metabolism are obviously prohibited with children but an alternative, non-invasive approach is to quantify the aerobic contribution to the test. This requires an estimate of the mechanical efficiency of supramaximal cycling. Unfortunately secure data are only available for submaximal exercise during which adult mechanical efficiencies of

20–25% have been estimated. The assumption of mechanical efficiency is particularly problematic with children where estimates have produced values ranging from 13–34% during submaximal cycling. A lower mechanical efficiency may be expected during a supramaximal effort[141] and is likely to lie somewhere between 15 and 25%.

Estimates for the aerobic contribution to the WAnT in adult subjects vary from 13–28%[749, 1366, 1426] according to the assumed mechanical efficiency. Comparable data for children are sparse. From expired air collection, Van Praagh *et al.*[1560] calculated that, on average, boys aged 7–15 years reached 60–70% of peak $\dot{V}O_2$ during the test. When expressed relative to external work and body mass $(mL \cdot kJ^{-1} \cdot kg^{-1})$ a 64% decline in oxygen consumption was observed between the ages of 9.5 and 15 years. In a small sample of late-adolescent hockey players, 44.3% of the total energy demand during the WAnT was reported to derive from aerobic sources.[1463] In our laboratory, using breath-by-breath expired gas analysis we have calculated the aerobic component of the WAnT, assuming a 25% mechanical efficiency, to be 33% and 36% in 10-year-old girls and boys, respectively. Calculations based upon a 15% efficiency reduced these values to 20% and 21% (unpublished data).

Despite the evident methodological problems associated with the quantification of the aerobic contribution to energy generation during the Wingate test, these studies are consistent in indicating a significantly higher aerobic involvement in children compared with adults. It remains to be demonstrated whether this arises due to true metabolic differences between children and adults or represents a limitation in the design or applicability of the test protocol, in its present form, to the assessment of young people's anaerobic performance.

The Margaria Step Test (MST)

Prior to the introduction of the WAnT, the Margaria Step Test (MST)[975] was the pre-eminent test of children's and adolescents' short-term anaerobic power.[401, 441, 975, 1462] Peak power scores obtained from the MST are highly correlated with WAnT estimated peak power with coefficients of $r = 0.77$ and $r = 0.84$ reported in untrained and trained boys, respectively.[71] In its original form, the MST required subjects to sprint, after an initial 2 m run up, up a staircase at maximal speed taking two 0.175 m steps at a time. Photocells placed on the first and final steps allowed the time (s) taken for the sprint to be measured. More recent adaptations have used pressure-activated switchmats linked to an electronic timer.[71] With the vertical height (m) between the switchmats, and the subject's body mass (kg) known, power (W) may be calculated from the equation,

$$Power = \frac{body\ mass \times 9.81 \times vertical\ height}{time}$$

where 9.81 is the acceleration due to gravity (m·s^{-2}). Subsequent modifications of the MST have shown that variations in the step height, length of run up, or use of external loading can increase the external power recorded in both adults and young people.[71, 289] With young people, we have identified a 5 m run-up as optimal.[71]

A problem with this test is the likelihood of a considerable learning effect, especially with younger children, as good motor co-ordination is essential to the successful completion of the test. In view of this, it is not surprising that the MST has generally been superseded by other tests.

The Force–Velocity Test

Although only recently introduced as a measure of peak anaerobic power, the Force–Velocity Test is being increasingly used in studies of both adults[1084, 1675] and children.[463, 532, 1025, 1561, 1653] The test involves a series of short (6–8 sec), maximal sprints on a cycle ergometer against a range of resistances applied in random order. Originally, eight sprints were included[1084] but recent modifications have recommended three or four.[1653, 1672] From the inverse relationship between force (resistance) and velocity (pedal revolutions) and the parabolic relationship between force and power derived, optimal peak power (OPP) and the force necessary to generate this may be interpolated (Fig. 2.1).

Published data reporting the reliability of the Force–Velocity Test with children do not appear to be available. In our laboratory (unpublished data) the test has proved moderately reliable in 9–10-year-old children for OPP with a reproducibility coefficient of $r = 0.80$. With the increasing popularity of this test, further data on its reliability with children and adolescents are urgently required.

Cunningham and Faulkner Treadmill Test

The Cunningham and Faulkner Treadmill Test[382] was designed to stress maximally the capacity of the anaerobic energy systems and is one of the few laboratory tests based upon running rather than cycle ergometry. With the gradient set at a constant 20%, belt speed may be adjusted according to the age or maturity of the child, for example 2.17 m·s^{-1} at age 10–11 years, 2.67 m·s^{-1} at 12–13 years, and 3.17 m·s^{-1} at 14–15 years—the aim being to elicit exhaustion within 80–120 sec.[1143] The obvious disadvantage of this lack of standardization is that growth-related changes cannot be precisely interpreted. Despite this, performance times have been shown to be moderately reproducible in 10- and 15-year-old children[1144] with test-retest correlation coefficients which exceed $r = 0.76$.

Successful performance on a maximal test of this duration relies heavily on subject motivation. Furthermore, in young people, the contribution

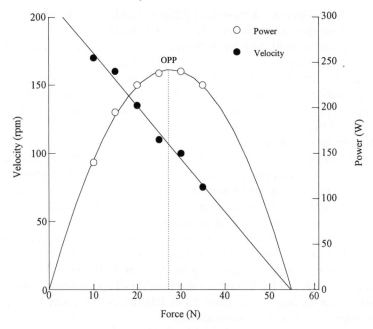

Fig. 2.1. The interpolation of optimal peak power (OPP) from force–velocity and force–power relationships.

from aerobic sources is likely to be considerable and raises questions regarding the test's validity as a measure of anaerobic capacity in this population. Supramaximal treadmill running is unsafe with young children and those inexperienced with treadmill running, and alternative tests may be preferable to determine their anaerobic performance.

Maximal accumulated oxygen deficit (MAOD)

This recently devised procedure attempts to estimate the maximal capacity of anaerobic energy systems via the measurement of the maximal accumulated oxygen deficit (MAOD).[1020] The rationale of the test is based upon two assumptions. First, that a linear relationship exists between steady-state oxygen uptake and exercise intensity at submaximal intensities and that this relationship can be extrapolated to estimate the oxygen demand of exercise at supramaximal intensities (i.e. exceeding peak $\dot{V}O_2$). Secondly, that the oxygen demand of a supramaximal exercise bout is constant throughout the duration of the effort.[650] The accumulated oxygen deficit for a particular supramaximal effort is thus the calculated accumulated oxygen demand minus the measured accumulated oxygen uptake.

Studies with adults have demonstrated that exhaustive exercise bouts lasting at least 2 min provide a reliable estimate of MAOD and have shown that it is independent of peak $\dot{V}O_2$ by demonstrating a reduction in peak $\dot{V}O_2$ but no change in MAOD under conditions of hypoxia.[1020]

Concerns with the validity of this technique centre on the two basic assumptions. It has been argued that the validity of extrapolating supra-maximal oxygen uptakes from submaximal measures is highly questionable as it has not been demonstrated that mechanical efficiency is constant with changes in exercise intensity.[650, 1315]

The technique has only recently been applied to children and adolescents and despite the attractions associated with the possibility of estimating total anaerobic capacity, the procedures required to achieve the necessary data render it an impractical proposition for regular assessment. It was originally shown that data from 10–15 submaximal exercise bouts were required to establish an appropriate linear equation describing the oxygen uptake-exercise intensity relationship at submaximal intensities. A further three or four laboratory visits are necessary to determine the MAOD. Although studies with children have reduced the number of submaximal bouts com-pleted to four or five[306, 307] as many as 12 laboratory visits may be required to complete the procedure satisfactorily.[307]

The results of studies with children using supramaximal exercise at intensities of 110%, 130%, and 150% peak $\dot{V}O_2$ have shown that the MAOD may be attained where exhaustion occurs within 60–90 sec in boys and in girls.[306, 307] This somewhat shorter period than suggested for adults is consistent with children's characteristically rapid adjustment of $\dot{V}O_2$ at the onset of exercise (see Chapter 4). Accumulated oxygen deficits approximating 35–37 mL·kg⁻¹·min⁻¹ in children[306, 307] compare with values of 45–60 mL·kg⁻¹·min⁻¹ reported for adults.[644, 710] These values are consistent with other physiological and biochemical evidence for reduced anaerobic capabilities during growth.

Obviously the non-invasive nature of the test is attractive but the limita-tions of the procedure must be emphasized. The variation in cycling effi-ciency observed in children and adolescents even during submaximal exercise may render the extrapolation to supramaximal intensities less secure than in adults. Successful determination of the MAOD is dependent upon the subject's determination to exercise maximally for longer time periods than usual in anaerobic tests, requiring highly motivated subjects if the procedure is to succeed. The available data reflect the responses of very limited sample sizes and are insufficient to confirm the test's re-liability. Although shown to be highly reproducible in 10–11-year-old boys ($r = 0.94$), only moderate reproducibility was reported by the same authors in a similar population of girls ($r = 0.57$).[307] Clearly, further research is required with larger and more diverse populations to substantiate the validity and reliability of the MAOD procedure.

Measurement of post-exercise blood lactate

Blood lactate sampling has become common practice in many paediatric physiology laboratories both during and after exercise performance tests. The lactate level measured provides an indication of the involvement of anaerobic (glycolytic) energy metabolism but does not directly reflect muscle lactate production.[253] When sampled during steady-state submaximal exercise, lactate may be used to provide an indication of aerobic fitness (see Chapter 4), with lactate levels at peak $\dot{V}O_2$ and following supramaximal exercise used to glean information regarding the development of energy metabolism during growth and maturation. Until recently, the methodological issues associated with sampling and assay of blood lactate, and their influence upon reported lactate values were neither well documented nor widely recognized. A lack of standardized techniques and inadequate description of sampling and analysis procedures in many published studies have confounded our understanding of children's metabolic responses to exercise. The following discussion highlights the main methodological considerations associated with blood lactate measurement and emphasizes their practical implications.

Sites of sampling

The majority of paediatric exercise studies measure lactate in capillary blood drawn from the fingertip[1028, 1657] or earlobe.[532, 534, 1561] Capillary sampling is recommended for children as it involves minimal trauma, is technically simple, and readily transferable to field situations. In addition, lactate levels are obtained which closely reflect those in arterial blood, provided that a good blood flow to the sampling site is ensured.[645, 1659] This is important given the close correspondence of arterial lactate levels with those in the femoral veins draining the active muscle which are reflective of lactate release from the muscle.[1102, 1317]

Although occasionally used with children[1021] the technical, ethical, and medical complications associated with arterial sampling have precluded its use from routine laboratory exercise assessments. As a result, some investigators have sampled venous blood.[849] The insertion of indwelling catheters into antecubital or dorsal veins is less hazardous than arterial cannulation and facilitates serial sampling. In adults, during steady-state submaximal cycle ergometer exercise, lactate levels in arterial blood are significantly higher than those in venous blood[1174] with the discrepancy becoming more marked at increasing exercise intensities.[1696, 1699] During comparable treadmill exercise, both significant[283, 498, 568] and non-significant [1659] differences in arterial-venous or capillary-venous lactate levels have been identified.

Table 2.4.   Blood preparations for lactate assay

Whole blood

Blood is collected into a capillary tube or cuvette coated with heparin to prevent clotting and is analysed, usually within minutes, without further treatment

Plasma

Blood is collected as above and centrifuged to separate the liquid (plasma) and solid constituents of the blood. Lactate is then assayed in the plasma

Serum

Blood is allowed to clot and then spun to separate the clear, straw-coloured serum which is assayed for lactate

Lysed blood

Blood is treated with chemicals which break open (lyse) the red blood cells releasing the intracellular lactate. The blood is not separated before assay

Protein-free preparation

The blood sample is chemically treated to break down blood proteins and then centrifuged to separate the solids and liquid. The liquid portion is then assayed for lactate

---

Methods of lactate assay

The specific blood handling and assay techniques used represent a further major source of variation in measured levels. As assay methodologies vary widely between laboratories, an awareness of the nature and extent of assay differences is essential to the valid interpretation of young people's lactate responses to exercise.

Once sampled, blood for lactate determination may be analysed immediately or undergo some preparation or chemical treatment prior to assay. The nature of treatment will be dictated by the specific analysis technique which may require either plasma, serum, lysed blood, or a protein-free preparation (Table 2.4). Many of the early studies which pioneered the use of blood lactate to evaluate exercise performance used an enzymatic-spectrophotometric type assay [e.g. 729] which forms the basis for several commercially available kits (e.g. Sigma and Boehringer) and analysers that measure lactate levels in protein-free preparations.[1639] Here, ice-cold perchloric acid is mixed with the blood to precipitate the proteins. Following centrifugation, the clear supernatant is assayed for lactate concentration. It is not uncommon for lactate levels obtained thus to be referred to as 'blood' or 'whole blood' lactates[1531] but these values are not comparable with assays (described below) that do indeed measure lactate in whole blood.

Modern, semi-automatic analysers are based upon an enzymatic electro-chemical (amperometric) assay. Such analysers have many advantages, not least that whole blood may be assayed within seconds of sampling, results are available within 60–90 sec and portable versions facilitate performance monitoring in the field or at the pool-side. If required, these analysers may also assay plasma, lysed blood, or serum.[1659] Even so, different analysers operating ostensibly upon the same principles may still produce results which differ systematically.[1659]

The two characteristics of the blood preparation which influence the measured lactate concentration are: (1) whether or not lactate from the red blood cells (erythrocytes) is included; and (2) whether the prepared sample contains solids. With whole blood as the assay medium, only the lactate in the plasma fraction is measured.[1076, 1611] The disruption of the red blood cell membrane, caused by the addition of perchloric acid or similar chemical lysing agents, releases lactate from the erythrocytes into the extracellular fluid, thus contributing an extra source of lactate. As a result lactate levels in lysed whole blood tend to be higher than those in whole blood, with the discrepancy increasing at higher lactate concentrations.[579, 1659] Inter-individual differences in haematocrit may contribute to variation in the determined lactate level and may need to be accounted for.[568, 1439]

It is the volume difference which perhaps causes the largest variation in measured lactate levels. In the blood of a normal individual with an haematocrit of 40%, approximately 88% of the volume is the aqueous phase with a non-aqueous phase of 12% consisting of cells, proteins, and cellular debris. Therefore, lactate determinations in whole blood are lower than those in preparations from which the solids have been removed (i.e. plasma, serum, or protein-free filtrates).

In view of the significance of these influences upon the interpretation of the lactate levels obtained, several studies have attempted to quantify the magnitude of the differences between the blood preparations. Lactate levels in protein-free filtrates and plasma have been reported to correspond closely[1639] or differ minimally.[1531] Due to the volume difference and inclusion of cellular lactate, lactate levels in protein-free samples are significantly higher than in whole blood.[579, 1604, 1076, 1611] Estimates vary as to the extent of the difference with some authors reporting a consistent 5% difference throughout a wide range of lactate levels[1611] with others noting a reduction in the magnitude of the difference with increasing lactate levels: 63.7% at submaximal exercise reducing to 20.4% at maximal exercise.[579] In the latter study, lysing the whole blood reduced the difference to 42.5% at sub-maximal exercise intensities. Plasma lactates are approximately 30% higher than levels in whole or lysed blood.[568, 1659]

These findings have implications for the interpretation of young people's blood lactate responses to exercise. It is clear that blood lactate measures are highly dependent upon the techniques used to sample and analyse the blood, therefore results from laboratories employing different measurement techniques cannot be compared directly. An awareness of these methodological considerations is critical where laboratory-based lactate determinations are used to set training intensities,[1213] or are extrapolated to field situations where different sampling and assay procedures are used to monitor exercise training.

Summary

The interpretation of the growth and maturation of aerobic and anaerobic performance is limited by ethical and methodological constraints. $\dot{V}O_{2\,max}$ is accepted as the criterion measure of aerobic fitness in adults and is objectively determined by the demonstration of a plateau in $\dot{V}O_2$ during incremental exercise. Only a minority of children and adolescents achieve the classical $\dot{V}O_2$ plateau therefore it is more appropriate to use the term 'peak $\dot{V}O_2$' to describe the highest $\dot{V}O_2$ elicited during a progressive exercise test to voluntary exhaustion in this population. The absence of a $\dot{V}O_2$ plateau in young subjects does not appear to be related to motivation, leg muscle mass, or indices of anaerobic metabolism. Peak $\dot{V}O_2$ may be accepted as a maximal index provided specific heart rate, respiratory exchange rate, and subjective criteria are fulfilled. The estimation of peak $\dot{V}O_2$ from submaximal responses or maximal field tests is not recommended with children and adolescents and such methods are not a valid substitute for direct determination of peak $\dot{V}O_2$ in the laboratory. The protocol independent nature of peak $\dot{V}O_2$ allows laboratory test protocols to be customized to accommodate ancillary measures such as cardiac output or blood lactate.

There is a lack of standardized, valid, and reliable methods of assessing anaerobic performance in young people. A variety of protocols are available to estimate peak and mean anaerobic power, the majority of which are based upon cycle ergometry and were originally designed to assess adult subjects. All anaerobic performance tests have methodological limitations which may not easily be overcome. Tests are reliant upon subject motivation and there are no physiological or biochemical markers which can be used to establish an objective endpoint. No single test can optimally estimate both peak and mean anaerobic power and standardizing appropriate resistances to accommodate body composition changes during growth and maturation has proved problematic. The recently introduced Force–Velocity Test has produced promising results but requires further validation with young people. Currently available tests of anaerobic 'capacity' are likely to elicit a significant contribution to energy supply from aerobic sources, particularly with young subjects. The development and refinement of valid and reliable techniques for estimating anaerobic performance indices in young people represents a challenging area for future research.

The measurement of blood lactate during and following exercise provides useful insights into energy metabolism and aerobic fitness. The site of blood sampling, blood preparation, and assay methodologies have a significant influence upon the actual level of lactate determined and are essential considerations in the interpretation of children's and adolescents' blood lactate responses to exercise. These preclude the direct comparison of data from laboratories whose analytical techniques differ and, for the same reasons, must be taken into account when extrapolating laboratory measures of blood lactate to field situations for training assessment purposes.

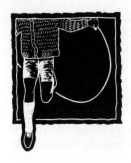

3

Scaling exercise data for body size differences during growth

Body size significantly affects physiological performance measures such as peak aerobic and anaerobic power and muscular strength. Therefore, in order to elucidate and interpret the changes which occur with growth and maturation, the data must be normalized or scaled for differences in body size.

Procedures to normalize performance data for body size differences have four main applications: (1) to compare an individual's performance against standards for assessment purposes; (2) to compare groups which differ in characteristics such as age, sex, or maturity; (3) in longitudinal investigations where training and growth effects need to be separated and quantified; and finally (4), in studies attempting to clarify the relationship between physiological variables and performance.[1673]

Techniques for accounting for body size in performance measures

Ratio standards

Performance variables such as peak $\dot{V}O_2$ are conventionally normalized for body size by expression in simple ratio with body mass (i.e. as $mL \cdot kg^{-1} \cdot min^{-1}$). These ratio standards are then used in further comparative or correlational analyses under the assumption that the influence of body mass has been appropriately and adequately removed. The caveats associated with the use of simple ratio standards are well documented.[793, 794, 976, 1096, 1673] First, ratio standards do not represent a dimensionless physiological performance variable: when peak $\dot{V}O_2$ expressed in $mL \cdot kg^{-1} \cdot min^{-1}$ is correlated with a body size dimension (e.g. mass), a negative correlation coefficient is invariably observed. Thus, the ratio standard may be seen to 'overscale' by converting the positive correlation between the absolute value of the physiological performance variable to a negative relationship.[1098] Secondly, the ratio method assumes a linear relationship between the body size and performance variables where the slope of the linear regression line passes through the origin (i.e. the intercept statistic is zero):

$$Y = a \cdot X + \varepsilon$$

Here, a is the constant derived from the means of the X and Y variables for the specific data set and ε is the additive, or constant, error term. To express how the validity of the ratio method may be determined in an alternative manner, Tanner demonstrated how the ratio standard is only applicable where the coefficient of variation (V) for the body size variable (X) divided by the V for the performance variable (Y) equals the Pearson product moment correlation coefficient between the two variables (i.e. VX/VY = rX,Y). Where this condition is not satisfied, the use of a ratio standard will distort the data with the size of the distortion increasing as the discrepancy between the two sides of the equation widens. The practical outcome of this will be that light individuals are advantaged whilst heavy subjects are penalized.[1673]

Least-squares linear adjustment (regression standards)

In relationships which can be demonstrated to be linear, Tanner[1502] recommended the use of a scaling method based upon least-squares linear regression. Here, the relationship between the performance variable and the body size variable within different groups is described by the equation:

$$Y = a + b \cdot X + \varepsilon$$

where a is the intercept of the regression line on the Y axis, b is the slope of the line of best fit and ε the error term which again is assumed to be additive (i.e. constant throughout the range of X and Y variables measured). Group comparisons, for example, by sex, age, or maturity, may be investigated using the statistical technique, analysis of covariance (ANCOVA).[1430] This procedure generates regression lines for each of the groups under investigation and compares their slopes and intercepts. Where the slopes are shown to be not significantly different (i.e. parallel) adjusted means are computed. These are means from which the influence of body size has been covaried out. Individual adjusted means are computed from the predicted value for the performance variable derived from the combined data of all groups in the comparison, to which is added the residual for that data point. Individual adjusted means are then averaged to produce an overall adjusted mean.

Linear adjustment scaling techniques have been shown to provide a better statistical fit for the interpretation of both peak aerobic and anaerobic data[1098, 1537] by a reduction in the residual error associated with the analysis. Consequently, some authors have strongly advocated their general application to the interpretation of exercise performance,[1537] a recommendation which has received equally strong criticism.[355] Several studies have demonstrated the pitfalls associated with linear-adjustment models and it appears that in certain situations they inadequately account for body size differences.[1096]

First, the derived regression line often has a positive intercept which suggests that for a body size of zero there still exists a physiological response—an obvious impossibility. Extrapolation beyond the data points to the axis is thus to be avoided. However, the phenomenon still 'creates unease'[1673] and has caused others to caution against indiscriminate use of empirically derived regressions to describe data.[826]

Perhaps of more significance is the problem associated with the assumption of an additive error term. It has been observed that this assumption is questionable where human physiological performance is being modelled[1096, 1098] as, more commonly, performance scores diverge with increasing body size.[1098, 1624] A linear model cannot adequately accommodate and control for this spread and a modelling technique which incorporates a multiplicative, rather than an additive, error term is indicated. In situations such as these a non-linear scaling model may be preferable.

Allometric modelling

Although widely used in the biological sciences to study structure/function relationships,[1340] allometric scaling techniques have rarely been applied to the interpretation of paediatric exercise data. In allometry, physiological variables are scaled in relation to body size according to the non-linear relationship:

$$Y = a \cdot X^b \cdot \varepsilon$$

Expression of the equation in its linear form, by fitting a least-squares linear regression line to data plotted on bi-logarithmic coordinates, facilitates the identification of the a (constant multiplier or proportionality coefficient) and b (exponent) parameters:

$$\ln Y = \ln a + b \cdot \ln x$$

The slope or mass exponent (b) can be either positive or negative according to the function under consideration and provides information as to the relationship between the dependent and independent variables. For example, a mass exponent equal to 1.0 indicates that the two variables increase in direct proportion with one another (i.e. in this case the simple ratio standard adequately describes the function–size relationship). Where the dependent variable increases at a slower rate than the increase in the independent variable a mass exponent of less than 1.0 will result. For example, some studies have shown mammalian metabolic rate to increase in relation to mass$^{0.75}$.[1340] Conversely, if the dependent variable increases at a faster rate than the independent variable then the mass exponent will be greater than 1.0, for example, in mammals, the skeleton increases to mass$^{1.08}$.[1340]

The constant multiplier or proportionality coefficient (a) is the other important numerical term in the allometric equation and indicates whether quantitative differences exist in the dependent variable for groups which share a common mass exponent. For example, in adult peak $\dot{V}O_2$ data,[1098] the identification of a common mass exponent of 0.66 demonstrated that peak $\dot{V}O_2$ changes with body size in the same way in both males and females. The significantly different proportionality coefficients indicated that the level of peak $\dot{V}O_2$ in each group differed systematically; in this case demonstrating lower levels of aerobic fitness in females.

Following logarithmic transformation of the data, group comparisons may be made using ANCOVA in the same way as described for the linear model above. Alternatively, by raising the body size variable to the power b identified (X^b) and dividing the resultant value into the absolute value of the performance variable (Y/X^b), power function ratios are derived. This approach still appropriately controls for body size differences[1096, 1098] but simplifies statistical comparisons as t-test or analysis of variance may be used to investigate group differences.[1624, 1673]

The mass exponent which best describes peak exercise performance in children and adolescents has, for many years, been a subject of interest for paediatric exercise scientists. Appropriate normalization of performance data for body size is fundamental to the accurate interpretation of changes in these parameters during growth. Traditionally, a mass exponent of 1.0 has been assumed (i.e. that variables such as peak $\dot{V}O_2$ increase in direct proportion with body mass) but theoretical arguments based upon geometric similarity and the surface law suggest that the mass exponent 0.67 is the appropriate scaling factor for physiological performance variables. The theoretical principles behind the derivation of this exponent have been expounded at length by other authors[102, 1340] hence only the basic principles will be outlined here.

The derivation of the mass exponent of 0.67 from geometric similarity is most often and simply described with reference to two cubes of similar dimensions but with the length of the side of one longer than that of the other. These two cubes are geometrically similar (or isometric) as corresponding linear dimensions are related in the same proportion and corresponding surface areas are related in the same proportion squared. The volumes of the cubes are related in the same proportion to the third power. These basic principles of isometric geometry can be summarized thus:

$$\text{surface area} \propto \text{length}^2$$
$$\text{volume} \propto \text{length}^3$$
$$\text{surface area} \propto \text{volume}^{2/3}$$

These principles will apply equally to animals and humans of different sizes if the proportion of the body's components (i.e. limbs, trunk, head) remain the same.

Assuming geometric similarity, it can be argued[102] that length (L) or stature (h) may be used as the basic unit against which body surface area, volume and mass can be compared. Therefore, body surface area is related to h^2, and the volumes of body components such as stroke volume, lung volumes, and total body mass are proportional to stature cubed (e.g. mass $\propto h^3$). If the body is considered as a dynamic system where peak aerobic power is a volume per unit time then peak $\dot{V}O_2$ should theoretically be proportional to $L^3 \cdot L^{-1} = L^2$, as from Newton's second law, in physiological systems, time is proportional to length.[102] Therefore, to be independent of size, peak $\dot{V}O_2$, for example, should be expressed as $mL \cdot m^{-2} \cdot min^{-1}$ or $mL \cdot kg^{-0.67} \cdot min^{-1}$, as $mass^{2/3}$ is analogous to $stature^2$ in geometrically similar bodies.[120]

The assumption of geometric similarity in growing children is a matter of contention. Some authors have argued that the theoretical exponent of $\frac{2}{3}(0.67)$ is plausible in children and adolescents as growth is isometric, at least from the age of 10 years after which age body proportions remain approximately the same.[94, 102] Others have suggested that allometric (non-isometric) scaling is particularly appropriate precisely because growth is not isometric and therefore theoretical exponents may not apply.[1673]

The surface law proposes an alternative derivation of the 0.67 exponent.[648] The principle is based upon the recognition that metabolic rate in smaller mammals is higher in relation to their body mass than in larger mammals. Heat production and heat loss must be carefully matched in order to maintain homeothermy. As heat loss is proportional to the surface area:body mass ratio, which itself is proportional to body $mass^{0.67}$, it follows that resting and peak oxygen uptakes should also correspond to $mass^{0.67}$.

This theoretical reasoning is somewhat at odds with the empirical data recorded by several investigators relating the resting metabolic rates to body size of mammals and birds. When plotted on logarithmic coordinates, metabolic rates fall along a straight regression line with a slope closer to 0.75 than 0.67[252, 825] suggesting that metabolic rates are not proportional to body surface area. In an attempt to ascribe a theoretical justification to the empirical observations, McMahon[1012] proposed a model of elastic similarity where biological proportions and metabolic rates are limited by the elastic properties of the animal. These properties ensure that bending and buckling forces during locomotion do not impair the structural integrity of the joints and limbs. In this schema, limb length is predicted to be proportional to the 0.67 power of its diameter. The cross-sectional area is thus proportional to the 0.75 power of mass as is peak $\dot{V}O_2$.[354] This mass exponent is analogous to stature raised to the power 2.25.

The concept of elastic similitude in animals has been disputed[715] and the 0.75 exponent dismissed as a statistical artefact caused by fitting the same allometric model to data obtained from a number of different species[714] which, when examined individually, have slopes of 0.67.[1340] Others have criticized the species selection from which the 0.75 exponent was derived.[290] Despite subsequent provision of a mathematical explanation for both 0.67 and 0.75 as valid exponents for intra- and inter-species energy metabolism data, respectively[543] others maintain that there is, as yet, no biologically meaningful explanation for the 0.75 exponent.[715] Furthermore, it is questionable whether this exponential relationship, derived as it is from resting oxygen consumption, is necessarily applicable to peak $\dot{V}O_2$.[120]

So how does the empirical evidence derived from determinations of peak $\dot{V}O_2$ in human subjects conform to the theoretical predictions? Allometric modelling of peak $\dot{V}O_2$ in groups of male and female adult athletes representing a diverse range of sports resulted in mass exponents ranging from 0.47–0.86.[179] When analysed together a mass exponent of 0.71 was derived which was interpreted as supporting a mass exponent of 0.67 for data normalization. The same exponent was derived for fat-free body mass in an early study of peak $\dot{V}O_2$ in physical education students.[1584] A recent study, including a much larger, and more representative sample has yielded mass exponents for peak $\dot{V}O_2$ and peak and mean anaerobic power of almost exactly 0.67 in male and female subjects.[1098] Similar results have been reported for rowers.[1097, 1353] There is, therefore, accumulating evidence to support the contention that the 0.67 mass exponent appropriately normalizes peak exercise performance data in adult subjects.

Data from children and adolescents are much less consistent and more difficult to interpret. The small sample sizes in some studies are unlikely to be sufficient to identify representative mass exponents and the mix of longitudinal and cross-sectional data further confounds the issues. Table 3.1 summarizes the findings of studies reporting mass exponents for peak $\dot{V}O_2$ in children and adolescents. What is immediately evident is that in the majority of these studies, the identified mass exponents exceed the theoretically derived values. As a result the recommendation that there is no sound reason to abandon the use of the simple ratio standard (mass$^{1.0}$) is wholly understandable.[138, 1377, 1383]

It has been postulated that theoretical principles fail to adequately reflect size-related function in children due to the use of cross-sectional data or effects associated with the pubertal growth spurt.[1377] An alternative explanation suggests that qualitative changes occur within muscles as part of the maturational process which results in increased force generation per cross-sectional area. This challenges an underlying assumption of geometric similarity that this should be independent of body size.[354]

Nevill[1095] has recently challenged the validity of the 0.75 exponent and provided a plausible explanation for how inappropriate statistical modelling of data from heterogeneous groups inflates the mass exponent. Nevill's thesis is based upon previous work[13] which demonstrated that within a

Table 3.1. Allometric scaling factors for peak $\dot{V}O_2$ in children and adolescents as a function of body mass

Study	Population age (yrs)	Sex (M/F)	n	Mass exponent
McMiken[1017]	7–13	M	50	0.88
McMiken[1017]	12–16	F	30	0.97
McMiken[1017]	10–15	M	14	1.07
Ross *et al.*[1246]	8–16	M	25	0.95
Ross *et al.*[1246]	8–16	M	25	0.76
Sjodin & Svedenhag[1411]	12–19	M	8 trained	0.78
		M	4 untrained	0.75
Paterson *et al.*[1147]	11–15	M	18	1.02
Welsman *et al.*[1624]	10–adult	M & F	156	0.80
Welsman & Armstrong[1621]	10–11	M & F	164	0.66
Rogers *et al.*[1227]	8.9	M & F	42	0.52
Cooper *et al.*[359]	6–18	M & F	109	1.01

range of mammal species, larger animals have a greater proportion of proximal leg muscle mass in relation to total body mass (i.e. mass[1.1]). A similar relationship has been confirmed in male adolescents with a mass exponent of 1.1 reported for leg volume.[1095] If the groups under consideration vary widely in size (as is likely in groups of children and adolescents ranging widely in age) and are thus characterized by an increasing proportion of muscle mass with increasing body size, the allometric equation will consequently be unable to separate the contribution from the individual's muscle mass, from the contribution that reflects the increasing proportion of muscle mass within the group. Assuming the peak performance measure is proportional to mass[0.67] the effect of the increase in muscle mass can be demonstrated thus:

$$Y = a_1(a_2 \cdot m^{0.67})^{1.1} = a_3 \cdot m^{0.74} \text{ (ref. 1095)}$$

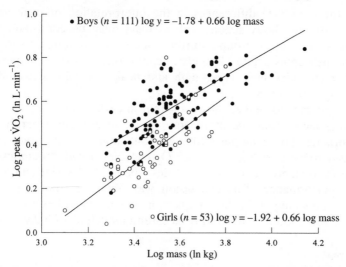

Fig. 3.1. The log-linear relationship between peak $\dot{V}O_2$ and body mass in pre-
pubertal children. Redrawn from Armstrong, N., Kirby, B.J., McManus, A.M. and
Welsman, J.R. (1995). Aerobic fitness of prepubescent children. *Annals of Human
Biology*, **22**, 427–44. Reprinted with permission.

Modelling data without consideration of this effect violates an important
assumption of the allometric model which assumes that muscle mass
represents a consistent proportion of body mass in all subjects. In heterogeneous groups, then, body size as well as body mass must be controlled for.
This can be achieved by incorporating stature into the allometric model as
a continuous covariate $Y = a(Z)m^b$.[1095] By doing so, any disproportionate
increase in muscle mass with increasing size will be controlled, allowing the
independent contribution from body mass to be identified.

Data from our laboratory[1624] clearly illustrate these principles. Allometric
modelling of data for body mass alone revealed a common mass exponent
of 0.80 in groups of prepubertal, pubertal, and adult males and females.
With stature incorporated as a continuous covariate, the mass exponent
was reduced to 0.71, a value not significantly different from 0.67. In what
appears to be the only published study of allometric modelling in a large
($n = 164$) well-defined (prepubertal), homogeneous sample of children,[72, 1621]
the identified exponent of 0.66 corresponded almost exactly to the
theoretically predicted value (see Fig. 3.1).

Recent research findings[1095, 1098, 1621, 1624] support the contention[1502] that ratio
standards appear to account inadequately for body size differences in
exercise performance variables such as peak $\dot{V}O_2$. There is compelling evidence that the theoretical mass exponent of 0.67 may more appropriately

control for body size differences in the interpretation of peak aerobic function although body size as well as mass must be controlled for in heterogeneous subject groups. Further studies are required to examine and establish appropriate allometric scaling factors for other performance characteristics such as strength and peak anaerobic power during growth and maturation.

It is important to realize, however, that in certain situations alternative scaling factors may be more appropriate to normalize performance characteristics. For example, although confirming the accuracy of the 0.67 mass exponent to describe peak $\dot{V}O_2$ data, Nevill *et al.*[1098] demonstrated that the ratio standard (mass[1.0]) best described actual sprint and 5000 m running performance. This conclusion was obtained from appropriate statistical modelling of the data in question and demonstrates how suitable scaling factors should be derived from careful modelling of individual data sets.

Multilevel modelling

The scaling methods described so far are most appropriate for cross-sectional comparisons, but where repeated measures are used, such as in longitudinal studies of physiological performance during growth, alternative modelling techniques are more sensitive and appropriate. Multilevel modelling[634] can be used to fit individual growth curves to performance data. The technique accommodates base lines that are not steady and can be used with both discrete and continuous responses. The technique has been used in recent longitudinal studies to investigate the effects of growth, maturation, and training upon peak $\dot{V}O_2$,[155] and the development of strength.[1249] Despite the complexity of the statistics, the sensitivity and flexibility of this modelling technique suggest it has considerable potential to clarify the development of physiological function during normal growth and with training.

Summary

The normalization of performance data to account for body size differences underpins the understanding of the growth and maturation of exercise performance. Unfortunately, the conventional method by which this is achieved—the construction of per body mass ratio standards (e.g. peak $\dot{V}O_2$ in mL·kg^{-1}·min^{-1}) is theoretically limited. The inability of ratio standards to partition out adequately body size has been demonstrated and their use may have clouded our interpretation of the growth of physiological function. Linear scaling techniques have been recommended but are unable to accommodate the spread in data (heteroscedasticity) which is often typical in physiological performance data from subjects of increasing size. Non-linear (allometric) scaling models have been demonstrated to account appropriately for body size differences in performance data from both adults and younger subjects. There is compelling evidence to recommend the normalization of peak aerobic performance by expression relative to $mass^{0.67}$. In subject groups representing a wide range of body size, the incorporation of stature as well as mass should be included in the allometric model. Multilevel modelling techniques are particularly appropriate for longitudinal performance data.

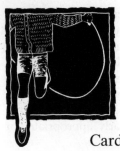

4

Aerobic exercise: growth and maturation

Cardiovascular responses to exercise

The main determinants of oxygen transport are cardiac output ($\dot{Q}$), ie the product of heart rate and stroke volume, and arteriovenous oxygen $[(a - \bar{v})O_2]$ difference,[1376] summarized in Fick's principle as:

$$\dot{V}O_2 = \dot{Q} \cdot (CaO_2 - C\bar{v}O_2),$$

where CaO_2 and $C\bar{v}O_2$ are the oxygen content of arterial and mixed venous blood, respectively. The way in which these components respond to exercise of increasing intensity in order to maintain the supply of oxygen to the exercising muscles is characteristically different in the exercising young person compared to the adult.

The estimation of cardiac output in the exercising individual is problematic, particularly at intensities close to peak $\dot{V}O_2$. The two most appropriate non-invasive methods for use during exercise are carbon dioxide (CO_2) rebreathing (indirect Fick method) and acetylene rebreathing. The methodological limitations associated with their use have been comprehensively reviewed elsewhere.[462] Accurate estimation of cardiac output with these techniques requires careful selection of rebreathing bag, appropriate concentration of rebreathing gas, and adequate emptying of the bag with each breath to ensure sufficient gas exchange between lung and bag. At high exercise intensities CO_2 rebreathing is likely to be uncomfortable and may produce dizziness or nausea. Even in experienced hands the variability within repeated measures is at least 10%.[462] As a result of these limitations, studies describing the cardiac output of the healthy child or adolescent during exercise are rare and much of our knowledge is based upon early studies where data were derived from invasive measures of cardiac output.

These studies have demonstrated that at any given level of oxygen consumption, cardiac output is as much as 1–2 $L \cdot min^{-1}$ lower in the young person than in the adult[510, 520, 523] largely as a result of a smaller stroke volume during both submaximal and maximal exercise.[512] When stroke volume is scaled to stature raised to the third power (h^3)[100, 102] the differences between young people and adults have been shown to disappear.[100, 512]

Children and adolescents compensate for their lower stroke volume by a higher heart rate at submaximal and maximal exercise intensities compared with adults.[512] Maximal heart rates are, on average, significantly higher in juveniles than in adults and remain fairly stable during childhood and adolescence. During childhood and adolescence, maximal values over 200 beats per minute (bpm) are common and often exceed 220 bpm.[80] After maturity, maximal heart rate declines by approximately 1 bpm per year and the formula, 220 minus age, represents an appropriate estimate of maximal heart rate from late adolescence. At submaximal exercise intensities children and adolescents also compensate for a lower stroke volume by increasing $[(a - \bar{v})O_2]$ difference, but at maximal exercise this ability is limited by the haemoglobin content of the blood. Haemoglobin levels increase slowly between the ages of 4–12 years from around 126–130 $g \cdot L^{-1}$. Concentrations then rise rapidly during puberty to approximate 140 $g \cdot L^{-1}$ in females and 160 $g \cdot L^{-1}$ in males. As blood volume remains constant at around 75–80 $mL \cdot kg^{-1}$ this represents a considerable increase in total haemoglobin mass relative to body mass.

Despite the lower cardiac output and oxygen-carrying capacity of the blood, the young person's oxygen transport system is not less effective than the adult's,[1377] because at maximal exercise, the $[(a - \bar{v})O_2]$ difference compares favourably with adults with almost all of the oxygen circulating through the working muscles extracted.[512, 1225]

Pulmonary responses to exercise

Children's and adolescents' pulmonary responses to exercise are less well documented than their cardiovascular responses. This is despite characteristic differences compared with adults which reflect both the simple quantitative changes taking place with growth and the modifications in ventilatory control which are present during this period.

Minute ventilation ($\dot{V}E$) is the product of respiratory frequency (f_r) and tidal volume (TV):

$$\dot{V}E = f_r \cdot TV$$

The pattern of the rise in $\dot{V}E$ during progressive exercise is essentially the same in adults and young people: At exercise intensities below 60–80% of peak $\dot{V}O_2$, $\dot{V}E$ is closely matched to the rise in exercise intensity. Beyond this, the rise in $\dot{V}E$ becomes non-linear, increasing disproportionately faster than exercise intensity.[1281] This point of the onset of the accelerated increase in $\dot{V}E$ tends to occur at a higher relative exercise intensity in children compared with adults.[138, 775, 1640] Some authors assume this 'ventilatory threshold' to reflect the lactate anaerobic threshold[406, 1601] as a marker of submaximal aerobic fitness. However, this issue remains controversial, particularly in view of the highly variable lactate response to exercise evident during childhood and adolescence and the unresolved issues relating to the maturation of the glycolytic energy system (discussed below).

Ventilatory parameters are related to anthropometric characteristics, particularly, stature, mass, and lean body mass.[96, 1026] Submaximal and maximal $\dot{V}E$ expressed in absolute terms ($L \cdot min^{-1}$) rise in parallel with the increase in stature.[1026, 1281] $\dot{V}E$ values at peak $\dot{V}O_2$ of 40–50 $L \cdot min^{-1}$ are typical of 8–10-year-old children,[1281, 1375] compared with values exceeding 150 $L \cdot min^{-1}$ in adults.[80] Expressed relative to body mass ($L \cdot kg^{-1} \cdot min^{-1}$), $\dot{V}E$ at peak $\dot{V}O_2$ has been reported as being both the same[138] or considerably higher than that observed in adults: 1.4–1.6 $L \cdot kg^{-1} \cdot min^{-1}$ vs. 1.0 $L \cdot kg^{-1} \cdot min^{-1}$, respectively.[1374] Results from our laboratory support the latter conclusion. Furthermore, our data set reflecting the responses of over 700 children and adolescents demonstrates values for boys aged 10–13 years (1.6–2.0 $L \cdot kg^{-1} \cdot min^{-1}$) which are consistently higher than those for similarly aged girls (1.4–1.6 $L \cdot kg^{-1} \cdot min^{-1}$). This interpretation of growth-related changes in ventilation may, however, be erroneous given the concerns raised in Chapter 3 regarding the validity of expressing size-dependent functions in ratio with body mass. In fact, allometric modelling of ventilatory responses to exercise in 11–15-year-old boys has yielded a mass exponent for peak $\dot{V}E$ of b = 0.68 not 1.0.[1026] It is unfortunate that these authors did not compare peak $\dot{V}E$ ($L \cdot kg^{-0.68} \cdot min^{-1}$) across the age groups examined as an allometric approach to the examination of growth-related changes may elucidate the maturation of pulmonary responses to exercise.

In contrast to adults, who increase $\dot{V}E$ by raising both tidal volume and breathing frequency, children predominantly increase breathing frequency[647, 1268] with mass-related tidal volume tending to be lower than in adults. This higher ratio of breathing frequency to tidal volume may reflect increased lung recoil forces in young people.[1709] At peak $\dot{V}O_2$ a breathing frequency greater than 60 breaths per min is not uncommon in children[84, 1267, 1281] compared with around 30–40 breaths per min in adults.[1267] As with other ventilatory parameters, breathing frequency is related to body size, although the correlation coefficients are somewhat weaker than for variables such as $\dot{V}E$.[1026]

The efficiency of exercising lung function is reflected by the ventilatory equivalent for oxygen ($\dot{V}E/\dot{V}O_2$). The higher the value, the less efficient the process. At any given level of exercise, the young person has a higher $\dot{V}E/\dot{V}O_2$ than the adult[98, 1267, 1269] and values decline gradually during growth. Explanations for this relative inefficiency have not entirely been resolved. The elevated breathing frequency described above may be a contributory factor by increasing the oxygen cost of respiration[138, 647] but, more importantly, data are accumulating which indicate that children's and adolescents' respiratory centres are more responsive to CO_2 than those of adults.[357, 647] It has been demonstrated that, although the same metabolic level of exercise produces comparable levels of end-tidal CO_2 in children and adults, this elicits a significantly higher ventilation in the younger subjects.[647] It would appear, therefore, that there is some maturation of the ventilatory control mechanisms during growth.

Gas exchange in the alveoli is determined by alveolar rather than pulmonary ventilation.[138] Despite the differences in young people's pulmonary responses to exercise compared with adults, particularly the reduced tidal volumes, alveolar ventilation is more than adequate to optimize gas exchange.[1384]

Aerobic fitness

Peak oxygen uptake and age

The aerobic fitness of children and adolescents has been extensively documented with peak $\dot{V}O_2$ determinations from children as young as 4 years of age recorded within the world literature. Some authors have questioned the validity of peak $\dot{V}O_2$ determinations in children younger than 8 years of age.[81, 967] Children younger than this often have short attention spans, poor motivation, and lack sufficient understanding of the procedures making it difficult to elicit maximal efforts.[1390] Reports of peak $\dot{V}O_2$ in very young children are difficult to interpret as termination criteria have not been made explicit[375, 1219, 1702] and subject numbers are generally small.[401, 1332] Some studies have pooled data from girls and boys[850, 1390] but the identification of significant differences in peak $\dot{V}O_2$ between boys and girls even in the prepubertal years[72] suggests that this approach may confound the interpretation of aerobic fitness during childhood and adolescence.

Data from young people aged from 8–16 years are more secure and we recently reviewed them elsewhere.[81] The graphs generated are reproduced in Figs 4.1 and 4.2 and represent 10 154 peak $\dot{V}O_2$ determinations. These graphs represent data drawn solely from untrained subjects. Because of the ergometer dependence of peak $\dot{V}O_2$ (see Chapter 2) data from treadmill and cycle ergometry are graphed separately rather than calculating an adjusted value for cycle values.[851] Even so, the data must be interpreted cautiously as both longitudinal and cross-sectional studies, with widely varying sample sizes, have been included. Sample composition may introduce some bias as random subject selection is not feasible and subjects in these studies were volunteers. As a result, very inactive or overweight individuals may have been excluded.

Regardless of the mode of exercise the figures clearly demonstrate a progressive, linear increase in peak $\dot{V}O_2$ with age in both males and females, although data for girls demonstrate notably more spread, particularly in later adolescence. Using the regression equations generated, treadmill determined peak $\dot{V}O_2$ increases from 1.23–3.06 L·min⁻¹ between the ages of

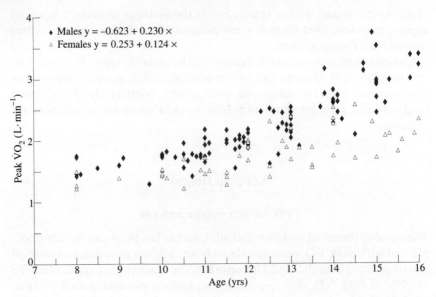

Fig. 4.1. Treadmill determined peak $\dot{V}O_2$ by age. Redrawn from Armstrong, N. and Welsman, J.R. (1994). Assessment and interpretation of aerobic fitness in children and adolescents. *Exercise and Sport Sciences Reviews*, **22**, 435–76. Reprinted with permission.

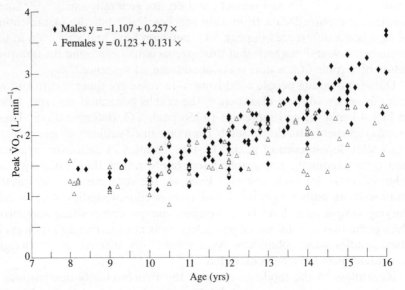

Fig. 4.2. Cycle ergometer determined peak $\dot{V}O_2$ by age. Redrawn from Armstrong, N. and Welsman, J.R. (1994). Assessment and interpretation of aerobic fitness in children and adolescents. *Exercise and Sport Sciences Reviews*, **22**, 435–76. Reprinted with permission.

8 and 16 years in boys and from 1.25–2.24 L·min^{-1} in girls over the same age span.

Longitudinal investigations with boys from Europe, Japan, and North America confirm a consistent increase in peak $\dot{V}O_2$ with increasing age. A large (n = 75) survey of 8–16-year-old Canadian boys[1041] reported an average yearly increase in peak $\dot{V}O_2$ of 11.1%. Between the ages of 12–13 years and 13–14 years the largest absolute increases of 0.31 and 0.32 L·min^{-1} respectively were observed.

Between the ages of 8 and 13 years a similar annual percentage increase (11.6%) has been recorded for 22 girls studied longitudinally.[1041] The highest absolute yearly increases of 0.25 and 0.23 L·min^{-1} were identified between the ages of 11–12 years and 12–13 years, respectively.

Despite the continued increase in peak $\dot{V}O_2$ suggested by this study and the data compiled in Figs 4.1 and 4.2, individual cross-sectional studies have suggested that girls' peak $\dot{V}O_2$ declines in the late teenage years or, at best, levels off.[327, 1083, 1700] For example, Yoshizawa recorded a drop in peak $\dot{V}O_2$ of 0.61 L·min^{-1} between the ages of 14–15 years in urban Japanese girls. Interestingly, this was not observed in their rural counterparts,[1700] perhaps indicating sociocultural influences upon aerobic fitness. Longitudinal studies of European girls, although limited by small sample sizes, indicate that peak $\dot{V}O_2$ reaches its highest value during the mid-teen years: 13.3 years in Norway and 14.7 years in Germany.[1280]

Sex differences in peak oxygen uptake

Using the linear regressions found to be the best fit for the data presented in Figs 4.1 and 4.2, we identified a 13% sex difference in treadmill determined peak $\dot{V}O_2$ in children as young as 10 years. By the age of 12 years, boys' peak $\dot{V}O_2$ was 23% higher than that of girls with the differential increasing to 31% at 14 years and 37% at 16 years of age. Analysis of the cross-sectional data obtained from cycle ergometry revealed a similar trend although the sex difference at 10 years (2%) was markedly lower than identified for treadmill exercise. The difference between male and female scores then increased to 17% at 12 years, 27% at 14 years, and 37% at 16 years. These findings are consistent with, although somewhat larger than, sex differences identified in individual longitudinal studies.[29, 1041, 1280]

Differences in haemoglobin concentration between boys and girls have been suggested to explain the sex difference in peak $\dot{V}O_2$ from the age of 11 years.[85, 810] A significant relationship has been shown to exist between haemoglobin and peak $\dot{V}O_2$ in 11–16-year-old males and females even with the common effect of age partialled out.[85] This provides credible evidence that the sex difference in haemoglobin concentration may well contribute to the observed sex difference in peak $\dot{V}O_2$. However, recent work from our laboratory has documented significant differences in peak $\dot{V}O_2$ in 10–11-year-old prepubertal children despite no significant differences in haemoglobin concentration.[72]

In young children, sex differences in peak $\dot{V}O_2$ have been attributed to differences in body composition; even during the prepubertal years boys have a higher percentage of lean body mass[1257] (and see Chapter 1). However, the results of a longitudinal investigation[811] relating peak $\dot{V}O_2$ to anthropometrically determined fat-free mass found that sex differences in peak $\dot{V}O_2$ remained throughout the age range examined, although the magnitude of the difference was reduced. Girls' lower peak $\dot{V}O_2$ during cycle ergometry has been ascribed to their smaller leg volume.[401] Studies from our laboratory have, however, failed to observe any relationship between peak $\dot{V}O_2$ and either leg volume or leg muscle volume, determined using anthropometric techniques or MRI in either boys or girls,[1625, 1671] once the effects of body size have been partitioned out appropriately.[1095]

Boys' higher peak $\dot{V}O_2$ has also been ascribed to their higher levels of habitual physical activity[851] but, as discussed in Chapter 7, the evidence relating habitual activity to peak aerobic fitness is inconclusive.[60, 106, 803] Well-controlled studies using objective measures of habitual physical activity indicate that as children rarely experience the levels of activity necessary to elicit improvements in aerobic fitness[60, 86] it is unlikely that differences in physical activity contribute significantly to the observed sex differences in peak $\dot{V}O_2$.

Peak oxygen uptake and maturation

The physiological responses of children and adolescents must be considered in relation to biological as well as chronological age. Although peak $\dot{V}O_2$ has been extensively documented in relation to growth, studies have rarely examined changes in aerobic fitness in relation to biological age. This is despite the recognition that peak $\dot{V}O_2$ is likely to be influenced by a body size–maturation interaction,[384] but is perhaps understandable in view of the problems associated with the ethics and practicalities of maturity assessment (see Chapter 1).

Few studies have investigated peak $\dot{V}O_2$ in relation to skeletal age, presumably due to the expense involved[1515] and the ethical issues the procedure engenders.[143] The finding of a skeletal age ranging from 9–16 years in a group of 13–14-year-old teenagers illustrates the wide variation in skeletal age evident in children of similar chronological age.[809] In this study, multiple regression analysis showed increases in peak $\dot{V}O_2$ to be highly related to skeletal age, but when the effects of chronological age, stature, and mass were controlled for, almost all of the variation in peak $\dot{V}O_2$ was shown to be explained simply by the increase in stature and mass. Similarly, a study of 770 children[1387] found that chronological age, stature, and mass explained the majority of the variance in peak $\dot{V}O_2$ scores with skeletal age failing to make a significant additional contribution.

Longitudinal studies permit the investigation of peak $\dot{V}O_2$ in relation to PHV,[385, 803, 834, 1041] but interpretation of the few data available is confounded by the lack, in some studies, of sufficient measurements to fit appropriate and meaningful mathematical models to individual growth curves. The Saskatchewan Growth Study found the greatest increase in peak $\dot{V}O_2$ to coincide with the year of PHV in both boys and girls,[1041, 1042] although it should be noted that PHV occurs early in adolescence in girls and much later in adolescence in boys. In contrast, an analysis of peak $\dot{V}O_2$ in boys from 3 years prior to 2 years after PHV[385] revealed a fairly consistent increase in values across this maturational age range. In a longitudinal study of young athletes a sex difference in the growth of aerobic power in relation to maturity status has been noted.[155] With confounding variables, such as age, stature, and mass, controlled for using multilevel modelling (see Chapter 3), peak $\dot{V}O_2$ increased with maturation in the boys, particularly towards the end of puberty but a similar relationship was not apparent in the athletic girls studied. Further studies with appropriate numbers of untrained subjects are required to elucidate the growth and maturation of aerobic power in the normal child and adolescent.

Despite the well-recognized limitations associated with their use, cross-sectional investigations of peak $\dot{V}O_2$ are restricted to the use of Tanner's indices to assess maturational status, particularly if comparisons between males and females are of interest. Several studies have used Tanner staging to classify individual subject groups as 'prepubertal' or 'pubertal'[85, 328, 1289, 1291] but only one major study appears to have considered peak $\dot{V}O_2$ by maturational stage,[85] probably because of the considerable numbers required to achieve a meaningful analysis. In both sexes a general trend towards an increase in peak $\dot{V}O_2$ with increasing maturity was noted although significant differences between groups were shown to be ergometer-specific. In treadmill-exercised girls, the only significant difference was noted between groups 4 and 2, whilst cycle ergometer testing revealed significantly higher mean peak $\dot{V}O_2$ in groups 4 and 5 than in the less mature girls in groups 1, 2, and 3. This latter finding was attributed to methodological artefact, with the less mature girls terminating exercise earlier due to peripheral muscle fatigue during cycle exercise (see Chapter 2). Results from boys were more consistent with the more mature boys (groups 4 and 5) having significantly higher peak $\dot{V}O_2$ than the less mature boys (groups 1, 2, and 3) regardless of the ergometer. It was inferred that this was probably due to higher haemoglobin concentration and to greater muscle mass in the mature boys, as indicated by a higher body mass but similar skinfold thickness compared with the less mature children. Sex differences within maturity groups were also noted with the absolute peak $\dot{V}O_2$ of boys in maturity groups 4 and 5 consistently higher than girls of comparable maturity. Within the cycle

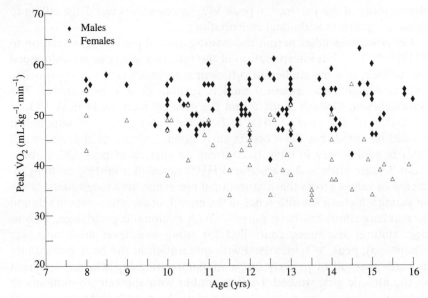

Fig. 4.3. Mass-related treadmill determined peak $\dot{V}O_2$ by age. Redrawn from Armstrong, N. and Welsman, J.R. (1994). Assessment and interpretation of aerobic fitness in children and adolescents. *Exercise and Sport Sciences Reviews*, **22**, 435–76. Reprinted with permission.

ergometer-tested subjects, boys also had significantly higher peak $\dot{V}O_2$ than the girls in maturity groups 2 and 3.

Using serum testosterone as a measure of maturity, Welsman *et al.*[1623] reported that testosterone made no significant contribution to the explained variance in the peak $\dot{V}O_2$ of 12–16-year-old untrained boys beyond the 74% accounted for by age, stature, and mass. These findings suggest that hormonal changes with puberty, *per se*, may not play a role in the development of aerobic power and that the effects of other growth-related factors predominate.

Peak oxygen uptake and body size

Mass-related peak $\dot{V}O_2$
The size-dependency of aerobic fitness is demonstrated by the consistently high correlation coefficients (typically exceeding $r = 0.7$) observed between peak $\dot{V}O_2$ and body mass or stature.[85, 1446] As most physical activity involves moving the body mass from one place to another, in order to facilitate comparisons between individuals of different body size, peak $\dot{V}O_2$ is conventionally expressed relative to mass (i.e. as $mL \cdot kg^{-1} \cdot min^{-1}$).[81] Figures 4.3 and 4.4 demonstrate that mass-related peak $\dot{V}O_2$ remains essentially stable

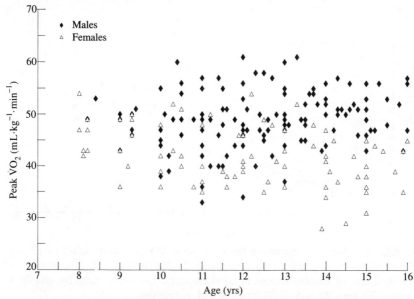

Fig. 4.4. Mass-related cycle ergometer determined peak $\dot{V}O_2$ by age. Redrawn from Armstrong, N. and Welsman, J.R. (1994). Assessment and interpretation of aerobic fitness in children and adolescents. *Exercise and Sport Sciences Reviews*, **22**, 435–76. Reprinted with permission.

with increasing age in boys, with values approximating 50 mL·kg⁻¹·min⁻¹, whilst in girls there is a tendency for values to fall with increasing age from around 45–35 mL·kg⁻¹·min⁻¹.[81] These trends are generally consistent with data from individual longitudinal studies[29, 126, 1041] although discrepant findings have been reported.[1280, 1446] Boys' mass-related peak $\dot{V}O_2$ is consistently higher than girls' throughout the age range 8–16 years with girls penalized by the expression of peak $\dot{V}O_2$ in mass-related terms due to their accumulation of body fat during puberty.

Alternative scaling methods

Compared with the large number of studies reporting mass-related peak $\dot{V}O_2$, studies examining age- or maturity-related changes in peak $\dot{V}O_2$ using alternative methods to partition out body size differences are sparse. However, the results of these have consistently diverged markedly from those indicated by conventional analyses. The theoretical and statistical principles behind the alternative linear adjustment and allometric scaling techniques were outlined in Chapter 3, therefore the discussion that follows is restricted to the results obtained from the use of these techniques to interpret the growth of peak $\dot{V}O_2$.

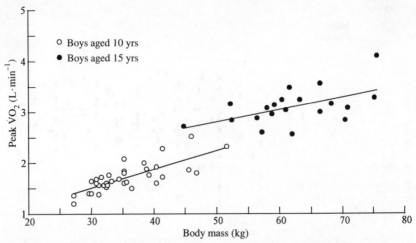

Fig. 4.5. The linear relationship between peak V̇O₂ and body mass in 10- and 15-year-old boys. Redrawn from Armstrong, N. and Welsman, J. Assessment and interpretation of aerobic fitness in children and adolescents. *Exercise and Sport Sciences Reviews*, **22**, 435–76. Reprinted with permission.

We used linear regression modelling to investigate changes in peak V̇O₂ by chronological age in two groups of boys aged 10 and 15 years.[1660] The mean values for mass-related peak V̇O₂ in the two groups were not significantly different whether examined by age or maturity. The regression lines describing the linear relationships between peak V̇O₂ and body mass for the two groups are illustrated in Fig. 4.5 and clearly denote two distinct populations. The results of the analysis of covariance comparing the two regression lines yielded a significantly higher adjusted mean for peak V̇O₂ in the older group. The same pattern of findings was obtained when results were analysed by biological age.

A subsequent development of the study to examine changes in peak V̇O₂ in groups of prepubertal, circumpubertal, and adult males and females[1624] confirmed the previous findings in boys and demonstrated a continued significant increase in peak V̇O₂ into adulthood. Analysis of female peak V̇O₂ using a linear model also produced challenging findings. Whereas a significant decline in aerobic fitness was indicated by a fall in mass-related peak V̇O₂ between puberty and adulthood, the linear adjusted means demonstrated a significant increase in peak V̇O₂ from prepuberty to puberty, with a maintenance of levels apparent into adulthood. In view of the well-recognized limitations of linear modelling, this study also examined changes in peak V̇O₂ using a log-linear (allometric) model. The results confirmed the progressive functional improvements in peak V̇O₂ in males and the increase into puberty and stability thereafter of peak V̇O₂ in females suggested by the linear model but the log-linear model was demonstrated to represent a better statistical fit for the data.

Similarly, using the theoretical mass exponent of 0.67 (see Chapter 3), Kemper and Verschuur[809] identified no significant relationship between peak $\dot{V}O_2$ normalized to $mL \cdot kg^{-0.67} \cdot min^{-1}$ and skeletal age in either boys or girls. This contrasted with the significant decline in mass-related peak $\dot{V}O_2$ observed with increasing chronological age.

Despite the discrepancies in the patterns of change in peak $\dot{V}O_2$ with maturation revealed by linear and log-linear scaling analyses compared with conventional analyses, studies which have concurrently examined sex differences in peak $\dot{V}O_2$ have shown that these remain when alternative scaling models are applied although the magnitude of the difference is marginally increased.[72, 1621, 1624]

Blood lactate as a measure of aerobic fitness

Although a high peak $\dot{V}O_2$ is a prerequisite for success in aerobic endurance activities and ultimately limits an individual's maximal aerobic performance, the measurement of peak $\dot{V}O_2$ is neither the best index of an individual's ability to sustain aerobic exercise at submaximal intensities nor the most sensitive means by which to detect improvements in aerobic endurance following training.

Despite its derivation from anaerobic metabolism, measures of blood lactate accumulation during submaximal exercise provide an accurate reflection of aerobic fitness[1632, 1698] and can be used to detect improvements in muscle oxidative capacity with training even in the absence of changes in peak $\dot{V}O_2$.[708, 1410]

The response of blood lactate to incremental exercise is illustrated in Fig. 4.6. With aerobic training, and the consequent changes in muscle metabolism which enhance oxidative energy generation (see Chapter 7), the entire lactate curve is shifted to the right (see Fig. 4.6). As a result, any given level of exercise elicits a lower level of blood lactate accumulation. This predictable and easily detectable change in the blood lactate curve can thus be used to monitor the submaximal aerobic fitness of individuals. The exact metabolic events reflected by blood lactate and how blood lactate responses should be standardized for performance assessment have been among the most contentious issues within the exercise sciences. The term 'anaerobic threshold' has become generic for submaximal measures of blood lactate but, as will be discussed, the use of this term in different studies does not necessarily imply the application of the same theoretical or practical measures and can lead to misinterpretation of data.

It is well documented that children typically respond to a given exercise bout with a lower blood lactate level than adults.[525, 896, 981] Therefore, it can be inferred that, during childhood and adolescence, some maturation of the

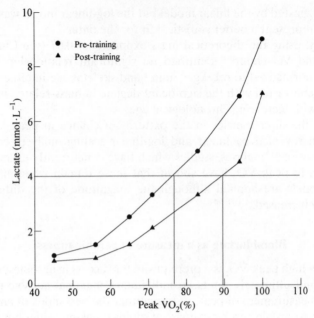

Fig. 4.6. Blood lactate responses to incremental exercise.

systems that regulate the predominance of a given energy system during exercise must occur. Physiological or metabolic explanations for the observed differences between young people and adults have proved elusive to establish, due both to methodological differences in blood analysis techniques (described in Chapter 2), and inconsistent lactate reference criteria.

Anaerobic threshold

The concept of 'anaerobic threshold' has been extensively debated and reviewed,[33, 253, 406, 1590, 1697] therefore only a brief discussion of the main issues follows to give context to the ensuing discussion of children's and adolescents' blood lactate responses to exercise.

In its original conception, the anaerobic threshold described specifically,

the level of work or O_2 consumption just below that at which metabolic acidosis and the associated changes in gas exchange occur.[1601, p. 236]

This onset of anaerobic metabolism or acidosis was assumed to reflect the point at which oxygen demand exceeded supply[1600] and thus could be identified during incremental exercise as the point at which blood lactate first increased above resting levels.[1601] Inherent to this theory was the assumption of a causal link between the onset of metabolic acidosis and the specific changes in ventilatory or gas exchange parameters (i.e. ventilation is stimulated by the increased CO_2 flux to the lungs arising from bicarbonate buffering of hydrogen ions dissociated from lactic acid). Thus, it was suggested, a non-invasive estimate of the lactate anaerobic threshold could be made from gas exchange markers, such as the initial departure of ventilation from linearity with exercise intensity (or $\dot{V}O_2$) or a consistent increase in the ventilatory equivalent for O_2 without a concomitant increase in the ventilatory equivalent for CO_2.[1601] The validity of the original anaerobic threshold concept has been disputed[253] and the argument presented that blood lactate levels reflect the balance between processes of lactate production and elimination rather than the onset of cellular anaerobiosis.

Several studies have provided credible evidence to suggest that the often observed coincidence of 'lactate' and 'ventilatory' thresholds is not causal and may be disrupted under a variety of experimental conditions. For example, with training a divergence of the two thresholds has been observed,[594] and in patients suffering from McArdle's disease, where a lack of the enzyme phosphorylase precludes lactate generation during exercise, a ventilatory threshold is still observed.[669] Although this evidence has been disputed on theoretical grounds[1009, 1590, 1697] there are sufficient data from normal subjects showing disparity of lactate and ventilatory thresholds[649, 1395, 1396] to question the validity of the proposed causal relationship.

Lactate reference levels

The theoretical and practical problems associated with the determination of the anaerobic threshold such as the identification of the threshold point and the influence of varying baseline lactate levels upon its determination[789] may be circumvented by the use of a fixed blood lactate reference level.[1408, 1631, 1633] The measurement of performance at a blood lactate of 4.0 mmol·L^{-1} has become the most widely accepted assessment criterion in adults.[675] Various terms have been used to describe this level, including anaerobic threshold[818] and onset of blood lactate accumulation.[1409, 1410] However, the rationale behind a 4.0 mmol·L^{-1} performance criterion is quite distinct from that proposed for the original anaerobic threshold and the two concepts should not be confused.

The highest level of blood lactate that can be sustained without a progressive accumulation has been defined as the maximal lactate steady-state (MLaSS).[693, 704] At this exercise intensity the processes of lactate accumulation and elimination are in equilibrium[704] permitting activity to continue for prolonged periods. Originally, the 4.0 mmol·L^{-1} level was hypothesized to reflect the maximal lactate steady-state and data have been provided to support this contention in adults[704] although wide inter-individual differences have been noted, particularly in athletes.[693, 1460]

Recognizing that many children can exercise close to exhaustion without exceeding a blood lactate of 4 mmol·L^{-1} [1658, 1701] some authors have expressed concern with the use of this level as an assessment criterion in young subjects.[1598, 1658] Based upon data collected in our laboratory from 103 12-year-old boys and girls, Williams *et al.*[1658] recommended the use of a lower criterion level of 2.5 mmol·L^{-1}. This recommendation was subsequently supported by the finding that the MLaSS occurred at 2.1 mmol·L^{-1} and 2.3 mmol·L^{-1} in 13-year-old boys and girls, respectively, with a corresponding exercise intensity of 78% peak $\dot{V}O_2$.[1656] Further analysis of the results revealed that cardiopulmonary responses at the MLaSS were not significantly different from those at the 2.5 mmol·L^{-1} determined during incremental treadmill exercise. Very few studies have examined the MLaSS in children so there is minimal corroborative evidence. Other studies of similarly aged children have reported lactate levels of 3.9 mmol·L^{-1} [189] and 5.0 mmol·L^{-1} [1047, 1048] at the MLaSS. The discrepancies between studies may be explained in part by the use of different assay methods, but also by the protocols used to estimate the MLaSS. In some studies the MLaSS may have been overestimated[1047, 1048] by the use of a discontinuous running protocol where children rested for 30 sec every 3.5 min during the exercise stage to permit blood sampling. This may have altered patterns of lactate production and elimination compared with continuous exercise. Billat *et al.*[189] did not measure the MLaSS directly but derived it mathematically from blood lactate responses measured during two 15-min exercise bouts at 64% and 74% peak $\dot{V}O_2$. As no more intense stages were completed, it is questionable whether the true MLaSS was established, particularly as the percentage peak $\dot{V}O_2$ cited for a blood lactate of 3.9 mmol·L^{-1} is markedly lower than that observed in other work.[1656] The validity of adopting for children an indirect assessment method of MLaSS originally derived and refined for adult élite athletes may be questioned and may have contributed to the discrepancies observed between this study and others. In prepubertal children even the 2.5 mmol·L^{-1} level may occur too close to peak $\dot{V}O_2$ to represent a suitable criterion for submaximal performance.[72]

Blood lactate responses to exercise and chronological age

Studies reporting a higher anaerobic threshold in children compared with adults[106, 1597, 1599] have often cited investigations which have used non-invasive measures to determine the anaerobic threshold[775, 1127, 1201, 1640] to support this conclusion. However, the concerns with the validity of the anaerobic threshold concept alluded to above, particularly when determined non-invasively suggest that child–adult differences in blood lactate responses cannot be reliably inferred from these studies.

The identification of age and maturational changes in blood lactate responses to exercise based upon direct measurements of a 'lactate threshold' or fixed lactate value is clouded by inconsistent methodologies which preclude inter-study comparisons. The effects of the analytical techniques used to sample and assay blood upon the lactate values obtained were discussed in Chapter 2, but in addition, definitions and methods of determining the anaerobic threshold vary between studies. For example 'anaerobic threshold' has been variously defined as the running velocity corresponding to the mathematically determined lactate inflection point,[1248] the running velocity which elicits a blood lactate slightly below 2 mmol·L^{-1} [1501] or the exercise intensity at a blood lactate of 4.0 mmol·L^{-1}.[598]

A complication of submaximal blood lactate responses in children and adolescents with reference to age is presented in Table 4.1. Age-related trends are difficult to discern with any accuracy due to methodological inconsistencies and a notable lack of data describing the responses of girls. In comparison with adults,[753] or when examined by chronological age during childhood and adolescence[1394, 1501] investigators have reported a decline in the heart rate or percentage peak $\dot{V}O_2$ at the lactate reference criterion with increasing age, perhaps indicative of a diminishing propensity for aerobic metabolism. Our study of performance at blood lactate reference values of 2.5 and 4.0 mmol·L^{-1} in 210 11–16-year-old subjects found no relationship between age and percentage peak $\dot{V}O_2$ at the 4.0 mmol·L^{-1} level. Significant coefficients were obtained when age was correlated with performance at the 2.5 mmol·L^{-1} level, however the biological significance of the very low coefficients ($r = -0.226$ in boys and -0.272 for girls) is questionable. Significant child–adult differences were observed consistently when percentage peak $\dot{V}O_2$ at 4.0 mmol·L^{-1} lactate was examined with values of 91% vs. 86% for boys and men, respectively, with comparable values for girls and women of 90% vs. 85%.[81] Although the boys retained a higher percentage peak $\dot{V}O_2$ than the men at the lower reference level (83% vs. 75%), the girls and women were not significantly different from one another (77% vs. 76%). These data indicate the post-adolescent period as significant for the maturation of blood lactate responses to exercise and further research efforts in this population are warranted.

Sex differences in submaximal blood lactate responses are difficult to establish as boys and girls have rarely been examined within the same study. Although there are indications of a higher anaerobic threshold in boys compared with girls[1598] other studies have not identified significant sex differences in performance at fixed reference levels.[1657]

Explanations for young people's lower blood lactates

Several lines of evidence have been examined in the search for an explanation for the observed differences in the blood lactate response to exercise in children and adolescents compared with adults. The main mechanisms proposed to account for the lower lactates are summarized in Table 4.2.

Table 4.1. Submaximal blood lactate variables in young people: lactate thresholds and fixed blood lactate reference values

Study[a]	Sex	n	Age (yrs)	Lactate variable	$\dot{V}O_2$ ($mL \cdot kg^{-1} \cdot min^{-1}$)	% peak $\dot{V}O_2$	Heart rate (bpm)	% peak $\dot{V}O_2$	Lactate ($mmol \cdot L^{-1}$)	Velocity ($km \cdot h^{-1}$)
Izumi & Ishiko[753]	M	11	13.3	LT[b]	35.8	72.7	164	85	3.84	
Tanaka & Shindo[1501]	M	15	8.8	LT			185	93		11.3
	M	11	10.9	LT			185	92		11.4
	M	11	12.7	LT			173	90		11.0
	M	19	14.6	LT			173	87		10.9
Atomi et al.[106]	M	11	10.4	LT	36.7	71	169	84	1.6	
Atomi et al.[104]	M	13	11.8	LT	33.2	63.7			1.9	
Atomi et al.[104]	M	11	19.6	LT	35.9	70.9				
Atomi et al.[105]	M	28	10.8	LT		82.24				10.04
Atomi et al.[105]	M	28	10.8	LT		85.07				10.36
Williams & Armstrong[1657]	M	84	11–16	2.5 mM	41	83	186	93		
	F	65	11–16	2.5 mM	32	77	184	92		
Tolfrey & Armstrong[1534]	M	26	11	2.5 mM		85				
	M	26	14	2.5 mM		85				
	M	26	11	4.0 mM		94				
	M	26	14	4.0 mM		92				
Keul et al.[814]	M		10–14	4.0 mM			190	97		
Williams & Armstrong[1657]	M	81	11–16	4.0 mM	45	91	195	97		
	F	81	11–16	4.0 mM	37	90	193	96		

[a] All studies reflect treadmill testing except Study 1 which used cycle ergometry.

[b] LT, lactate threshold (i.e. point of onset of rapid increase in blood lactate concentration).

Reproduced from Armstrong, N. and Welsman, J. (1994). Assessment and interpretation of aerobic function in children and adolescents. *Exercise and Sport Sciences Reviews*, **22**, 435–76. Reprinted with permission.

Table 4.2. Proposed explanations for young people's lower blood lactate responses to exercise

Explanatory factor	Proposed mechanism
Circulatory factors	Faster oxygen on-transients
	Smaller body size and circulation time
Muscle metabolic characteristics	Higher proportion of type I fibres
	Preponderance of oxidative enzymes
	Substrate utilization—increased metabolism of fat
Hormonal differences	Subdued catecholamine response to exercise
	Low levels of testosterone
Higher levels of habitual physical activity	Increased aerobic fitness

Muscle metabolic characteristics

Pioneering studies using invasive techniques, now generally proscribed, observed lower rates of glycogen usage and lower maximal muscle lactate concentrations in 11–15-year-old boys[521, 525] compared with adults suggesting a compromised ability to generate energy from glycolysis. The significantly lower levels of phosphofructokinase (PFK), the rate-limiting enzyme for glycolysis, observed in a parallel study of five 11-year-old boys was proposed as a causative factor[518] although the author himself, in acknowledgement of the small sample size stated 'the results must therefore be interpreted with caution and no general conclusions may be drawn'.[512, p. 18] Despite this note of caution these data have been frequently, and largely uncritically, cited in explanation for observed low levels of blood lactate in young people.[373, 1027, 1676]

Evidence from subsequent investigations has provided limited support for lower levels of PFK in male adolescents compared with adults,[562] but studies comparing the maximal activities of various glycolytic enzymes including PFK have failed to detect significant or consistent child–adult differences.[172, 683] The source of ATP for muscle contraction depends upon the intensity and duration of exercise and a constant supply is ensured by a complex interplay of anaerobic and aerobic provision. Therefore, the metabolic potential of children's muscle may be better understood if the functional capacity of the aerobic energy system is examined alongside the mechanisms which regulate glycolysis. Whereas the evidence for inferior glycolytic potential is ambiguous, studies have consistently observed elevated levels of oxidative enzymes, for example, succinic dehydrogenase

(SDH) and isocitric dehydrogenase (ICDH).[518, 562, 683] Differences in the ratio of PFK to ICDH in children (0.884) compared with adults (1.633) reflect an enhanced ability for pyruvate oxidation[683] and provide evidence that children are preferentially equipped for aerobic energy production.

Although data are limited, there are indications that children have a higher proportion of slow twitch (type I) fibres in the vastus lateralis muscle compared to untrained adults and, in fact, are more typical of adult endurance athletes.[165, 525, 635] The higher mitochondrial volume, ratio of mitochondria to myofibrillar volume, and intramuscular lipid storage observed in 6-year-old children compared with untrained men and women[165] provide additional indications that children have an enhanced ability to generate energy from aerobic metabolism. Recent investigations with adults have used MRI to determine muscle fibre type.[735, 864, 1134] The extension of this technique to children and adolescents may help resolve some of the key issues regarding the maturation of muscle metabolic characteristics.

Increased fat utilization during exercise

An increased availability of fat as an energy substrate may alter the pattern of the blood lactate response to exercise by delaying anaerobic metabolism, resulting in a lower lactate level for a given exercise intensity.[752] A significantly lower RER during submaximal exercise in boys compared with men has been a common finding[89, 1052, 1267] and is indicative of increased fat utilization. However, studies which have directly measured blood levels of energy substrates reflective of increased FFA utilization are sparse and their results contradictory. Blood free glycerol levels reflect the extent of lipolysis.[943] During prolonged exercise no significant differences between glycerol levels in children compared with adults have been identified.[524, 943] Similarly, no differences have been observed between prepubescent boys and adult men in changes in the fat-mobilizing GH during exercise at 70% peak $\dot{V}O_2$.[1122] Neither have relationships been observed between GH and blood lactate levels or any significant differences in FFA levels during exercise at 70% peak $\dot{V}O_2$, in prepubertal, pubertal, and postpubertal boys and girls.[1676] Contrasting results are available from a recent, well-controlled investigation into child–adult differences in substrate utilization during exercise at the same relative intensity.[981] These authors found a significantly lower RER during a 30-min exercise bout at 70% peak $\dot{V}O_2$ in girls compared with adults. Changes in FFA and glycerol levels corrected for changes in plasma volume were not significantly different between prepubertal girls and women. Girls were characterized by a significantly higher fat contribution to total energy expenditure throughout the exercise and a significant increase in the relative contribution of fats and accompanying decline in carbohydrate utilization was observed in the younger subjects, whilst no significant changes were observed in the adults. Further well-controlled studies with broader subject populations are required to clarify the validity of altered substrate utilization as an explanatory mechanism for children's lower lactate responses to exercise.

Faster oxygen on-transients

One frequently suggested explanation of young people's lower blood lactate is a faster circulatory adjustment following the onset of exercise resulting in the rapid attainment of a $\dot{V}O_2$ steady-state. In adults, faster oxygen on-transients during exercise occur with aerobic training[673, 718, 1643] and are associated with a reduced lactate accumulation.[322, 673] Thus, by increasing the availability of oxygen to the muscle, a faster oxygen on-transient is suggested to contribute to the lower blood lactate response in children.[937, 941]

In a carefully controlled study[1290] the time taken for $\dot{V}O_2$ to reach 50% of its asymptotic value, the t½ $\dot{V}O_2$[1156, 1289] did not differ significantly in adults (17.4 sec) from children (18.5 sec) during submaximal exercise at 40% peak $\dot{V}O_2$. Neither were any differences noted between children and adults in the oxygen on-transients to short bursts of exercise at intensities ranging from submaximal to supramaximal.[1708] In comparison, the results from several studies have supported a faster oxygen adjustment to exercise in children at maximal or supramaximal exercise intensities compared with adults. After 30 sec of maximal exercise children have been shown to attain a higher percentage of peak $\dot{V}O_2$ than adults.[940, 941, 1219] Similarly, significantly shorter t½ $\dot{V}O_2$ times have been observed in children[1156, 1289] with, for example, a mean value of 11.7 sec in boys, compared with 29.1 sec in adults, associated with lower blood lactate levels.[942]

Clearly, there are as yet, insufficient data derived from consistent methodologies to support or refute the hypothesis that oxygen on-transients and blood lactate responses are causally linked in children, particularly at submaximal exercise intensities. Further studies using more refined technologies, such as mass spectrometry, are required to clarify the nature and extent of the influence of such circulatory factors on blood lactate accumulation during exercise.

Higher levels of habitual physical activity

The inference that children naturally display high levels of habitual physical activity[139, 384] has been used to explain the minimal increases in peak $\dot{V}O_2$ often observed following a period of aerobic training in children.[138, 139, 680] It would appear reasonable, therefore, to suggest that this training effect extends to a reduction in the blood lactate response at a given level of exercise. The available evidence refutes any such linkage; children and adolescents are characteristically sedentary[57, 60, 64] and no significant relationships have been found between objectively measured physical activity and percentage peak $\dot{V}O_2$ at submaximal blood lactate reference values in prepubertal and pubertal children[73, 1620] (and see Chapter 7).

Catecholamine responses to exercise

Several studies have implicated catecholamine responses to exercise as a mediating influence upon children's and adolescents' lower blood lactates during incremental exercise. That incremental exercise elicits changes in adrenaline and noradrenaline that closely parallel those observed in the blood lactate response is well documented in both adults[895] and young people.[836, 838, 896] As noradrenaline initiates vasoconstriction[402] and adrenaline stimulates glycolysis in muscle[1101, 1204] it is plausible that the subdued catecholamine response to exercise observed in boys compared with adults[202, 896] is linked to the lower blood lactates via reduced vasoconstriction enabling the maintenance of a higher blood flow to the liver which is one of the major clearance sites for lactate.[937]

Despite much investigation, the available data are either insufficient or methodologically flawed to enable any one of these proposed mechanisms to be identified as the primary cause of young people's lower blood lactate responses to exercise. It is possible that a combination of these factors is contributory and further research in this area is required.

Maturation and blood lactate responses to exercise

There has been a long-standing hypothesis that the ability to generate energy from glycolytic processes is dependent upon sexual maturation. This theory originated from the work of Eriksson and co-workers[521] whose results indicated a relationship between sexual maturation in boys as indicated by testicular volume and lactate metabolism. These findings have frequently been used as evidence for a maturity-dependence of lactate metabolism despite the fact that the relationship was very clearly stated as an 'almost significant' ($r = 0.67$, $P > 0.05$) correlation derived from a sample of eight 13–15-year-old boys. Also frequently cited to reinforce the maturity-dependence hypothesis are the results of studies which have demonstrated the necessary role of testosterone in the maturation of glycolysis in rat skeletal muscle.[479, 480, 858] However, the available research evidence is insufficient to substantiate the existence of a similar causal relationship in children and adolescents.

Significant, although moderate ($r \approx 0.4$), correlations between testosterone levels and blood lactate responses to exercise at a wide range of intensities have frequently been reported[533, 1027, 1028] and cited as evidence for an androgenic influence upon glycolysis. Similarly, a significant relationship between skeletal age, which closely reflects androgen levels in boys, and performance at the lactate threshold has been observed.[1501]

These data appear to support the contention that maturation and blood lactate responses are causally linked but there are several conceptual problems with this interpretation. All of the subjects in these studies were prepubertal with testosterone levels considerably lower than would be expected to have significant metabolic effects. Indices of anaerobic performance have, in fact, been shown to increase prior to puberty and in the absence of any significant changes in testosterone levels.[532]

Several studies can be criticized for failing to adequately control for the confounding influence of the intercorrelations between testosterone, other growth indices, and the performance variable under consideration. Testosterone levels are highly correlated with stature and body mass during the adolescent period therefore any examination of the independent effect of testosterone upon blood lactate responses should use statistical techniques which allow these confounding relationships to be controlled for.

Using regression analysis to investigate the contribution of body size and testosterone to the variance in submaximal and peak blood lactate responses, we identified no significant independent effect of the hormone upon lactate measures over and above the effects of stature and body mass in 12–16-year-old boys whose maturational status ranged from pre- to post-puberty.[1623] A similar analysis failed to identify any relationship between testosterone and blood lactate following a 30 sec supramaximal effort in 12–13-year-old boys.[1622]

Additional evidence to refute an independent effect of sexual maturity upon blood lactate responses to exercise is available. Despite a two year differential in biological age, Paterson and Cunningham[1143] failed to identify significant differences in the post-exercise blood lactates in children of the same chronological age classified as early or late maturers. Our investigation of changes in submaximal and peak exercise blood lactate levels by maturity stage in 11–16-year-old boys and girls[1657] revealed no significant changes with increasing maturity in either sex.

Finally, despite widespread documentation and discussion of the effect of testosterone upon the development of glycolysis, there has been a notable failure to address the nature of this relationship in females. Girls have only minimal levels of testosterone throughout maturation yet their ability to produce lactate during exercise is clearly not compromised.[1622, 1657] In fact, girls have occasionally been shown to attain higher levels of blood lactate accumulation than boys.[378, 1332] This provides compelling evidence that factors other than hormonal adjustments with maturity mediate the development of energy metabolism.

Summary

Cardiovascular and pulmonary responses to exercise in children and adolescents appear typically different from adults, although methodological constraints have hindered the precise quantification of measures, such as cardiac output and stroke volume. Ventilatory function is somewhat less efficient in young people compared with adults, perhaps due to increased sensitivity to CO_2. Peak $\dot{V}O_2$ has been extensively documented in children and adolescents and data compiled from 8–16-year-olds indicate a linear increase in peak $\dot{V}O_2$ in both sexes over this period. Peak $\dot{V}O_2$ is consistently higher in boys than in girls and has been attributed to their increased muscle mass and haemoglobin levels, although these factors do not adequately explain the observed sex difference in peak $\dot{V}O_2$ in prepubertal children. Boys may experience a growth spurt in peak $\dot{V}O_2$ with PHV but this appears unrelated to the increase in testosterone levels. Expressed relative to body mass, boys' peak $\dot{V}O_2$ remains consistent throughout childhood and adolescence whilst a decline in peak $\dot{V}O_2$ is observed in girls. The inadequacy of ratio standards to normalize peak $\dot{V}O_2$ data during growth has been demonstrated, and linear and log-linear scaling methods have shown size-related peak $\dot{V}O_2$ to increase throughout adolescence in boys and increase into puberty before levelling out in girls as they approach adulthood.

Blood lactate measured during incremental exercise provides an estimation of aerobic fitness which is, in adults, more sensitive to training than peak $\dot{V}O_2$. Blood lactate levels at any given exercise intensity are lower in children and adolescents than adults, but methodological and theoretical issues regarding the standardization of lactate criteria have hindered our understanding of the growth and maturation of blood lactate responses. Objective reference criteria may be more appropriate to assess changes with growth than use of the 'anaerobic threshold' but the adult derived 4.0 mmol·L^{-1} reference criterion is too high to consistently reflect submaximal aerobic fitness in young people. The 2.5 mmol·L^{-1} level may be more appropriate and has been shown to approximate the maximal lactate steady-state in teenagers. Age-related changes in blood lactate responses have been difficult to discern from compiled data due to methodological inconsistencies but the post-adolescent period may be significant for the transition to adult responses. Many explanations have been proposed to explain children's and adolescents' lower blood lactate responses to exercise but data are insufficient to confirm hormonal differences, muscle metabolic differences, faster oxygen transients, or increased habitual physical activity as explanatory factors.

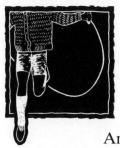

5

Anaerobic exercise: growth and maturation

Anaerobic performance and age

As demonstrated for peak aerobic power (Figs 4.1 and 4.2), peak and mean anaerobic power share a strong positive relationship with chronological age in both males and females. These relationships are summarized in Figs 5.1 and 5.2 which collate published anaerobic performance data from subjects aged 8–16 years. A few studies have measured the anaerobic characteristics of children as young as 7 years old[532, 1561] but these results have been excluded from the graphical presentation. This has been done to be consistent with the summarized aerobic data (Figs 4.1 and 4.2) and in view of concerns with the validity and reliability of the WAnT as a measure of anaerobic performance in very young children (see Chapter 2). The graphed data reflect peak and mean anaerobic power assessed using the WAnT (see Chapter 2). Care has been taken to exclude any data reported in more than one paper, and as far as it has been possible to determine from subject descriptions, data are drawn from healthy, untrained children and adolescents.

The relative lack of documentation of young people's anaerobic performance is highlighted by the number of subjects represented in these figures. For example, Figs 5.1 and 5.2 summarize the data from fewer than 650 boys and fewer than 300 girls, a poor comparison to the more than 10 000 data points represented in the comparable graphs for peak $\dot{V}O_2$ (Figs 4.1 and 4.2) These values also emphasize the dearth of data describing the anaerobic performance of girls, who have participated in far fewer experimental studies than boys, with a particular lack of information available for the 13–16-year-old age range.

Caution must be applied to the interpretation of these graphs as the methods used to obtain the data have varied considerably among studies. In contrast to the protocol-independent nature of peak $\dot{V}O_2$ determinations, values for anaerobic performance parameters will vary according to factors such as the relative resistance applied, the nature of any warm-up prior to the test, and any variation in the administration of the test such as the use of a rolling or static start.

Figures 5.1 and 5.2 indicate that age-related patterns of change in anaerobic performance differ from those in aerobic power. One immediately striking feature is the differential pattern of increase in peak and mean power between the sexes. Although individual studies have found exponential

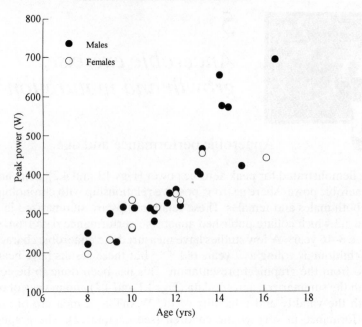

Fig. 5.1. Peak anaerobic power by age.

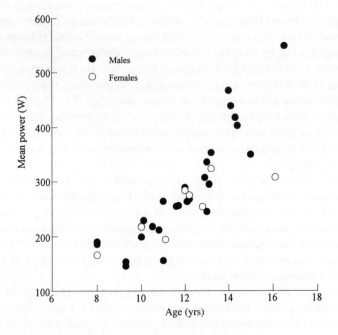

Fig. 5.2. Mean anaerobic power by age.

terms to best describe age-related changes in aerobic parameters,[532] no attempt has been made to generate curves to fit the data presented here because of the variation in methodology. The data for boys do, however, suggest an accelerated increase in peak and mean anaerobic power apparent from the age of 12–14 years. This compares with a consistent, progressive increase in peak $\dot{V}O_2$ over this period. In contrast, peak and mean power data for girls suggest a fairly linear increase with age reaching a plateau around the mid teens, although this interpretation is limited by the lack of data points from 13 years onwards.

In contrast to the growth of peak aerobic power, boys do not demonstrate consistently higher values for absolute peak and mean anaerobic power than girls throughout childhood. Sex differences are minimal until the onset of the accelerated growth of anaerobic power indices in boys.

There are remarkably few substantial studies reporting age-related trends in anaerobic performance in normal, untrained subjects. The vast majority of these are cross-sectional and report data exclusively from boys.[373, 532, 1025] Longitudinal data are reported in only one study[535] and, again, are derived from boys.

Despite the paucity of data, results from individual studies conform broadly to the picture presented by the data compiled in Figs 5.1 and 5.2. Both cross-sectional and longitudinal studies have consistently confirmed, in boys at least, an increase in peak and/or mean power of at least 150% between the ages of 8–16 years.[373, 532, 535, 1025] Studies examining annual changes in anaerobic performance report a maximal annual increase in peak and mean power of 30–40%. The age at which this is reported to occur varies from 11–12 years[532] to 12–13 years.[1025] This supports the spurt in anaerobic performance indicated at these ages in Fig. 5.1. The precise magnitude of annual change between other ages is difficult to determine due to methodological differences and/or inconsistent age increments between the subject groupings used for comparison.[532]

Individual studies have indicated the presence of a period in late childhood to early teen years where girls' anaerobic performance is superior to that of boys. Unpublished longitudinal data from our laboratory show a 2% higher peak and mean power in girls ($n = 60$) at the age of 12.2 years falling to 2% lower than boys ($n = 70$) 12 months later. Similarly, in cross-sectional studies of 10-year-old children we have observed values about 6% higher in girls than in boys. A study of anaerobic performance during maximal knee flexions and extensions for 10 and 30 sec has reported significantly higher values in boys throughout the age range 13–19 years.[1288]

Anaerobic performance and maturation

Given the indications that the sexual dimorphism in patterns of growth in anaerobic performance originates at around 12–14 years of age, further examination of performance in relation to a biological rather than chrono-logical time base is critical to the interpretation of the underlying physio-logical characteristics.

Unfortunately, although several studies have used skeletal,[535] secondary sexual characteristics,[1106] and hormonal[1562] indices of maturity to charac-terize their subject groups, studies examining anaerobic performance in relation to a broad spread of biological age are rare. The largest published database of cross-sectional data collected within a single study is restricted to boys[532] as are the two published longitudinal studies.[535, 1143] A study of 144 boys aged 6–15 years noted that peak and mean anaerobic power, expressed in ratio with body mass ($W \cdot kg^{-1}$), increased by 52% and 58%, respectively, between the ages of 10–15 years in association with an almost two-fold increase in testosterone levels over the same period.[532] The large increase in both peak and mean power between the groups with mean ages of 13.1 and 14.4 years was associated with a similar increase in testosterone over the same period. Although this was not the greatest inter-group increase in testosterone, it represents the transition between early puberty (Tanner stages 2–3 for pubic hair/genitalia) and late puberty (stage 4),[285] a period which is characterized by significant developmental events such as the attainment of PHV and subsequent accelerated growth of muscle mass (see Chapter 1). These findings concur with the observation of marked increases in peak power during the growth spurt[1025] and, in conjunction with the significant correlations observed between mass-related peak ($r = 0.45$) and mean ($r = 0.47$) power and testosterone levels,[532] are indicative of the significance of boys' sexual maturation in the development of anaerobic performance. In this latter study, the common influence of the much higher correlation coefficients also noted between age, stature and body mass, and testosterone ($r = 0.61–0.71$) was not partialled out of the testosterone–performance relationship[1623] leaving it open to question whether testoster-one actually exerts a significant and independent effect upon anaerobic performance over and above simple growth-related factors. Furthermore, large increases in peak and mean power were observed between much younger age children in the absence of notable increases in testosterone. The influence upon anaerobic performance of other non-androgenic hormones which mediate growth (e.g. thyroxine and growth hormone), may be of significance and warrants further investigation.[532]

The peak anaerobic power of 36 boys measured four times over an 18-month period and summarized by pubertal stage assessed by pubic hair development[1503] also indicated an acceleration of peak mass-related anaer-obic power between Tanner stages 3 and 5 although the nature of the experimental design precluded statistical analysis.[535] We have examined WAnT-determined peak and mean power aligned by stage of maturity in data generated in our laboratory. These cross-sectional data support an acceleration in peak and mean power between maturity stages 3 and 4 in boys, whereas in girls more consistent increments with increasing maturity are evident.

Contrasting results are evident from a longitudinal study of the anaerobic 'capacity' of 19 boys who completed a supramaximal treadmill test to exhaustion every year between the ages of 11 and 15 years.[1143] Performance data examined relative to PHV in groups classified as early or late maturing according to skeletal age in relation to chronological age, showed no difference in the pattern of increase in anaerobic capacity, as reflected by oxygen debt and post-exercise blood lactates, between the two groups. In other words, anaerobic capacity was similar in early and late maturers at any given age suggesting that maturative events are unrelated to the growth of anaerobic performance. However, the small sample sizes in the early and late maturity groups, combined with the problems of determining accurately PHV from one annual measurement, the necessary modification of the test protocol according to age, and the questionable validity of O_2 debt and blood lactate as indices of anaerobic capacity, may partially account for these discrepant findings.

Anaerobic performance and body size

Mass-related anaerobic performance

Peak and mean anaerobic power are highly correlated with body size[532] and are conventionally expressed in ratio with body mass (i.e. as $W \cdot kg^{-1}$) to facilitate comparisons between individuals of different size. Figures 5.3 and 5.4 illustrate the growth of mass-related peak and mean power as reflected by data compiled from the extant literature. With absolute and mean peak power expressed in relation to body mass, sex differences in the growth of these characteristics remain. In striking contrast to the static nature of mass-related peak $\dot{V}O_2$ across this same age range, Fig. 5.3 indicates that boys' mass-related peak and mean power continue to increase significantly throughout childhood and adolescence with the pattern of progression seemingly more linear than observed for absolute measures. Again, in contrast to the decline in mass-related peak $\dot{V}O_2$ observed in girls, mass-related peak power increases linearly until the mid teen years. Data for girls' mass-related mean power suggest a similar pattern of increase but data are too dispersed to allow firm conclusions to be drawn. In accordance with data from individual studies[1170, 1288] mass-related peak and mean power appear consistently higher in boys than in girls at all ages represented.

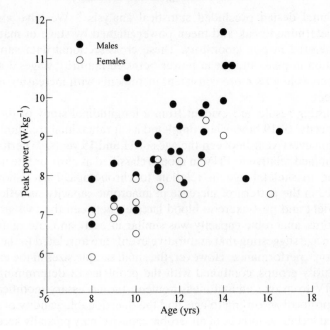

Fig. 5.3. Mass-related peak anaerobic power by age.

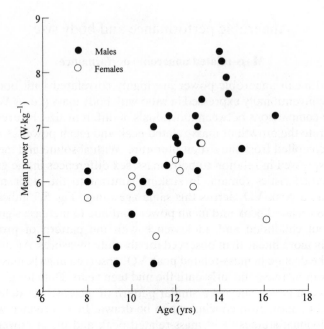

Fig. 5.4. Mass-related mean anaerobic power by age.

Several studies have expressed anaerobic power variables in relation to lean body mass (LBM) or lean leg or arm volume[1025, 1288, 1562] in order to examine whether male–female differences in performance are related simply to body composition differences during puberty or whether the existence of qualitative differences in muscle metabolic characteristics with growth is indicated.

In boys, peak anaerobic power expressed relative to anthropometrically estimated LBM evolves in a similar fashion to that observed for total body mass.[1025] Furthermore, in the same study, LBM was shown to explain 88% of the variance in peak power. In pubescent boys and girls significant sex differences in mass-related peak power ($W \cdot kg^{-1}$) have been shown to disappear when power is expressed relative to LBM.[1562] A similar, although not statistically significant, trend was observed for mean power. However, expression of peak power in relation to lean thigh volume, determined using the Jones and Pearson anthropometric technique,[771] substantially increased the magnitude of the sex difference for both peak and mean power respectively compared with simple mass-related comparisons. This suggests that qualitative differences may indeed contribute to the observed sex differences, particularly as these differences remained even when a linear scaling model was used to examine the data. Data from other studies showing higher total work outputs observed in boys during 10, 30, and 90 sec maximal leg extensions and flexions relative to thigh cross-sectional area lend support to this conclusion.[1288]

Alternative scaling methods

Using a linear regression scaling technique to partition out body size differences from the examination of adult sex differences in peak power relative to lean leg volume, Winter *et al.*[1674] noted that for a given leg volume, power output was significantly higher in males than females. This suggests that a qualitative difference exists between the metabolic characteristics of male and female muscle. This difference was masked when the analysis was based upon a per-body-mass ratio and emphasizes the necessity for exploring the use of alternative scaling techniques to interpret anaerobic performance.

Whilst rapidly gaining momentum as a tool for understanding aerobic fitness (see Chapter 3), these methods have, as yet, been largely neglected in the interpretation of the growth and maturation of anaerobic power. Linear regression models have been employed in two studies to examine sex differences within restricted age groups. In a study of late adolescents the use of ANCOVA to partial out the influence of body mass, fat-free mass, and muscle cross-sectional area from peak and mean power, increased the magnitude of male–female differences in these variables.[1106] In contrast, data from another study[1562] have indicated a reduction in the sex difference in peak and mean power in relation to both total body mass and lean thigh volume when ANCOVA formed the basis of the comparisons in 12- and 13-year-old subjects.

The results of using allometric techniques to model the anaerobic characteristics of 372 12- and 13-year-old boys and girls tested in our laboratory (unpublished data) support the indications of the latter study. Examined in simple ratio with body mass, our data indicate a consistent 4% higher peak power in boys than girls at both 12 and 13 years of age. Sex differences in mean power rise from 6% at 12 years to 11% at age 13 years. Allometric modelling reduced all sex differences to a non-significant 1–2%. Initial allometric modelling revealed mass exponents of $b = 1.02$ and $b = 0.91$ for peak power at 12 and 13 years, respectively, and $b = 0.82$ and $b = 1.20$, respectively, for mean power; values which considerably exceed the theoretical mass exponent of 0.67 for maximal power outputs.[1098] As discussed in Chapter 3, the search for theoretical mass exponents in groups of subjects of diverse body size can lead to artefactually elevated exponents if stature is not taken into account. Within the groups of 12- and 13-year-old children studied here, the full maturational range was represented. Consequently, a substantial range of body mass and stature was evident despite the defined chronological age. Subsequent incorporation of stature into the allometric model substantially reduced the mass exponents for peak power to $b = 0.78$ and $b = 1.09$ for 12- and 13-year-olds, respectively, with values of $b = 0.55$ and $b = 0.64$ for mean power. The deviation of the observed exponents from theoretical values may, in part, reflect concerns with the test's ability to represent a valid measure of both maximal peak and mean power discussed in Chapter 2.

Maturational stage was determined using Tanner's indices for pubic hair (see Chapter 1) in 159 of the 13-year-old children allowing anaerobic performance in relation to body size and sex to be examined by maturational age. Sufficient numbers were obtained to enable comparison between maturity groups 2–5. Using a conventional mass-related analysis, peak power ($W \cdot kg^{-1}$) increased by 25% in boys and 12% in girls between these two stages. Over the same maturational range, mass-related mean power ($W \cdot kg^{-1}$) increased by 17% in boys but did not change in girls. Appropriate allometric modelling reduced the maturity-related changes in peak and mean power to insignificance in both boys and girls.

These results provide further insight into the development of anaerobic performance in children and, as demonstrated for aerobic power, indicate how the use of alternative scaling techniques may present a different picture of the development of these characteristics.

Anaerobic performance and exercise training

Children's inferior power outputs measured using currently accepted criterion tests of anaerobic performance support indications that their ability to generate energy from these systems during high-intensity exercise is deficient when compared to adults. This deficiency may, in part, be attributable to concerns with the validity of the criterion tests to adequately isolate and quantify anaerobic energy production, in particular their lack of reliable and objective endpoints and reliance upon the subject's motivation to perform maximally. Despite this, there is consistent evidence to suggest that children's energy metabolism is preferentially geared towards aerobic rather than anaerobic energy provision (see Chapter 4). It is, however, also apparent that under certain testing conditions children appear capable of generating and tolerating high levels of blood lactate.[84, 378, 1622]

Early studies using invasive techniques to examine training responses in young and adolescent boys provided evidence of biochemical and metabolic adaptations indicative of an enhanced ability for anaerobic energy generation. In muscle biopsies taken from the vastus lateralis, significantly increased resting glycogen stores and a greater rate of glycogen utilization during exercise have been observed in eight 11–15-year-old boys following an 11-week training programme which included interval running, basketball, and soccer.[518] A parallel study of five 11-year-old boys revealed significant increases in muscle PFK levels after just 2 and 6 weeks of cycle ergometer training which involved three 20–50 min periods per week at 70–85% peak $\dot{V}O_2$.

Similar findings have been reported in 12 boys aged 16–17 years[562] subsequent to a 3-month sprint-training programme. Significant increases in PFK were identified in biopsy samples although there were no concurrent changes in either fibre type distribution or cross-sectional area. A second experimental group whose training was aerobic endurance-based showed improvements in biochemical indices associated with aerobic metabolism suggesting that biochemical changes are consistent with the training modality.

These lines of evidence suggest that potential for improving young people's anaerobic capabilities exists. However, these data must be interpreted cautiously as only small, single-sex subjects groups have been studied thus precluding more generalized extrapolation.

Studies demonstrating significantly better anaerobic performance in trained children and adolescents compared with age-matched controls provide indirect support for the hypothesis that appropriate training can enhance anaerobic metabolism during growth and maturation. The effects of growth, maturation, and athletic training upon anaerobic performance in young boys have been examined in a series of studies.[1027, 1028, 1029] Total work done during two bouts of maximal cycle exercise lasting 15 and 30 sec, respectively, separated by a 30 min rest was significantly higher in the athletic group compared with the non-athletic controls at the initial examination. These differences persisted after 1 and 3 years of further training and with the progression of the children into puberty. Similarly, 10-year-old élite male prepubertal cross-country runners have been reported to perform significantly better during a 30 sec modified WAnT test compared with an age-matched control group.[989] However, given the significant aerobic contribution to the Wingate test, apparent even in untrained children (see Chapter 2), the possibility that this discrepancy in performance reflects enhanced aerobic performance in the highly trained subjects cannot be discounted.

In contrast to this pattern of findings, no significant differences in either peak or mean power have been observed between groups of prepubertal swimmers, 'active', or 'non-active' boys,[534] although these results are confounded by the unquantified anaerobic component of the swimmer's training programme and the use of a non-sports-specific lower limb assessment of anaerobic performance.

Notwithstanding the methodological limitations emphasized, these biochemical and performance modifications suggest that young people's anaerobic performance may be enhanced through participation in structured exercise training programmes. Unfortunately, there exists limited experimental evidence to support this contention.

The problems intrinsic to the design and implementation of aerobic training studies with children (see Chapter 7) are similarly applicable to the design of anaerobic training studies. Additional factors which specifically complicate the evaluation of anaerobic training responses in children include the methodological concerns with anaerobic tests described in Chapter 2, and the difficulties of sustaining children's and adolescents' motivation and interest in a strenuous training programme which requires consistent near-maximal or maximal effort. It is also difficult to regulate and monitor objectively exercise intensity on an individual basis.

Exercise prescriptions for improving anaerobic performance in adults are well established[563] but whether or not these are applicable to children and adolescents has not been ascertained. Tables 5.1 and 5.2 summarize a prudent approach to the training of young people's phosphagen and glycolytic systems.[79]

Tables 5.3 and 5.4 summarize the results from studies drawn from the literature which have examined changes in anaerobic performance, specifically peak and mean power, in adolescents and children respectively and compared results with an age-matched control group. As few studies have assessed the maturational age of their subjects, for the purposes of Tables 5.3 and 5.4 children and adolescents are defined as those under and over 11 years of age, respectively. Direct comparisons between the results of different studies are impossible due to inconsistent methodologies

Table 5.1. Guidelines for training the phosphagen system

Frequency	3 times per week				
Intensity	Maximal				
Time	5–10 sec exercise period with a work–rest ratio of 1:5; 5 repetitions per set, 3 sets with a recovery of 5–10 min between sets*				
Type, e.g.	*Exercise*	*Repetitions*	*Sets*	*Intensity*	*Rest recovery*
	50 m run	5	3	Maximal	40 sec walk between repetitions, 5 min jog between sets

* The rest recovery is extremely important if the quality of work is to be maintained.
From Armstrong, N. and Welsman, J. (1993). Training young athletes. In M. Lee (Ed.), *Coaching Children in Sports*. London, Spon, pp. 191–203.

Table 5.2. Guidelines for training the glycolytic system

Frequency	Not more than 3 times per week				
Intensity	Not less than 90% of maximum				
Time	20–30 sec exercise periods with a work–rest ratio of 1:3 (this can be reduced to 1:2 as training progresses); 5 repetitions per set, 2 sets with up to 10 min jogging between sets				
Type, e.g.	*Exercise*	*Repetitions*	*Sets*	*Intensity*	*Rest recovery*
	150–200 m run	5	2	90%	90 sec jog between repetitions, 10 min jog between sets

From Armstrong, N. and Welsman, J. (1993). Training young athletes. In M. Lee (Ed.), *Coaching Children in Sports*. London, Spon, pp. 191–203.

including the mode and type of training, the overall duration of the training programme and the nature and administration of the criterion tests used to assess anaerobic performance pre- and post-training. Furthermore, the lack of data describing the training responses of girls in early puberty and boys in late puberty is immediately apparent so extrapolation from these results is limited.

Small, but significant, improvements in peak power have been noted in adolescent boys following a training programme of sprint-running.[660] Although a second cycle ergometer-trained group completed a similar volume of exercise, peak power did not change significantly, perhaps

Table 5.3. Exercise training and anaerobic performance: studies with adolescents

Study	Subjects Experimental (E)	Control (C)	Training protocol Frequency (per wk)	Intensity	Time (at start of training)	Length (wks)	Type	Peak power (W) Pre	Post	Change (%)	Mean power (W) Pre	Post	Change (%)
Grodjinovsky et al.[660]	E₁ $n=17$ B, 11–13 yrs; E₂ $n=17$ B, 11–13 yrs	$n=14$ B, 11–13 yrs	3	Max	E₁ 3 × 8 s + 3 × 30 s; E₂ 3 × 40 m + 3 × 150 m	6	E₁ cycle; E₂ sprint-running	E₁ 295.1; E₂ 324.5; C 347.0	310.8; 339.2; 337.2	5.3; 4.5; –2.8	250.7; 274.2; 288.4	262.6; 287.7; 279.5	4.7; 4.9; –3.1
Docherty et al.[451]	2 groups; E₁ $n=11$ B, 12 yrs; E₂ $n=12$ B, 12 yrs	$n=11$ B, 12 yrs	3	E₁ high resist./low velocity; E₂ low resist./high velocity	2 × 20 s at an unspecified number of stations	4	Isokinetic resist. training	E₁ 330.0; E₂ 339.0; C 342.0	386.9; 377.8; 363.2	17.2; 11.4; 6.2	305.4; 313.8; 335.1	310.6; 342.0; 346.9	1.7; 9.0; 3.5
Adeniran & Toriola[8]	E₁ $n=22$ G, 15.4 yrs; E₂ $n=23$ G, 15.6 yrs	$n=23$ G, 15.8 yrs	3	E₁ 80–85% max HR; E₂ 90% max HR	E₁ 4.8 km; E₂ 4 × 240 s	8	Running	E₁ 682.3; E₂ 671.6; C 664.7	772.4; 769.7; 680.7	13.2; 14.6; 2.4			

B, boys; G, girls; HR, heart rate.

Table 5.4. Exercise training and anaerobic performance: studies with children

Study	Subjects		Training protocol					Peak power (W)			Mean power (W)		
	Experimental (E)	Control (C)	Frequency (per wk)	Intensity	Time (at start of training)	Length (wks)	Type	Pre	Post	Change (%)	Pre	Post	Change (%)
Rotstein et al.[1248]	E₁ n = 16 B, 10.8 yrs	n = 12 B, 10.8 yrs	3	Unknown	3 × 600 m + 5 × 400 m + 6 × 150 m	9	Running	E 255.6 C 267.1	289.2 267.3	13.1 0	225.4 228.3	245.8 233.7	9.1 2.4
Williams et al.[1654]	2 groups E₁ n = 13 B, 10.1 yrs E₂ n = 12 B, 10.1 yrs	n = 14 B, 10.1 yrs	3	E₁ 80–85% max HR E₂ max	E₁ 20 min E₂ 3 × 10 s + 3 × 30 s	8	E₁ cycle E₂ sprint-running	E₁ 309.7 E₂ 317.7 C 318.0	369.9 399.8 379.0	19.4 25.8 19.2	221.2 245.6 232.1	258.9 287.2 265.1	17.0 16.9 14.2
McManus et al.[1016]	E₁ n = 10 G, 9.3 yrs E₂ n = 10 G, 9.8 yrs	n = 7 G, 9.6 yrs	3	E₁ 80–85% max E₂ max	E₁ 20 min 3 × 30 s	8	E₁ cycle E₂ sprint-running	E₁ 219.8 E₂ 291.4 C 297.5	264.1 319.8 304.3	20.2 9.7 4.0	175.1 245.6 210.7	174.3 287.2 205.7	-0.5 16.9 -2.4

B, boys; G, girls; HR, heart rate.

indicating the effect of keeping training and testing exercise modes consistent. However, the absence of significant changes in mean power in this study and both power indices in another study of adolescent boys[451] may be in part at least due to the abbreviated duration of the training programme. The only study located of late-adolescent girls[8] also observed significant increases in peak power measured during a Sargent jump test[563] following either continuous or interval running training. However, these results provide limited evidence of the trainability of anaerobic power as both experimental groups had followed essentially aerobic training programmes —the duration of the intervals and work–rest ratio of 1:1 in the interval training group being more likely to stress aerobic energy systems—whilst the criterion test used to measure peak power reflects energy generation from the phosphagen system.

The results from studies with children are also inconsistent. Training programmes used with these younger subjects largely conform to the guidelines described in Tables 5.1 and 5.2, although the work–rest ratio cannot be determined in one study[1248] and in another study[1016] the work–rest ratios of 1:4 and 1:5 differ from those recommended to represent an optimal overload for training the glycolytic system.[79] Although both of the studies with boys observed apparently high increases in peak and mean power only the one using the most intensive training programme yielded statistically significantly changes.[1248] The improvements in both power indices noted in our laboratory[1654] failed to achieve significance due to the concurrent changes shown by the control group.

Significant training-induced improvements in the ability to derive energy from glycolysis as indicated by a 20% increase in endurance time during a treadmill run to exhaustion were observed in 10–11-year-old boys following a 12-week interval running programme.[1072] These results have been excluded from Table 5.2 as power outputs were not measured and, despite the magnitude of the improvement with training, the significance of the results is diminished by the non-random assignment of two 'premier' soccer teams to be experimental and control groups and the continuation of the latter group with their normal training and competition regime.

In girls, interval running training designed to overload both the phosphagen and glycolytic systems yielded a significant increase in peak power despite the attenuated work–rest ratio but failed to change mean power.[1016] In the same study, a second experimental group who followed a cycle ergometer training protocol designed to enhance aerobic fitness also significantly increased peak power although the increase was somewhat less than that observed in the sprint-trained group.

This latter study highlights an interesting feature of the data presented in Tables 5.1 and 5.2 in that improvements in peak and mean power have been reported in both control groups[451, 1654] and those trained using aerobic prescriptions[8, 1016, 1654] that would minimally overload anaerobic metabolism.

This opens up some intriguing physiological and methodological questions, particularly as there were no significant changes in body size over the period of the studies which could account for these improvements. Although there is some evidence to suggest that high-intensity interval or resistance training might improve aerobic metabolism (see Tables 7.2 and 7.3) there is no firm theoretical basis for suggesting the reverse to occur. Increased anaerobic performance post-aerobic cycle ergometer training could perhaps be explained by improved cycling efficiency.

One further confounding factor common to the majority of the training studies summarized here, which may prove more difficult to resolve in the immediate future, is the use of criterion tests and training programmes that employ different exercise modalities. The specificity of training effects indicates that significant improvements are more likely to be demonstrated when the criterion test simulates the training activity as closely as possible.[935] It is conceivable that the absence of consistent anaerobic training effects in children and adolescents is a consequence of a mismatch between testing and training exercise modes.

In view of the available data and the methodological problems highlighted the extent to which anaerobic performance can be enhanced through training in children and adolescents must remain conjectural. Currently available guidelines reflect a prudent approach to training anaerobic characteristics in children and adolescents[79] although their efficacy will not be established until further research evidence has been gathered. Furthermore, the recommendation that training to improve glycolytic energy provision is not introduced until late adolescence[79] seems reasonable as, until then, individuals are unlikely to have developed the psychological as well as physiological maturity required to sustain such repetitive, high-intensity training. Intensive anaerobic training rapidly depletes glycogen stores therefore attention to the young person's diet is essential to ensure adequate carbohydrate replenishment.

Interrelationships between aerobic and anaerobic performance

Many active adults and particularly élite athletes demonstrate what has been termed 'metabolic specialization'.[138] This encompasses the morphological, biochemical, and performance characteristics that predispose individuals towards success in a given sporting event. Thus, an ectomorphic physique, high aerobic power, and predominance of type I muscle fibres typify the marathon runner, whilst sprinters are characterized by high explosive strength, a muscular physique, but not necessarily high aerobic fitness.

Bar-Or[138] speculated that, in contrast to adults, children were 'metabolic non-specialists'. This theory was supported by data showing that children who performed well on aerobic tests were also rated as above average when their anaerobic performance was assessed.[149, 749] Indeed, even in élite child cross-country runners a significant correlation coefficient ($r = 0.82$) was observed between performance on the WAnT and peak $\dot{V}O_2$; results indicative of a lack of metabolic specialization.

Blimkie *et al.*[207] introduced the concept of an anaerobic to aerobic power ratio to examine the relative evolution of the energy systems during growth and maturation. Using aerobic and anaerobic data compiled from two different studies, a progressive increase in the anaerobic to aerobic ratio from 1.87–3.21 was observed in girls between the ages of 8–14 years with values for similar-aged boys increasing from 1.90–2.83. A preliminary investigation of aerobic and anaerobic data drawn from the same subjects demonstrated that the power ratio levelled out over the period 14–19 years, indicating mid to late puberty as a critical period for metabolic specialization.[207] These findings have been supported subsequently with a significant increase in the anaerobic to aerobic ratio from 1.7–2.8 and from 1.3–1.9 for peak and mean power, respectively, in 6–15-year-old boys.[532]

Although not widely documented, studies have consistently shown moderate but significant correlations between peak $\dot{V}O_2$ and indices of anaerobic performance in children.[450, 534, 989] Some authors[450] hesitate to suggest that their results support non-specialization arguing that the common variance of 22–32% demonstrated by their findings is too low to have great biological significance.

Expressed in absolute terms, when correlated with peak $\dot{V}O_2$, data from our laboratory yielded coefficients exceeding $r = 0.69$ for peak power (WAnT) and $r = 0.75$ for mean power in 12- and 13-year-old boys and girls (unpublished data). These coefficients became non-significant when correlations were based upon mass-related scores. These findings highlight the need to account appropriately for anthropometric and maturity characteristics in subjects of the same chronological age. Scaling power outputs for body size using the alternative scaling methods described in Chapter 3 may more accurately represent the development of metabolic potential.

The biochemical characteristics of children, such as an increased number of transitional (undifferentiated) muscle fibres[562] and an enzyme profile which favours aerobic metabolism,[518, 683] are suggestive of a malleable and changing metabolic potential during growth. Although these characteristics would tend to support the hypothesis of non-specialization, the results from the bioenergetic profiling studies described above are confounded further by methodological issues. As previously discussed, the WAnT has a considerable aerobic component, particularly in pre- and early-pubertal children. In this respect it is not surprising that the results from peak $\dot{V}O_2$ and WAnTs (particularly mean power) are correlated. This does not, however, adequately explain the correlation between peak power, which can be assumed to have minimal aerobic contribution, and peak $\dot{V}O_2$. Results may be confounded by the use of a single resistance determined as a fixed proportion of the subject's total body mass (e.g. 0.75 g·kg^{-1}). Peak power derived from the force–velocity test may, therefore, be more appropriate to examine aerobic–anaerobic relationships. Using this test significant relationships between mass-related peak power and peak $\dot{V}O_2$ have been observed (ref. 534, Armstrong and Welsman unpublished data) although with shared variance of 13.6–34% in the respective studies, these data provide only limited support for a lack of metabolic specialization.

Clearly, despite the indications from biochemical markers, data from performance measures are insufficient, in terms of subject numbers and composition, to support firmly or refute the hypothesis that children are non-metabolic specialists. In addition, methodological problems with the criterion measures of anaerobic performance and methods used to interpret the results confound the picture. The refinement of testing protocols for the measurement of anaerobic power and the use of appropriate statistical procedures are required to clarify the development of muscle–metabolic profiles in children and adolescents.

Summary

Anaerobic performance characteristics are less well documented than aerobic power and data for girls, particularly in later adolescence, are particularly sparse. As with peak $\dot{V}O_2$, peak and mean anaerobic power are highly correlated with chronological age in both males and females although the pattern of increase in anaerobic performance is different. Collated data from published studies indicate an exponential increase in boys' peak and mean power with a notable acceleration in values around 12–14 years and coincident with PHV and the spurt in muscle growth. Girls' peak and mean power increase more linearly, reaching a plateau in the mid teens. Sex differences in absolute power indices are minimal until the period of rapid growth occurs in boys. Expressed relative to body mass, boys' peak and mean power continue to increase progressively from 8–16 years in contrast to the static nature of peak $\dot{V}O_2$. Girls' data are too few to establish age-related change in mass-related power indices with certainty but a linear increase into the mid teenage years is indicated. Relative power indices are consistently higher in boys than in girls. The trainability of children's and adolescents' anaerobic performance is not well established. Studies have noted improvements in biochemical markers of anaerobic energy provision and anaerobic performance but data are inconsistent and confounded by methodological problems. Observed correlations between indices of aerobic and anaerobic performance have led to the hypothesis that, in contrast to adults, children are 'metabolic non-specialists'. However, the explained variance is typically low at around 30% and the relationship may be spurious given the high aerobic component to the WAnT demonstrated in young subjects. Data based upon more refined testing protocols are required to evaluate further changes in bioenergetic profile with growth and maturation.

PART III
Physical activity and health

In adult life the effect of regular physical activity in promoting aerobic fitness,[22, 1316] increasing muscular strength,[103, 440] lowering blood lipids,[478, 1678] reducing high blood pressure,[668, 1533] countering obesity,[243, 1458] retarding osteoporosis,[1425, 1432] improving blood glucose control,[852, 1589] and increasing psychological well-being[257, 1111] is extensively documented. There is a growing conviction that adults' health and well-being has its origins in behaviour established during childhood[6, 368, 926] and there is general agreement that young people should be encouraged to adopt active lifestyles which can be sustained into adult life.[51, 1309] However, despite the general acceptance of the desirability of promoting physical activity with young people understanding of the potential of physical activity to confer health benefits during childhood and adolescence is limited.[52, 1302]

The primary focus of Part III is to examine the effects of physical activity, including exercise training, on aspects of young people's health. In addition, we will explore the current physical activity patterns of children and adolescents and analyse the evidence which suggests that physical activity habits persist (track) into adult life. But first we need to clarify terms and concepts.

Health-related physical activity is physical activity of the appropriate type, intensity, duration, and frequency to improve or maintain health.[61] Despite the problems involved in monitoring habitual physical activity the physical activity patterns of youngsters have been well-documented.[53, 1206] The data are remarkably consistent but until recently they were difficult to interpret because widely recognized physical activity guidelines for young people were not readily available.

Exercise training is the systematic use of exercise of specific intensities, durations and frequencies to attain a desired effect, often the improvement or maintenance of one or more of the components of physical fitness. Research concerned with the response of the growing child to exercise training is accumulating but knowledge of children's and adolescents' responses to exercise training remains fragmentary. One reason for this lack of understanding is the confounding problem that children grow at their own rate and it is often difficult to separate the relative contributions of growth and exercise training to observed changes. Furthermore, researchers are loathe to expose children to invasive techniques, such as muscle biopsies, in order to monitor subcellular changes. The increasing availability of techniques such as magnetic resonance imaging (MRI) may provide new insights but few studies have been published.[1161, 1707]

The exercise training principles upon which programmes should be based are applicable to both adults and children (Table III.1). It is necessary to overload habitually a system to cause it to respond and

Table III.1. Principles of exercise training

Overload	Exercising against a resistance greater than that which is normally encountered
Progression	The frequency, duration, and intensity of exercise training should be gradually increased over time
Specificity	Exercise training induced changes are stimulus-specific
Reversibility	Exercise training effects are reversible
Adaptability	Exercise training programmes must be flexible
Periodization	An organized division of the training year (or several years) in pursuit of optimal improvements in performance and peaking at specific times
Evaluation	Exercise training effects should be monitored periodically in order to evaluate the success of the programme.

Adapted from Armstrong, N. and Welsman, J. (1993). Training young athletes. In M. Lee (Ed.), *Coaching Children in Sport*. London, Spon, pp. 191–203.

adapt but gradual progression is particularly important with young people. Elucidating the effects of de-training (reversibility) on young people is confounded by the youngster's continued growth and maturation during the de-training period. However, it appears that adaptations to exercise training are transient and will steadily decay once training ceases. Long-term benefits, therefore, depend upon the continuance of exercise training through adolescence and into adult life.

Sport is a subcategory of physical activity that includes activities that are structured, organized, rule-governed, competitive, and involve gross motor actions. Training for sport must adhere to the principle of specificity to obtain optimum benefits. A particular form of physical activity may induce a change in one tissue or organ but not in another, therefore training programmes for sport should reflect the specific requirements of the sport. All exercise training programmes should be adaptable with allowances being made for injury and illness. With adolescent sports persons individual growth and maturation rates must be considered in relation to training demands, particularly in fixing appropriate overloads. Because of largely unpredictable rates of growth and maturation it is extremely difficult to periodize

Table III.2. Components of health-related fitness

Aerobic fitness	The ability of the cardiac, circulatory, and pulmonary systems to supply fuel and to eliminate waste products during exercise
Muscular strength	The ability of a muscle group to exert force against a resistance in one maximal effort
Muscular endurance	The ability of a muscle group to perform repeated contractions against a light load for an extended period of time
Flexibility	The range of motion around a joint
Body fatness	Percentage of body mass that is fat

programmes for young athletes to peak at specific times. Periodization techniques are therefore probably of limited value with young athletes.[1467] It is, however, important for young athletes to evaluate periodically their training programmes so that appropriate modifications can be made where necessary.[82]

Health-related fitness has been defined as, 'the ability to perform daily tasks with vigour and manifestation of traits and capacities that are associated with minimal risk of developing hypokinetic diseases'.[1136, p. 174] The components of health-related fitness are defined in Table III.2.

The World Health Organization (WHO) define health as, 'a state of complete physical, mental and social well-being and not merely the absence of disease or infirmity'.[1685, p. 1] Positive health is associated with a capacity to enjoy life and to withstand challenges, whereas negative health is associated with morbidity and, in the extreme, with mortality.[228] The term 'wellness' is often used to describe a state of positive health in the individual and it comprises both biological and psychological well-being.[1378]

The complex relationships between physical activity, physical fitness, and health have been discussed at length[228, 1136, 1378] and they are illustrated, in a simplified manner, in Fig. III.1. The model indicates that physical activity can influence both physical fitness and health. Aspects of physical fitness may influence health status and may also be related to the level of habitual physical activity (i.e. fitter individuals may be more likely to engage in physical activity). Similarly,

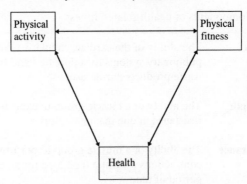

Fig. III.1. The relationships among physical activity, physical fitness, and health.

health status influences both habitual physical activity and aspects of physical fitness. The precise interrelationships among health, physical activity, and physical fitness are further complicated by factors such as genetic characteristics, environmental conditions, and personal attributes.

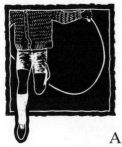

6
Physical activity patterns

Assessment of physical activity

The measurement of adults' habitual physical activity is one of the most difficult tasks in epidemiological research,[28, 474, 1054, 1058] and the assessment of the habitual physical activity of young people is even more problematic.[46, 133, 1325, 1326] The technique used must be socially acceptable, it should not burden the subject with cumbersome equipment, and it should minimally influence the subject's normal physical activity pattern. Ideally the intensity, frequency, and duration of activities should be monitored and if a true picture of habitual physical activity is required some account should be taken of any day-to-day variation. A minimum monitoring period of three days has been recommended.[138]

A range of methods for estimating adults' physical activity has been developed[473, 873, 1596] and several of these methods have been used to assess young people's habitual physical activity, without due consideration being taken of factors that may limit their feasibility and validity when used with the paediatric population. More than 30 different methods of assessing physical activity have been identified[876] but the available techniques can be grouped into four categories: (1) self- and/or proxy-report; (2) observation; (3) motion sensor monitoring; and (4) physiological analyses (see also Table 6.1).

Self-report and/or proxy-report

Self-report of physical activity is the most widely used method in epidemiological research due to the ease and low cost of implementation. Self-report methods include retrospective questionnaires, interview-administered recall, activity diaries, and mail surveys.[1299, 1596] Proxy reports by parents and/or teachers have been employed in studies with children[1078, 1109, 1330, 1514] and some studies have estimated level of physical activity through self-report of surrogate measures such as sports participation.[707, 995, 1438]

Concern has been expressed over the imprecision of self-report methodology.[474, 877, 910, 1401] Actual behaviour is not directly assessed by self-reports. The data obtained are,

memories of the behaviour of interest that have decayed, been filtered through perceptions and biases, and have been tainted by competing memories, social desirability and misunderstanding of instructions.[1299, p. 215]

Physical activity and health

Table 6.1. Methods of assessing habitual physical activity

Objective instruments	Subjective instruments
Pedometers	Recall questionnaire
Electronic motion sensors	Recall interview
Accelerometers	Proxy-report
Indirect calorimetry	Activity diary
Doubly labelled water	Observation
Heart rate monitoring	Dietary intake

Considerable demands are placed on the child's cognitive abilities to recall specific events from the past.[132, 1399] The self-recall of the intensity, frequency, and duration of bouts of activity by children is therefore even more problematic than with adults. In addition, children are less time-conscious than adults and tend to engage in physical activities at sporadic times and intensities rather than in consistent bouts.[573] The problem is further compounded by leisure time activity, which is more difficult to quantify than occupational activity, making up a greater proportion of total habitual physical activity in children.[388]

Self-administered questionnaires are believed to be less accurate than those administered by an interviewer[1058] and large discrepancies have been demonstrated between the two methods.[1603, 1635] Physical activity diaries have been reported to be superior to retrospective questionnaires[132, 1514] but some studies have found that the quality of completed diaries is inconsistent with children.[1324, 1604] Diary measures place a heavy burden on the subjects[1299] and keeping a diary may in itself influence physical activity habits.[1314] Parents and teachers can only give secondary information, especially when it concerns activities outside home or school, and proxy-reports therefore tend to be unreliable.[1325, 1330, 1514]

Several research teams have attempted, on the basis of self-report data, to classify activities according to their estimated energy expenditure[232, 472, 476, 807, 1574] using physiological data from elsewhere.[28, 347, 477, 627, 1135] This approach is fraught with inaccuracies due to the methodological limitations of directly determining the energy expenditure of children outside a laboratory and the inappropriateness of extrapolating data obtained from adults to children. The economy of movement varies between people and the use of energy costs of activities determined on adults to estimate energy expenditure in children introduces substantial errors. In young children, relative energy costs may be underestimated by up to 40% using adult values. At 10 years of age the underestimation is about 20% decreasing to about 5% at the age of 16 years.[1137, 1304, 1536]

The major advantage of self- and proxy-report measures of physical activity is low cost. These measures can be used easily with large numbers of subjects and, consequently, despite the well-documented methodological problems concerned with young people's self-reported physical activity the vast majority of available data have been generated in this manner. Self-report measures do not appear to be useful with children under 10 years of age[1137, 1299, 1308, 1326] and with older children and adolescents results must be interpreted with caution. Converting self-report measures of physical activity into predicted energy expenditure is not tenable.

Observation

The assessment of physical activity through the use of observation has inherent appeal and recent technological advances permitting complex observational codes to be entered, stored and analysed by microcomputers have stimulated research into children's physical activity patterns using observational techniques.[1003, 1004] Children's physical activity levels can be observed reliably, and observers can be quickly trained to record accurate information. A comprehensive review of the literature[1003] identified eight sophisticated recording techniques but they were all designed for studying the physical activity of young children and none appear to have been tested for use with older children and adolescents. Although instruments, such as the Children's Activity Rating Scale (CARS)[1187] (see Table 6.2) and the Fargo Activity Timesampling Survey (FATS),[828] have the potential to provide valuable information about children's physical activity patterns, comparisons of different systems have not been conducted. Insufficient information exists to indicate which systems are the most accurate and reliable. The extent to which even well-trained observers affect subject behaviour (subject reactivity) has not been demonstrated.[1114]

Observation studies are labour-intensive, time-consuming and therefore costly. Events studied must be observable and codeable and observers or video cameras need to be in the same environment as the subject. Early research utilized film to monitor the activity levels of obese and non-obese children over short time periods.[273, 365] Subsequent work often focused on the observation of children during structured situations such as at summer camps, in physical education lessons, or in precise locations such as the home or school playground.[369, 653, 738, 848, 860, 1312] Few longer-term observational studies have been undertaken with children.[122, 134, 135, 468, 1416, 1417]

Table 6.2.　A scale for rating children's activity (CARS)

Level/description	Expected heart rate (bpm)	Representative activities
1. Stationary: no movement	<100	Lying Sitting
2. Stationary: with movement	100–119	Standing/Colouring Standing/Ball activity
3. Translocation: slow/easy	120–139	Walk 0% grade
4. Translocation: medium/moderate	140–160	Walk 5% grade Walk 10% grade
5. Translocation: fast, very fast/strenuous	>160	Walk 15% grade

From Puhl, J., Greaves, K., Hoyt, M. and Baranowski, T. (1990). Children's Activity Rating Scale (CARS): Description and Calibration. *Research Quarterly for Exercise and Sport*, **61**, 26–36. Reprinted with permission.

Motion sensors

Movement counters

As almost all forms of physical activity require movement of the trunk or limbs the measurement of activity with movement counters is appealing. Until recently the most common mechanical device for measuring movement was the pedometer which was first used in this context by Lauter[889] in 1926, although Leonardo da Vinci designed a pedometer to measure distance by counting steps somewhat earlier.[1054, 1325, 1326] Pedometers were used widely in early studies of children's physical activity[805, 1328, 1329] then gradually replaced by more sophisticated mechanical, electronic, and magnetic counters such as the actometer,[1346] the Large Scale Integrated Motor-Activity Monitor (LSI)[875] and the biomotometer.[1347] Careful and extensive field validation of these instruments has not been carried out.[574, 1058]

Accelerometers

Electronic motion sensors, known as accelerometers, which measure both frequency and intensity of movement in the vertical plane have largely replaced movement counters in physical activity research.[760, 1022, 1060] The most popular instrument is the Caltrac accelerometer which is about the size and weight of a pocket calculator and can be enclosed in a locked pouch secured to the waist.[827, 831, 970] The validity and reliability of the Caltrac have been studied in children and although its use has been supported it have been suggested that sporadic activity patterns may not be adequately represented by a simple unidimensional device.[244, 396, 495, 1305] The Tritrac-R3D activity monitor has been recently developed to correct some of the limitations of the Caltrac monitor. The Tritrac is based on the same accelerometry principles as the Caltrac but it is capable of assessing activity in three dimensions rather than in one. Early trials have been promising but the instrument requires further evaluation before full acceptance as a valid means of measuring young people's physical activity.[1616]

Both Caltrac and Tritrac can be programmed to estimate energy expenditure using basal metabolic rate estimated from stature, body mass, gender, and age, plus total caloric expenditure estimated from activity. This methodology makes a number of unsubstantiated assumptions and for research purposes it is advisable to use activity 'counts' as the criterion measure.[574, 1137] Nevertheless, accelerometers have developed into useful tools, although the time and expenses of using the devices may be prohibitive in large-scale epidemiological studies.

Physiological analyses

Energy intake

As young people are subject to the law of conservation of energy, if energy intake is measured over an extended period of time (at least 7 days) and changes in body mass are taken into account, physical activity (energy expenditure) may be quantified in terms of energy intake. There is an extensive literature concerned with the methodology of determining energy intake.[208, 606] Methods can vary from weighing and analysing the energy content of duplicate food portions to 24 h recall techniques. As self-report methods are the only feasible techniques for large studies accuracy depends upon the subject's ability to recall and describe the kind and amount of food eaten. A further limitation of dietary estimates is the inability to identify the frequency, duration, and intensity of physical activity.[233, 1186, 1324]

Energy expenditure

Energy expenditure can be directly measured by determining oxygen uptake (indirect calorimetry), if it is assumed that daily physical activity is almost entirely aerobic. The measurement of $\dot{V}O_2$ requires a means of assessing expired respiratory gas volume and analysing it for oxygen and carbon dioxide content. Early studies required subjects to have a Douglas Bag fixed to their back[161] and although recent technology has alleviated the problem, the wearing of a facemask or a mouthpiece and noseclip is still obligatory. These requirements make this method unsuitable for assessing young people's physical activity patterns.

The recent development of the technique of using stable isotopes (doubly labelled water to estimate oxygen consumption has overcome the restrictions of wearing a facemask and provided an unobtrusive and non-invasive means of measuring energy expenditure.[370, 1342, 1343] The technique was developed in the 1950s by Lifson and colleagues[903] but it was 1975 before the feasibility of using it with humans was described.[904]

The method depends upon the kinetics of two naturally occurring, stable isotopes of water [^2H_2O] (deuterium-labelled water) and [$H_2^{18}O$] (oxygen-18-labelled water), with no known toxicity or side-effects at the low doses used.[769] Following an oral dose, the isotopes mix in the body water pool and reach equilibrium after about 4 h. Deuterium-labelled water is lost from the body through urine, sweat, and evaporative losses with a half-life in young children of about 7 days.[638] Oxygen-18-labelled water is lost from the body at a faster rate since, in addition to all routes of water loss, the isotope is also lost in carbon dioxide production. The difference in the rate of loss between the two isotopes is therefore a function of the rate at which the body produces carbon dioxide.[637] Using an estimated RER and standard indirect calorimetric calculations $\dot{V}O_2$ and therefore energy expenditure can be calculated.[432, 1179, 1441]

The doubly labelled water technique makes several assumptions, some of which are violated in human studies and accounted for, using modelling refinements,[637, 1179, 1441] but the technique has been quite extensively validated in comparison with indirect calorimetry.[770, 1216, 1217, 1343, 1344, 1638] The method appears to be accurate to within 5% relative to data derived by indirect calorimetry for subjects living in metabolic chambers.[1327]

The use of stable isotopes to estimate energy expenditure provides a powerful tool for the accurate measurement of daily energy expenditure. However, because of the cost of the isotopes, the scarcity of deuterium-labelled water, and the need for sample analysis by sophisticated isotope ratio mass spectrometry, the technique is unlikely to be used in large-scale studies in the near future. Furthermore, the data obtained only provide a measure of total energy expenditure over the period of study and no information is provided on the subject's physical activity pattern.

Heart rate monitoring

A number of self-contained, computerized telemetry systems have been developed for the unobtrusive measurement of heart rate. Typically, these systems consist of a lightweight transmitter, which is fixed to the chest with electrodes, and a receiver/microcomputer which is worn as a watch on the wrist. They are socially acceptable, they permit freedom of movement, they are not immediately noticeable, and therefore should not unduly influence the child's normal physical activity pattern. Some systems are capable of

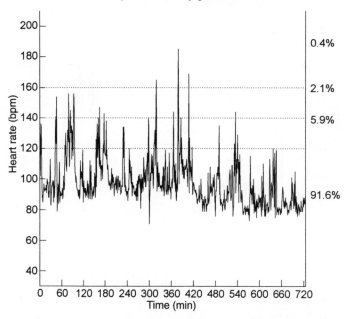

Fig. 6.1. A 12 h heart rate trace with no sustained periods of physical activity.

storing minute-by-minute heart rates for up to 16 h and therefore allow long duration monitoring of physical activity. The Polar Sport Tester (Quantum XL) is currently the instrument of choice as it provides excellent validity and stability and it permits almost total freedom of motion.[893] The instrument has been extensively analysed and found to be reliable and valid with both adults and children.[790, 791, 1541, 1544]

Because of the ease of measuring heart rate and the problems encountered in measuring $\dot{V}O_2$ in field conditions several investigators have chosen to monitor heart rate to predict young people's energy expenditure.[1324, 1331, 1573, 1575] The use of heart rate to estimate energy expenditure derives from the work of Bergen and Christensen[175] who demonstrated, under laboratory conditions, a linear relationship between heart rate and $\dot{V}O_2$ (energy expenditure) over most of the range, for walking, running, and cycling. Subjects are normally brought into a laboratory and an oxygen uptake–heart rate calibration curve is determined during steady-state cycle ergometry or treadmill exercise. The calibration curve is then used to convert heart rates recorded in the field into $\dot{V}O_2$, and subsequently into energy expenditure.[386, 1208, 1440, 1449, 1572, 1574] There are several problems with this methodology, notably the fact that steady-state exercise in a laboratory is somewhat different from the intermittent physical activity experienced in real life situations. Stroke volume and arteriovenous oxygen difference are

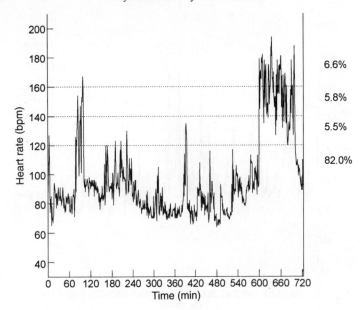

Fig. 6.2. A 12 h heart rate trace illustrating a sustained period of physical activity.

not constant at different levels of $\dot{V}O_2$ and, especially at the extremes of the range, the heart rate–oxygen uptake relationship departs significantly from the linear model.

A careful study using a whole body calorimeter clearly illustrated the limitations of the heart rate–oxygen uptake relationship and demonstrated that, as the average 24 h heart rate is low the use of heart rates to accurately estimate daily energy expenditure is not tenable.[397] Even within the range where heart rate and $\dot{V}O_2$ are linearly related during controlled, incremental treadmill exercise the sometimes rapid changes of intensity of activity in the real life situation will dissociate the relationship between the two variables.[876] In addition, heart rate may be more affected than $\dot{V}O_2$ by different modes of activity (static vs. dynamic),[138, 991] activity with different muscle groups (arms vs. legs),[1582] the ambient environment,[1364] fatigue,[891] emotional stress,[102] and state of training.[787] It is therefore questionable to extrapolate individual heart rates recorded in the field to estimates of energy expenditure on the basis of regression equations determined during controlled laboratory tests.

Several investigators[107, 296, 616, 1362] have simply reported totalized time or percentage of time heart rates were above certain criteria during the period studied. Others have argued that in addition to noting total time in specific heart rate bands the number and length of sustained periods above threshold heart rates should be monitored.[45, 56, 64, 758] This technique may present a more informative picture of physical activity patterns.

The interpretation of heart rate is complex because it not only reflects the metabolism of the subject but also the transient emotional state, the prevailing climatic conditions, and the specific muscle groups which perform the activity. However, in comparison with other forms of physiological analysis heart rate monitoring is the most suitable single method for use in large-scale physical activity studies with children.[500, 911, 1325, 1326] It provides an objective assessment of physical activity patterns and an estimation of total energy expenditure of population groups, although its value in predicting individual energy expenditures remains to be proven.

Combining methods of assessment

Physical activity is a behavioural characteristic but it can occur only as a result of skeletal muscle activity that is supported by cellular level energy transformation processes. Physical activity is therefore interrelated with energy expenditure but it may cause an elevation in metabolic rate that persists long after cessation of observable movement. Different techniques may therefore be measuring different dimensions of physical activity and this could, at least in part, account for the often weak relationships between different measurement techniques used on the same subjects.

Low to moderate relationships have been reported between self-report measures and heart rate,[188, 1208] and with monitoring using motion sensors,[282, 830, 1306] and observational techniques.[132, 1588] Similarly, only low to moderate relationships have been demonstrated between Caltrac scores and both heart rate monitoring[129, 1304] and observation.[1075, 1109] Comparison of heart rate monitoring with doubly labelled water has resulted in a close estimation of total energy expenditure in one study[911] and a 12% overestimation of energy expenditure in another.[500]

The assessment of young people's habitual physical activity is extremely complex and all current methods have deficiencies. Comparing data generated using different methods is simplistic and, ideally, a combination of different techniques should be used. For example, simultaneous use of doubly labelled water, heart rate monitoring, and structured observation would yield information on total energy expenditure, pattern of relative physiological load (intensity) on the cardiopulmonary system, and frequency, duration, and type of physical activity experienced. Unfortunately, the choice of method in large scale epidemiological studies is likely to continue to be dictated largely by practical, logistic, and financial considerations. (Table 6.3.)

Table 6.3. Ideal combination of methods to evaluate young people's physical activity patterns

Method	Role
Observation	To note frequency, duration, and type of physical activity
Heart rate monitoring	To note pattern of relative physiological load on the cardiopulmonary system
Doubly labelled water	To note total energy expenditure

Physical activity patterns

Despite the problems involved in monitoring habitual physical activity the physical activity patterns of young people in the United Kingdom,[46, 292] Europe,[53] and North America[1139] have been well documented. Because of the variation in methodology estimates of physical activity levels across studies are often difficult to interpret and compare, but it is possible to examine age- and gender-related trends within and across studies.[1139]

Self-report studies

Large-scale, national surveys of young people's physical activity patterns have been carried out in Canada (sample size 4756),[299, 300, 1380, 1381] the United States (sample size 8800),[1235–1239] Northern Ireland (sample size 3211)[1205, 1208] and Wales (sample size 6581).[701, 702] Further self or parental/teacher report data on the activity patterns of young people are available from North America,[1041, 1267, 1310, 1398, 1530] Belgium,[1640] Finland,[1512, 1514] Sweden,[502, 503, 1494] Norway,[1516] Czechoslovakia,[1362] Italy,[974] Germany,[590, 747, 1282] the Netherlands,[408, 805, 1331] and the United Kingdom.[434, 435, 625, 1522, 1651] Levels of physical activity cannot be confidently compared across studies, but age- and gender-related trends are remarkably consistent.

Significant numbers of children appear to have adopted sedentary lifestyles. Boys are more physically active than girls, and younger children tend to be more active than adolescents. Gender differences in level of physical activity start early in childhood but the differences are greater among older children and adolescents.

A multinational WHO study[820] illustrated the trends quite elegantly. In each of 11 countries, target groups representative of the national population in terms of age, gender, and geographic distribution were recruited. Three age groups were selected to simulate a longitudinal study, the median

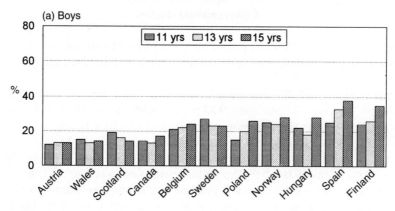

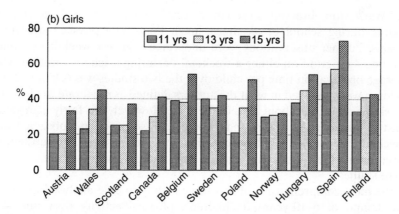

Fig. 6.3. Percentage of young people who exercise less than once a week outside school: (a) boys; (b) girls. Figures drawn from data reported by King, A.C. and Coles, B. (1992). *The Health of Canada's Youth*. Canada, Minister of Supply and Services.

ages of which were set at 11, 13, and 15 years. Substantial sample sizes ranged from 2984 subjects in Austria to 6498 subjects in Hungary. The young people were asked how often per week they exercised, outside school hours, to the point they got out of breath or sweated. The percentages of boys and girls who exercised once a week or less are illustrated by age and participating country in Fig. 6.3. The decrease in exercise participation with age, especially for girls, is readily apparent and consistent across countries. Fewer girls than boys exercised at least once a week at all ages studied.

Observational studies

Few studies have observed young people's physical activity for extended periods of time and all published studies appear to have focused on young children.[122, 134, 135, 468, 1416, 1417]

Baranowski and his associates[135] observed 24 third- and sixth-grade children for periods averaging 9.83 h per child and concluded that their results, 'contradict the common perception of children being very active' (p. 205). The same research group assessed the level of physical activity of 191 3- and 4-year-old children by observation with the CARS for up to 12 h, from 07.00–19.00.[134, 468] The children were observed up to four times in the course of a year over a 3 year period. Boys were shown to be significantly more active than girls and the researchers concluded that their study, 'contradicts the myth that young children 3–5 years of age are always moving or active'.[468, p. 1419]

Using similar techniques with English children (age 5–11 years) Sleap and Warburton observed, on separate occasions, 64 children[1417] and 56 children[1416] during school break times, lunch times, and physical education lessons. Further observations were undertaken on one weekday evening and one 4 h period on either a weekend or during a school vacation. The average observation time per child over the two studies was 6.45 h and the children were engaged in what the authors defined as moderate to vigorous physical activity, for about 30% of the time. However, this fairly high value must be placed in the context that classroom lessons were not observed and the children were likely to have been inactive at these times. No substantial variation in physical activity between boys and girls was noted in either of these studies.

The most comprehensive observational study to date analysed the level and tempo of 6–10-year-old children's physical activity over nine 4 h observation blocks, encompassing the period from 08.00–20.00 and involving three observation periods within each time block: 08.00–12.00, 12.00–16.00, and 16.00–20.00.[122] Despite the small sample size (8 boys and 7 girls) this study is of interest because of the high resolution with which physical activities were observed. The data indicated that children engage in very short bursts of intense physical activity interspersed with varying intervals of activity of low and moderate intensity. No period of intense activity lasting 10 consecutive minutes was ever recorded, and 95% of intense periods of physical activity lasted less than 15 sec. The medium duration of an activity lasted less than 15 sec. The medium duration of an activity at any level (low, medium, or high) was 6 sec and the median duration of an intense activity was only 3 sec.

The limited data available from observational studies indicate that children spend most of their time engaged in activities of low intensity interspersed with very short bursts of high intensity physical activity. Baranowski

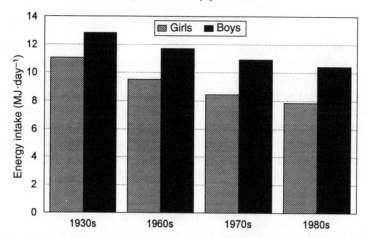

Fig. 6.4. Energy intakes of 14–15-year-olds in the United Kingdom. Figure drawn from data reported by Durnin, J.V.G.A. (1992). Physical activity levels – past and present. In N. Norgan (Ed.), *Physical Activity and Health.* Cambridge University Press, pp. 20–7.

et al.'s[134] finding of gender-related differences at an early age is of interest but requires confirmation.

Motion sensor studies

Little information on children's and adolescents' physical activity patterns has been obtained using motion sensors. The data are, however, consistent and indicate that boys are more active than girls and that the level of physical activity of both sexes declines from childhood through adolescence.[805, 1494]

Energy intake studies

Studies of energy intake provide little insight into young people's physical activity patterns but an analysis of historical data provided by Durnin[475] is of interest. Durnin pooled data collected from the 1930s to the 1980s[351, 416, 476, 1646] and demonstrated a progressive decrease in the energy intake of adolescents in the United Kingdom (Fig. 6.4). The body mass of both boys and girls was almost identical within each sex for all four groups and the methodology was the same on each occasion. The only conceivable explanation for the very marked reduction in energy intake, which must reflect diminished energy expenditure, is that adolescents' physical activity has radically decreased over the last 50 years.

Energy expenditure studies

Bedale's analysis of the energy expenditure ('heat production') of Hampshire schoolchildren during selected activities was probably the first attempt to classify the daily energy expenditure of young people.[161] She collected expired respiratory gases in Douglas bags and analysed the gases for oxygen and carbon dioxide content using a Haldane apparatus. Subsequent research, often with small sample sizes, has relied upon energy expenditure predicted from heart rates[1324, 1440, 1574] or doubly labelled water[911] but the results have been consistent. At all ages from 6–17 years boys appear to have a higher total energy expenditure than girls.

Heart rate monitoring

A number of investigators have monitored the heart rates of young people for up to 12 h and reported the cumulative time with heart rates above predetermined thresholds.[58, 107, 236, 296, 616, 618, 619, 758, 933, 1207, 1362] Although small sample sizes are common the data unequivocally support the premise that children, and especially adolescents, are engaged primarily in low-intensity or sedentary activities.

To obtain a true picture of habitual physical activity a minimum monitoring period of 3 days is required.[138] A series of studies from our laboratory therefore used the Polar Sports Tester to monitor the heart rates of 743 10–16-year-olds from 09.00–21.00 over three normal schooldays.[57, 64, 188, 1013, 1620] In order to interpret the heart rate data a representative sample of 40 youngsters exercised at various speeds on a horizontal treadmill. It was noted that brisk walking at 6 km·h^{-1} (1.67 m·s^{-1}) elicited steady-state heart rates averaging 146 beats per minute (bpm). The mean heart rate of the subjects at peak $\dot{V}O_2$ was 200 bpm. For the present purpose we have re-analysed the data on the basis of primary schoolchildren (165 girls, mean age 10.9 years; 167 boys, mean age 10.9 years) and secondary schoolchildren (243 girls, mean age 13.1 years; 168 boys, mean age 13.0 years) and used the heart rate threshold of 140 bpm to represent brisk walking. The primary schoolboys spent a significantly greater percentage of time with their heart rate above 139 bpm (9.2%) than both primary schoolgirls (7.7%) and secondary schoolchildren (boys, 6.3%; girls, 4.7%). The younger girls spent significantly longer above the threshold than the older girls.

Because of the limitations of simply reporting percentages of time above a threshold value and to provide a clearer picture of the youngsters' physical activity patterns the number of 10 min periods with heart rate sustained above 139 bpm was calculated. The data, which are shown in Fig. 6.5, demonstrate that significant numbers of young people seldom experience the equivalent of a 10 min brisk walk.

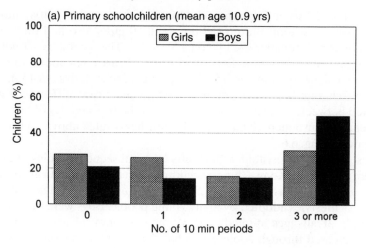

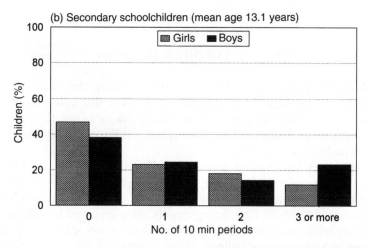

Fig. 6.5. The percentage of young people sustaining 10 min periods with their heart rate above 139 bpm during 3 day monitoring: (a) primary schoolchildren; (b) secondary schoolchildren. Figures drawn from data reported by Armstrong, N. *et al.* (1990–95).[56, 57, 63, 64, 73, 188, 1013, 1620]

These studies were carried out throughout the school year, but in order to investigate whether there was any difference between physical activity levels during the autumn and summer terms, 24 children were monitored for 3 days during each term. No significant differences were detected.[63] Young people's physical activity during the summer vacation does not appear to have been studied using heart rate monitoring, probably because of the logistics involved.

A total of 252 secondary schoolchildren (115 boys and 137 girls) and 119 of the primary schoolchildren (59 boys and 60 girls) also had their heart rates monitored from 09.00–21.00 on a Saturday. The secondary schoolgirls spent significantly less time (2.8%) with their heart rates above 139 bpm than secondary schoolboys (5.5%), primary schoolboys (6.4%), and primary schoolgirls (5.9%). Interestingly, no significant differences were detected between the primary schoolgirls and the two samples of boys. The frequency of sustained 10 min periods with heart rates above 139 bpm is illustrated in Fig. 6.6.

These data are consistent with results from subsequent studies of Singaporean and Hong Kong Chinese children which used identical methodology and analytical techniques,[613, 1015] and they clearly illustrate the sedentary lifestyles adopted by many young people. Boys were more active than girls at all ages studied. The volume of physical activity of both sexes decreased through adolescence but the decline was more marked in girls.

Tracking of physical activity

The view that high levels of physical activity during childhood increase the likelihood of such participation as an adult has often been proposed.[629, 642, 961, 1567] The hypothesis is intuitively plausible but the definitive study of physical activity tracking from childhood through adult life has yet to be carried out.

Early studies of physical activity tracking focused on the habitual physical activity of former college athletes. Several studies indicated that former college athletes were no more likely to be active in later life than non-athletes.[265, 443, 1059, 1461] Conflicting results were reported by others who found that active men were more likely than sedentary men to have been members of high school or college athletic teams.[536, 685, 1176]

Data generated from college students, however, are not representative of the population and they provide limited insight into children's behaviour as physical activity patterns are likely to be well established before college entrance. The comparison of 'athletes' with 'non-athletes' introduces further selection bias, for example, on the basis of genetic endowment.[966] The generic use of the term 'athlete' probably confounds the analysis as activities that do not require a team may be more easily sustained into adult life. Similarly, the specialization of successful young athletes may be achieved at the expense of developing a broader use of fundamental motor skills, which in turn may affect adult participation.

National adult fitness surveys have been conducted in England[6] and the United States[270, 338] and, through retrospective questionnaires, both surveys

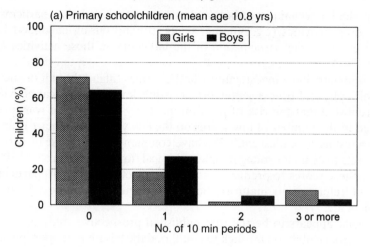

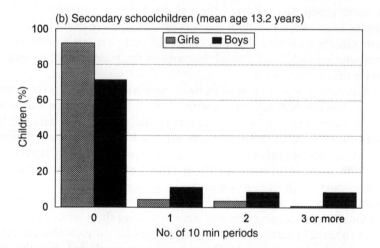

Fig. 6.6. The percentage of young people sustaining 10 min periods with their heart rate above 139 bpm during 12 h of Saturday monitoring: (a) primary schoolchildren; (b) secondary schoolchildren. Figures drawn from data reported by Armstrong, N. *et al.* (1990–95).[56, 57, 63, 64, 73, 188, 1013, 1620]

indicated that lifelong physical activity behaviour is likely to begin during childhood and adolescence. The English study of adults reported that,

25% of those who said they were very active aged 14–19 were very active now, compared with only 2% active now who were totally inactive at that early age.[6, p. 64]

Using similar techniques other studies have concluded that participation in outdoor activities (e.g. hunting, skiing, fishing) during childhood has a direct effect on the participation of the individual in those activities as an adult.[1433, 1695]

Researchers have investigated whether males' high school[414] or medical school[578] physical fitness scores predict adult levels of physical activity. It was reported that the risk of physical inactivity in adulthood was linearly related to the number of low scores on the 600 yard (548.6 metre) run and sit-ups test as an adolescent.[414] We have commented on the use of performance tests to estimate young people's physical fitness elsewhere[40, 41, 43, 1168] and to use these scores to predict future physical activity patterns, particularly without reference to maturity, body mass, and body fatness is at best problematic.

In what appears to be the first published prospective study of physical activity from childhood through to adulthood the leisure time sporting activities of 2464 randomly selected Swedish 15-year-olds was investigated.[502, 503] The same group was followed through mailed questionnaires 5, 10, and 15 years later and a full data set was obtained on 1675 individuals. The results clearly indicated the importance of early experiences of physical activity during childhood and adolescence in the maintenance of an active lifestyle during adulthood.

Two recent prospective studies have supported physical activity tracking.[626, 862] The physical activity patterns of more than 3300 men and women aged 36 years, and who were members of the 1946 British national birth cohort study, were examined. It was reported that adolescent characteristics which were positive predictors of high sporting activity during adult life included above average ability at school games and teacher-assessed (proxy-report) high energy expenditure at age 13 years.[862] In a smaller Swedish study, 62 males and 43 females were required to complete a questionnaire concerning physical activity during their leisure time at the ages of 16 and 27 years.[626] At the age of 16 years the subjects also underwent a series of physiological tests. The investigators concluded that, the major portion of the variation in level of physical activity in the women, but not in the men, could be predicted from physical characteristics, physical performance, and activity level at 16 years of age.

Perhaps the most persuasive evidence in support of physical activity tracking has emerged from a recent study of 961 Finnish youngsters, aged 12, 15, or 18 years at baseline, who were followed for 6 years.[1193] Physical activity was assessed with a standardized questionnaire and an index was derived from the product of intensity, frequency, and duration of leisure time physical activity. Significant tracking of physical activity was observed with 3 year correlations of the index ranging from 0.35–0.54 in boys and from 0.33–0.39 in girls. Tracking was better in older age groups. Approximately 57% of those initially classified as inactive remained inactive after a

6 year follow-up. The authors concluded that the level of physical activity tracks significantly from adolescence to young adulthood and that physical inactivity shows better tracking than does physical activity.

Summary

Physical activity is a complex phenomenon with different dimensions and the assessment of young people's physical activity patterns is difficult. A number of techniques have been developed and all have both merits and limitations. No single 'gold standard' has emerged and ideally a combination of methods should be used. The ideal combination of techniques required for a comprehensive evaluation of youngsters' physical activity patterns is likely to remain impractical for use with large numbers of young people in the foreseeable future. The variation in methodology across studies often precludes valid, comparative analyses but it is possible to examine trends within studies with confidence. The available data are remarkably consistent. Sedentary lifestyles are common. Males between the ages of 6 and 17 years have been estimated to be 15–25% more physically active than females of the same age.[1300] During childhood and adolescence both boys and girls reduce their physical activity as they grow older but the rate of decline is 2.5 times greater in girls than in boys.[1300]

Although data have been collected for over 70 years, methodological problems prevent any meaningful analysis of whether youngsters' habitual physical activity has declined over time. However, Durnin's[475] review of adolescents' energy intakes over the period 1930s–1980s suggests a reduction in energy expenditure over this period.

Adult physical activity patterns may be established during childhood and adolescence. No prospective study has followed children into middle age and beyond, but the available data support the premise that inactive young people are unlikely to become physically active adults.

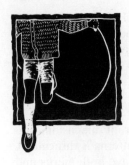

7

Physical activity and aerobic fitness

Aerobic fitness

Aerobic exercise is dependent upon pulmonary, cardiovascular, and haematological components of oxygen delivery and the oxidative mechanisms of the exercising muscles. As maximal exercise is limited by the individual's peak $\dot{V}O_2$ this variable is widely recognized as the best single index of aerobic fitness. In Part II we discussed peak $\dot{V}O_2$ in detail and expressed our reservations about the use of ratio standards (e.g. mL·kg^{-1}·min^{-1}), however, in order to interpret the extant literature we will in this section need to refer to peak $\dot{V}O_2$ in this manner.

The first laboratory-based studies of children's aerobic fitness were carried out by Robinson,[1219] Morse *et al*,[1071] and Astrand[98] and the findings of these pioneer workers have since been supplemented by data from most parts of the world.[138, 851, 1375] In a recent review,[81] we analysed aerobic fitness data on untrained subjects, aged 8–16 years, from studies representing 10 145 peak $\dot{V}O_2$ data points (see Figs 4.1 and 4.2). The data provided a consistent picture of a progressive rise in boy's peak $\dot{V}O_2$ from 8–16 years with girls' data showing a similar but more varied trend. At 10 years of age, boys' peak $\dot{V}O_2$ was observed to be 13% higher than that of similarly aged girls (1.68 vs. 1.48 L·min^{-1}) increasing to 37% higher at 16 years of age (3.06 vs. 2.24 L·min^{-1}). However, the aerobic fitness of young people appears to have remained remarkably consistent over almost six decades, with current data closely reflecting the findings of earlier studies.

Members of the European Pediatric Work Physiology Group[164] have expressed the view that a low mass-related peak $\dot{V}O_2$, in the absence of other health-related problems, may constitute a health risk. Risk levels of 35 mL·kg^{-1}·min^{-1} for boys and 30 mL·kg^{-1}·min^{-1} for girls were proposed. A reworking of data on children and adolescents who had their peak $\dot{V}O_2$ determined
in our laboratory has revealed that only about 2% of young people aged 9–16 years could be classified as at risk.[58, 70, 73, 85] There is therefore little evidence to suggest that young people have low levels of aerobic fitness.

Habitual physical activity and aerobic fitness

The relative importance to short- and long-term health of aerobic fitness and habitual physical activity has been widely debated.[44, 47, 576, 910] The evidence linking young people's aerobic fitness to their level of physical activity is, however, conflicting and must be interpreted in the light of the problems associated with assessing both physical activity and aerobic fitness.

Several studies have relied upon self-report data and submaximal predictions of aerobic fitness.[702, 1311, 1496, 1516] Other investigations have used field test scores as their criterion measure of aerobic fitness.[1, 456, 1138, 1140, 1306] The results have been equivocal but any significant correlations between physical activity and aerobic fitness have been low in magnitude.

A high level of physical activity has been related to high peak $\dot{V}O_2$ scores[810, 811, 1042] but other studies have concluded that young people with different levels of peak $\dot{V}O_2$ do not differ substantially in their daily physical activity.[27, 1323]

Most studies using peak $\dot{V}O_2$ as the criterion measure of aerobic fitness have only monitored physical activity for a limited period of time, usually only part of one day. Results have been conflicting with significant relationships observed between aerobic fitness and physical activity in boys,[14, 1493] in girls,[758] and in a mixed group[545] in some studies but not in either boys[386, 758, 875, 1362] or girls[1493] in others. Correlations have, at best, been small to moderate and typically about $r = 0.16$.[1070]

In two studies carried out in our laboratory we monitored the heart rate of 85 boys and 111 girls, aged 11–16 years,[60] and 86 prepubescent boys and 43 prepubescent girls, aged 10–11 years,[73] for at least three 12 h periods, to estimate habitual physical activity. Peak $\dot{V}O_2$ directly determined on either a cycle ergometer or a treadmill was used as the criterion measure of aerobic fitness. We detected no significant relationship between physical activity and aerobic fitness in either study. In a third study we used the same methodology for estimating daily physical activity but the percentage of peak $\dot{V}O_2$ at the 2.5 mmol·L^{-1} blood lactate reference level was utilized as a criterion of aerobic fitness.[1620] No significant relationships were revealed with a sample of 73 young people, aged 11–16 years.

A unique study of the recovery of peak $\dot{V}O_2$ of five children after 9 weeks of bedrest following femoral fractures is also of interest.[1265] From the extremes of normal physical activity to prolonged total immobilization the children lost only an estimated average of 13% of their peak $\dot{V}O_2$, which was regained within 3 months following bedrest. These findings indicate that daily physical activity makes only a very limited contribution to peak $\dot{V}O_2$.

The evidence relating habitual physical activity to peak $\dot{V}O_2$ in children and adolescents is equivocal, perhaps because most studies have involved small sample sizes, limited periods of monitoring physical activity, or predictions of aerobic fitness from field tests or submaximal data. That a relationship between peak $\dot{V}O_2$ and habitual physical activity remains to be proven is not unexpected, given the complexity of any relationship that may exist. Peak $\dot{V}O_2$ is a physiological variable whereas habitual physical activity is a behaviour, and although it has been suggested that high levels of aerobic fitness may encourage individuals to engage in strenuous leisure time activities this has yet to be established.[388] The evaluation of any relationship between level of physical activity and peak $\dot{V}O_2$ is further confounded by the presence of an as yet unquantified genetic component of peak $\dot{V}O_2$.[225, 226, 966]

However, the simple explanation for the lack of relationship between habitual physical activity and aerobic fitness probably lies in the low level of physical activity of most young people. The vast majority of children and adolescents rarely experience physical activity of sufficient intensity and duration to increase peak $\dot{V}O_2$, and structured exercise training programmes appear to be necessary for the improvement of aerobic fitness.

Exercise training and aerobic fitness

Exercise training-induced adaptations in adults' aerobic fitness have been studied extensively[340, 546, 1427] and it is well documented that the rate and magnitude of increase in maximal oxygen uptake is related to the level of aerobic fitness prior to the commencement of training, and the frequency, duration, and intensity of the exercise training programme.[209, 1173, 1197] Exercise prescriptions for improving adults' aerobic fitness are well established[23, 24, 1634] and some authorities have recommended their application to young people.[22, 1253] However, despite an abundance of research on the topic, the issue of children's and adolescents' responses to exercise training is controversial.

Numerous reviews have been compiled to synthesize the literature on young people's trainability[69, 100, 121, 127, 222, 235, 380, 385, 851, 1257, 1261, 1290, 1400, 1554, 1618, 1693, 1711] but the evidence remains equivocal. The effects of exercise training on prepubescent children are particularly debatable and several reviews have specifically targeted this population.[143, 1142, 1149, 1253, 1382] Few studies, however, have reported the responses of children or adolescents to carefully controlled and well-defined exercise training programmes.

Factors to be considered in the design of exercise training studies

The ethical issues concerning the involvement of young people in research, the use of techniques of negligible risk, and the problems of using equipment and protocols designed for the determination of adults' maximal

Table 7.1. Factors to be considered in designing a training study with children and adolescents

---

• Ethics

• Criterion tests

• Habitual physical activity

• Pre-training aerobic fitness

• Recruitment of experimental subjects

• Recruitment of control subjects

• Adherence to the programme

• Subject attrition

• Genetics

• Maturity

• Exercise prescription

• De-training

---

oxygen uptake have been discussed in Chapter 2. It has been suggested that children's and adolescents' high inherent level of habitual physical activity may confound their responses to exercise training,[18, 680] but we demonstrated in Chapter 6 that few children experience the volume of physical activity associated with improvements in aerobic fitness.

Several authors have hypothesized that young people might be less trainable than adults because of their relatively high initial fitness level.[931, 1290] These comments were based on the use of ratio standards and we have addressed what may be more valid methods of interpreting children's and adolescents' peak $\dot{V}O_2$ in Chapter 3. Nevertheless, subjects used in some published studies did in fact have a high level of initial fitness[151, 375, 492, 1049] and others were specially selected or already belonged to athletic clubs.[256, 394, 522, 800] In cases such as these a substantial increase in volume of exercise may be necessary to induce improvements in peak $\dot{V}O_2$.

Young people who volunteer for exercise training studies may possess characteristics that are atypical of the population and they must be willing and able to devote sufficient time and effort to the programme. The commitment required may lead to poor adherence and a large drop-out rate, both of which cloud the interpretation of the results[1290] but few studies have commented upon sample attrition.[492, 1372] It has been suggested that the attrition rate may be less in studies involving children than in those involving adults[1382] but it is important to note whether those subjects with poor adherence and those who drop out differ on important characteristics from those who complete the study.

The interaction between the effects of exercise training and growth and maturation on aerobic fitness is controversial but some allowance must be made for it within the experimental design of all training studies with young people. An adequate control group is therefore of paramount importance when studying children and adolescents as it allows the investigator to tease out changes in aerobic fitness which result from growth and maturation alone.[1554] What constitutes an adequate control group is not altogether clear. Subjects can be matched for biological age, anthropometric characteristics, habitual physical activity, and pre-training aerobic fitness, but one is still left with accounting for any genetic influence on aerobic trainability.[226]

Bouchard[224] noted a substantial variation in the response of children to a well-standardized training programme. Some individuals appear to exhibit a high response to exercise training (e.g. a significant increase in peak $\dot{V}O_2$) whereas others are almost non-responders to training. Bouchard's work with monozygotic twins[678, 1184] has suggested that the sensitivity of peak $\dot{V}O_2$ to exercise training may be largely genotype-dependent. This work requires further exploration[224] but as a problem in experimental design the optimum solution would be to use non-training identical twins as control subjects.[1610] This is, however, not normally feasible. Rowland[1273] has used a time series design in which each subject serves as his/her own control by measuring peak $\dot{V}O_2$ changes over a period of time immediately prior to the exercise training programme. The use of a matched control group, however, remains the method of choice despite the inability to account for genetic influences.

The use of an appropriate control group can help to compensate for any changes in aerobic fitness which may occur with repeated exposure to the testing procedures independent of any exercise training effect.[1290, 1341] There is, of course, always the problem of contamination of control subjects by personal contact with experimental subjects but this is probably slight[1377, 1382] although in at least one study there was some exchange of subjects between control and experimental groups.[492]

Exercise training and maturation

Several of the studies which have reported no significant increase in mass-related peak $\dot{V}O_2$ with exercise training have involved young children[65, 166, 1465] and this finding is consistent with other studies involving a wider age range which have observed no increase in the mass-related peak $\dot{V}O_2$ of their younger subjects.[835, 1002, 1042] These results led Gilliam and Freedson[615] to hypothesize that a maturational threshold exists whereby prepubescent children are unable to elicit physiological changes in response to training. Katch[795] proposed that there is one critical time period in a child's life (a 'trigger point') below which the effects of training will be minimal, or will not occur at all. He suggested that,

this trigger phenomenon is the result of modulating effects of hormones that initiate puberty and influence functional development and subsequent organic adaptations.[795, p. 241]

In a study which is often used in support of the critical period hypothesis Kobayashi and his associates[834] followed a group of seven boys from the age of 9.7–15.8 years and determined their peak $\dot{V}O_2$ annually. The boys trained for 1–1.5 h per day, four to five times per week throughout the period of observation. No control group was available in the early part of the research. Peak $\dot{V}O_2$ was observed to increase slowly until 1 year prior to PHV after which 'training effectively increased aerobic power above the normal increase attributable to age and growth'.[834, p. 666] In a conflicting report, Weber and his associates[1610] studied 12 pairs of identical twins, four sets aged 10 years, four sets aged 13 years, and four sets aged 16 years. One twin from each set followed a 10 week exercise training programme. The results suggested that the 10- and 16-year-old twins experienced greater relative increases in their peak $\dot{V}O_2$ than the 13-year-old twins, and this was interpreted by the authors to demonstrate that children are less trainable around the age of puberty.

We examined the physiological responses of 18 10-year-old and 16 22-year-old females to an 8 week cycle ergometer training programme involving three 20 min sessions per week with the heart rate maintained between 160 and 170 bpm.[65] The young women's peak $\dot{V}O_2$ demonstrated a small but significant increase of 4.3% whereas no significant change in the children's peak $\dot{V}O_2$ was noted. A control group of 16 10-year-old girls also exhibited no significant change in peak $\dot{V}O_2$ over the 8 week period. A similar study[490] compared the exercise training response of eight girls, aged 12–13 years, to that of eight young women following the same 14 week training programme and reported that the magnitude and rate of increase of peak $\dot{V}O_2$ were identical in both groups.

Savage et al.[1336] described the effects of a 10 week exercise training programme on the peak $\dot{V}O_2$ of eight prepubescent boys and eight men who trained at 40% of peak $\dot{V}O_2$, and 12 prepubescent boys and 12 men who trained at 75% of peak $\dot{V}O_2$. Significant increases in peak $\dot{V}O_2$ were limited to the high-intensity training groups but did not differ between men and boys. It must therefore be concluded that the case for a critical period for enhanced responses to exercise training remains to be proven.

Cross-sectional studies

Several researchers have adopted an approach in which comparisons are made between trained and untrained young people. These cross-sectional analyses have consistently demonstrated that trained children and adolescents have higher peak $\dot{V}O_2$ than untrained youngsters.[90, 101, 382, 387, 596, 989, 1292, 1407, 1485, 1553, 1556] We have reported a mean peak $\dot{V}O_2$ of 67 mL·kg^{-1}·min^{-1} in a group of highly trained 14-year-old male swimmers two of whom attained values in excess of 75 mL·kg^{-1}min^{-1}.[67] These values are 40% higher than the mean value for untrained boys of the same age.[81] Whether this high peak $\dot{V}O_2$ was induced solely by exercise training is, however, impossible to deduce. Evidence does exist that young athletes beginning serious training already have functional advantages[515] and the interpretation of such studies is further confounded by the finding that boys participating in regular sports training are generally more advanced in maturity.[245, 951]

Longitudinal studies

Several comprehensive reviews have tabulated details of the large number of training studies which have used adolescent subjects[235, 384, 851, 1142, 1290, 1554, 1618] but in the light of the information in the previous section we will restrict our discussion to the better controlled studies. Few investigations have classified subjects according to maturation[65, 931, 1016, 1629, 1654] so we have, for our current purpose, defined adolescents as aged 11 years and above.[1302]

Studies with adolescents

In a study of adolescent girls' response to training a 16.1% increase in the mass-related peak $\dot{V}O_2$ of the experimental group was observed following a four times a week, 7 week swim training programme. The peak $\dot{V}O_2$ of the control group remained unchanged.[1470] Two studies of adolescent boys[451, 983] reported significant increases in peak $\dot{V}O_2$ following short duration programmes, whereas a third study[1465] failed to induce a significant change in peak $\dot{V}O_2$. The range of change in mass-related peak $\dot{V}O_2$ in the six experimental groups was –0.6–18.4% (weighted mean, 8.6%) with the higher-intensity experimental groups experiencing the greater change. (Table 7.2.)

Studies with children

Tabulated details of exercise training studies with young children are available in several reviews.[143, 1142, 1149, 1253] Table 7.3 summarizes nine of the better controlled studies involving children aged less than 11 years. Although maturational status was only assessed in six of the studies[65, 931, 1016, 1336, 1629, 1654] it is likely that the vast majority of subjects were prepubescent as, with the exception of the 8-year-old girls in one study,[615] those whose maturity was not assessed were boys under the age of 11 years.

Table 7.2. Exercise training and aerobic fitness: studies with adolescents

| Study | Subjects | | Training protocol | | | | | Peak $\dot{V}O_2$ (L·min⁻¹) | | | Peak $\dot{V}O_2$ (mL·kg⁻¹·min⁻¹) | | |
	Experimental (E)	Control (C)	Frequency (per wk)	Intensity	Time	Length (wks)	Type	Pre	Post	Change (%)	Pre	Post	Change (%)
Stransky et al.[1470]	n = 16 G, 15.8 yrs	n = 14 G, 15.9 yrs	4	Unknown	12 800 yds/week	7	Swim training	E 2.45 C 2.46	2.80 2.50	14.3 1.6	E 41.6 C 42.9	48.3 42.9	16.1 0
Docherty	2 groups E₁ n = 11 B, 12 yrs E₂ n = 12 B, 12 yrs	n = 11 B 12 yrs	3	E₁ high velocity E₂ low resist./high velocity	2 × 20 sec at an unspecified number of stations		Isokinetic resist. training	E₁ 2.06 E₂ 1.90 C 2.12	2.43 2.31 2.22	18.0 21.6 4.7	47.0 E₂ 46.2 C 47.0	55.1 54.7 49.0	17.2 18.4 4.3
Massicotte & Macnab[983]	3 groups n = 9 B in each, 11–13 yrs	n = 9 B, 11–13 yrs	3	E₁ HR 170–180 E₂ HR 150–160 E₃ HR 130–140	12 min	6	Cont. cycling	E₁ 2.0 E₂ 1.8 E₃ 1.7 C 2.0	2.3 1.9 1.8 1.9	15.0 5.6 5.9 –5.0	E₁ 46.7 E₂ 47.4 E₃ 46.6 C 45.7	51.8 48.0 48.2 44.2	10.8 1.3 3.4 –3.3
Stewart & Gutin[1465]	n = 13 B, 10–12 yrs	n = 11 B, 10–12 yrs	4	90% max HR	14–21 min	8	Interval running	E – C –	– –	– –	E 49.8 C 48.4	49.5 49.2	–0.6 1.7

B, boys; G, girls; HR, heart rate.

Table 7.3. Exercise training and aerobic fitness: studies with children

Study	Subjects Experimental (E)	Control (C)	Training protocol Frequency (per wk)	Intensity	Time	Length (wks)	Type	Peak V̇O₂ (L·min⁻¹) Pre	Post	Change (%)	Peak V̇O₂ (mL·kg⁻¹·min⁻¹) Pre	Post	Change (%)
Lussier & Buskirk[931]	n = 16 11 B 5 G, 10.3 yrs	n = 10 9 B 1 G, 10.5 yrs	4	92% max HR	45 min	12	Cont. running & games	E 1.76 C 1.83	1.96 1.96	11.4 7.1	E 55.6 C 53.1	59.4 53.9	6.8 1.5
Becker & Vaccaro[158]	n = 11 B, 9.9 yrs	n = 11 B, 10.0 yrs	3	50% of the way between AT and peak V̇O₂	40 min	8	Cont. cycling	E – C –	– –	– –	E 39.0 C 41.7	47.0 44.0	20.5 5.5
Rotstein et al.[1248]	n = 16 B, 10.8 yrs	n = 12 B, 10.8 yrs	3	Unknown	45 min	9	Interval running	E – C –	– –	– –	E 54.2 C 57.1	58.6 58.3	8.1 2.1
Savage et al.[1336]	2 groups E₁ n = 12 B, 8.0 yrs E₂ n = 8 B, 8.5 yrs	n = 10 B, 9.0 yrs	3	E₁ 75% peak V̇O₂ E₂ 40% peak V̇O₂	2.4–4.8 km	10	Interval running	E₁ – E₂ – C –	– – –	– – –	E₁55.9 E₂52.2 C 57.0	58.5 54.6 55.7	4.7 4.6 –2.3
Weltman et al.[1629]	n = 16 B, 8.2 yrs	n = 10 B, 8.2 yrs	4	Unknown	45 min	14	Resist. training	E 1.39 C 1.48	1.66 1.44	19.4 –2.7	E 46.8 C 54.6	53.2 51.7	13.7 –5.3

cont'd

Table 7.3. *cont'd*

Study	Subjects Experimental (E)	Control (C)	Training protocol Frequency (per wk)	Intensity	Time	Length (wks)	Type	Peak $\dot{V}O_2$ (L·min⁻¹) Pre	Post	Change (%)	Peak $\dot{V}O_2$ (mL·kg⁻¹·min⁻¹) Pre	Post	Change (%)
Williams et al.[1654]	2 groups E_1 $n=13$ B, 10.1 yrs E_2 $n=12$ B, 10.1 yrs	$n=14$ B, 10.1 yrs	3	E_1 80–85% max HR E_2 max sprints	E_1 20 min E_2 8–16 min	8	E_1 Cont. cycling C running E_2 Interval	E_1 1.80 E_2 1.84 C 1.92	1.93 1.91 1.97	7.2 3.8 2.6	E_1 54.7 E_2 54.8 C 56.4	57.5 56.2 56.7	5.1 2.6 0.5
Gilliam & Freedson[615]	$n=11$ B & G, 8.5 yrs	$n=12$ B & G, 8.5 yrs	4	84% of max HR	25 min	12	Enhanced PE programme	E 1.29 C 1.34	1.34 1.40	3.9 4.5	E 43.4 C 40.5	42.9 40.9	-1.2 1.0
McManus et al.[1016]	2 groups E_1 $n=12$ G, 9.3 yrs E_2 $n=11$ G, 9.8 yrs	$n=7$ G, 9.6 yrs	3	E_1 80–85% max HR E_2 max sprints	E_1 20 min E_2 8–16 min	8	E_1 Cont. cycling E_2 Interval running	E_1 1.30 E_2 1.54 C 1.49	1.43 1.67 1.46	10.0 8.4 -2.0	E_1 45.4 E_2 48.3 C 44.9	48.7 50.3 43.8	7.3 4.1 -2.4
Armstrong et al.[65]	$n=17$ G, 10.1 yrs	$n=16$ G, 10.2 yrs	3	80–85% max HR	20 min	8	Cont. cycling	E 1.74 C 1.72	1.77 1.72	1.7 0	E 52 C 49	52 48	0 -2.1

B, boys; G, girls; AT, anaerobic threshold; HR, heart rate.

In two studies with girls we used cycle ergometry to maintain heart rates in the range 160–170 bpm for three 20 min sessions per week over a period of 8 weeks. In one study[1016] a small but significant increase in peak $\dot{V}O_2$ was noted whereas in the other study[65] no significant change in peak $\dot{V}O_2$ was detected.

Two studies[615, 931] used mixed groups of prepubescent boys and girls and reported conflicting results. One study observed no significant change in peak $\dot{V}O_2$ following a 12 week enhanced physical education programme[615] whereas the other study, which used a more intense and longer duration exercise training programme reported a significant 6.8% increase in mass-related peak $\dot{V}O_2$ despite the high initial aerobic fitness of the subjects.[931]

Five studies reported data on young boys[158, 1248, 1336, 1629, 1654] and although the range of increase in mass-related peak $\dot{V}O_2$ in the seven experimental groups was 2.6–20.5% (weighted mean, 8.7%) only three studies[1248, 1336, 1629] observed statistically significant increases in peak $\dot{V}O_2$.

Adaptations to exercise training

Well-controlled, prospective studies of exercise training with children and adolescents are sparse and virtually all suffer from small sample sizes and short duration training programmes. However, the available evidence does suggest that young people's peak $\dot{V}O_2$ increases with appropriate exercise training, although changes in peak $\dot{V}O_2$ are relatively small to moderate when compared to those often observed in adult subjects. Very few data are available from girls but gender does not appear to be an important determinant of trainability.[1142, 1149] Similarly, the experimental evidence does not support the view that prepubescent children cannot respond to exercise training.[1142, 1382] Studies which have used several experimental groups have observed greater changes in peak $\dot{V}O_2$ in their high intensity group than in other groups.[983, 1336] The effects of long-term exercise training studies (>12 weeks) on young people's peak $\dot{V}O_2$ remain to be seen.

Exercise training induced changes in variables other than peak $\dot{V}O_2$ are summarized in Table 7.4 but evidence is sparse, often based on cross-sectional studies, and sometimes equivocal. Cross-sectional studies indicate that young endurance athletes experience an increase in cardiac output at a given exercise intensity,[1437] elevated blood volume, elevated plasma volume, and an increase in total haemoglobin.[522, 839] A reduced heart rate and enhanced stroke volume response to submaximal exercise following training is well documented.[138, 151, 1465] Myocardial mass and heart volume are higher in trained young people.[492, 523, 897] Trained young swimmers have been reported to have higher pulmonary capillarization and pulmonary diffusing capacity than untrained children and adolescents,[1703] although others have observed no change in pulmonary diffusing capacity with training.[837] The effects of exercise training on static and dynamic lung volumes

Table 7.4. Exercise training induced changes related to improved aerobic fitness

Variable	Change
Heart volume	Increase
Blood volume	Increase
Total haemoglobin	Increase
Heart rate	
(submaximal)	Decrease
(maximal)	Decrease or no change
Stroke volume	
(submaximal)	Increase
(maximal)	Increase
Cardiac output	
(submaximal)	Decrease or no change
(maximal)	Increase
Arteriovenous oxygen difference	
(submaximal)	No change
(maximal)	No change
Minute ventilation	
(submaximal)	Decrease
(maximal)	Increase
Respiratory rate	
(submaximal)	Decrease
Tidal volume	
(maximal)	Increase
Blood lactate concentration	
(submaximal)	Decrease or no change
(maximal)	Increase or no change
Peak oxygen uptake	Increase

Adapted and further developed from: Armstrong, N. (1992). The development of training programmes for children. *Athletics Coach*, **26**, 5–9, and Bar-Or, O. (1989). Trainability of the prepubescent child. *The Physician and Sports Medicine*, **17**, 65–82.

are equivocal[501, 835, 1552, 1710] but maximal ventilation and respiratory rate appear to increase[1448] and submaximal ventilatory function is more efficient[1711] following training. Neither submaximal[608] nor maximal[522] arteriovenous oxygen difference change with exercise training, probably because of the relatively high arteriovenous oxygen difference even in the untrained child.

The effects of exercise training on blood lactate concentration are difficult to interpret because of the methodological issues discussed in Chapter 2. There is some evidence to suggest that blood lactate concentration at peak $\dot{V}O_2$ increases following exercise training[983] although conflicting data are also available.[948] Blood lactate indices of submaximal performance have been reported to improve with exercise training[104, 597, 598, 1248] but between-study comparisons are problematic due to the wide range of techniques employed (see Chapter 2). Reductions in blood lactate concentrations at submaximal exercise intensities following training have been observed with both increases in peak $\dot{V}O_2$[983] and no change in peak $\dot{V}O_2$.[65] Another study reported a significant 11% increase in peak $\dot{V}O_2$ following a 14 week training programme but no change in submaximal blood lactate concentration.[948] The responses of blood lactate to exercise training are intriguing but further research is required to clarify any relationship.[81, 1622]

Adaptations to de-training

Elucidating the effects of de-training on children and adolescents is confounded by the youngster's continued growth and maturation during the de-training period. No well-controlled studies of the problem are available but it appears that adaptations to exercise training are transient and will steadily decay once training has stopped.[1031, 1372] It has been demonstrated that if adolescent athletes with high aerobic fitness are retested a few years after ceasing training their peak $\dot{V}O_2$ is similar to that of those who were never athletes.[526, 1077]

Perhaps the best example of the lack of permanency of adaptive responses to even long-term training during childhood and adolescence is provided by the Swedish girl swimmers studies.[101, 516, 517] Astrand and his colleagues[101] observed high levels of peak $\dot{V}O_2$ in a group of 30 girls engaged in long-term strenuous swim training. When the study was followed up 10 years later[516] it was found that all the girls had stopped their regular training and most did not engage in any specific exercise in their spare time. The mean value of the girls' peak $\dot{V}O_2$ had decreased by 29%. Four of the girls were persuaded to undertake a new swim training programme at the ages of 29–31 years and their resultant increase in peak $\dot{V}O_2$ was similar to that of women with no previous training history.[517] It appears that long-term benefits of exercise depend upon the continuance of training sessions into adult life.

Table 7.5. The FITT principle

F	Frequency	How often?
I	Intensity	How hard?
T	Time	How long?
T	Type	What to do?

Exercise prescription

The American College of Sports Medicine (ACSM) define exercise prescription as, 'the process whereby a person's recommended regimen of physical activity is designed in a systematic and individualized manner'.[24, p. 93] All exercise prescriptions should adhere to the principles of training described in Table III.1 and include both a warm-up and cool-down period. The frequency, intensity, time (duration), and type (mode) of exercise required should be designated. The FITT taxonomy is often used (Table 7.5).

Recommending an exercise prescription which is based on sound experimental evidence and is appropriate for all children and adolescents is not possible. A consensus exists concerning the type of exercise most likely to increase aerobic fitness and although terminology may vary exercise that requires rhythmic movement of the large muscle groups (e.g. running, swimming, skipping, skating, cycling) is generally recommended.[79, 1400] Nevertheless, at least two well-controlled studies have demonstrated a significant increase in peak $\dot{V}O_2$ through reciprocal, concentric resistance training using either hydraulic or isokinetic devices.[451, 1629] Other studies employing traditional isotonic weight training programmes have been less successful.[200, 999] Recommendations for frequency of exercise range from three to five times per week[1253, 1290] and suggestions for the duration of each exercise session range from 20–30 min.[1290, 1400] However, there is a need to consider children's attention span when determining the optimum length of exercise training sessions, especially when young children are involved. There is some evidence of beneficial effects on aerobic fitness from exercise sessions of short duration.[407, 840] The optimum intensity of exercise for the promotion of aerobic fitness remains to be established but it may well be towards the upper end of recommendations for adults.[1290]

Adherence to the exercise prescription described in Table 7.6 for a period of not less than 12 weeks would be likely to induce an increase in aerobic fitness in both boys and girls. An enhanced response may be achieved by maintaining an exercise intensity close to the top of the recommended range.

Table 7.6.   Exercise prescription

Frequency	3–5 times per week
Intensity	80–90% of maximal heart rate*
Time	20–30 min at the above intensity
Type	Rhythmic exercise using large muscle groups (e.g. running, cycling, swimming)

* Although there are individual variations in maximal heart rate a value of 210 bpm with children and 200 bpm with adolescents can be assumed for the design of exercise training programmes.

Summary

There is little evidence to suggest that young people have low levels of aerobic fitness and it appears that the peak $\dot{V}O_2$ of children and adolescents has remained remarkably consistent over the last 50 years. Habitual physical activity has little or no relationship with peak $\dot{V}O_2$ probably because young people rarely experience the amount of physical activity associated with the promotion of aerobic fitness.

Few studies have reported the responses of young people to carefully controlled and well-defined exercise training programmes. Studies with girls are sparse. The optimum exercise prescription for children and adolescents is yet to be designed and reliable dose–response data are not available. Nevertheless, the weight of evidence suggests that exercise training programmes of the appropriate frequency, intensity, duration, and mode of exercise will induce, in both boys and girls, increases in peak $\dot{V}O_2$ and other beneficial adaptations. The size of the changes, however, may be less than those expected with adult subjects. The hypothesis that there is a critical period of enhanced responses to exercise training remains to be proven.

Exercise training during childhood and adolescence does not induce permanent increases in aerobic fitness and once training stops its effects begin to decay. In this context it may therefore be more important to engender positive attitudes to physical activity and to encourage young people to adopt more active lifestyles than to promote exercise training programmes exclusively devoted to the improvement of aerobic fitness.[49, 51, 1415]

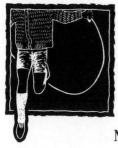

8

Physical activity and muscular strength

Muscular strength and health

This chapter will focus specifically on muscular strength, although reference will be made to the closely related health-related fitness component of muscular endurance which is also addressed in Chapter 5. The health-related benefits of muscular fitness are not as readily apparent as those of aerobic fitness but adequate muscular strength and endurance are necessary to perform a wide range of daily tasks without undue fatigue. High levels of muscular strength are advantageous in many recreational and sporting activities[197] and early maturing boys are therefore more likely to experience success in school sport than their late maturing peers.[245]

The development of appropriate muscular strength linked with adequate joint flexibility (see Chapter 14) may help to prevent muscular, joint and connective tissue injuries,[286, 705] and avoid or alleviate lower back pain in adults.[362] Resistance (strength) training is often used in the rehabilitation of musculoskeletal injuries.[1296] There is some evidence to support the view that resistance training may have beneficial effects during childhood and adolescence on blood lipids,[1630] the blood pressure of hypertensives,[670] and aerobic fitness[451, 1629] but this remains to be substantiated (see Chapters 7 and 9).

Resistance training may be an effective form of therapy in young people with neuromuscular diseases, provided they are able to perform this activity.[1576] The effectiveness of resistance training for increasing bone density in adult women has been demonstrated[333] and it has therefore been recommended to girls as a means of preventing osteoporosis in adult life.[926]

Assessment of muscular strength

To produce tension the muscle can shorten (concentric contraction), lengthen (eccentric contraction), or remain unchanged (isometric contraction) and to accomplish normal daily tasks all three types of muscular contraction occur. A fourth type of contraction, requiring a special dynamometer, is isokinetic, meaning constant velocity.[726, 1157] Both concentric and eccentric contractions may be isokinetic and isometric contractions may be considered a special case of isokinetic contraction in which the velocity

Table 8.1.   Types of muscular contraction

Concentric contractions	The muscle shortens while developing tension
Eccentric contractions	The muscle lengthens while developing tension
Isometric contractions	There is no change in muscle length while developing tension
Isokinetic contractions	The muscle shortens at constant velocity while developing tension
Isotonic contractions	The muscle develops tension against a resistance that remains constant throughout a range of motion

remains constant at zero.[1297] Normally, however, isokinetic contractions refer to constant velocity concentric and eccentric contractions. Contractions against a resistance that remains constant throughout the range of motion are known as isotonic (Table 8.1).

The assessment of adults' muscular strength is well documented and the force (peak tension) produced by each type of contraction can be measured.[1297] Research with children has focused on isometric and isokinetic contractions and field tests of muscular fitness.

Isometric contraction strength is determined using isometric dynamometers[219, 1056] or cable tensiometers.[311, 1133] Much of the available data on young people's muscular strength have been obtained using handgrip dynamometry.[198] The measurement of isokinetic contraction strength requires isokinetic dynamometers[279, 1632] and despite the high cost of these machines data on children's and adolescents' isokinetic contraction strength are accumulating.[1628] Field tests traditionally involve resisting or moving part or all of the body mass. Examples include sit-ups, flexed arm hangs, and pull-ups.[1141, 1397]

The extent to which one measure of muscular strength can be interpreted as an indicator of the strength of other types of contraction or muscle groups is unclear. Even measures of composite strength (strength scores from several different muscle groups) which are claimed to provide an assessment of overall or general muscular strength must be viewed cautiously.[198]

The assessment of young people's muscular strength can be problematic and modification of adult testing equipment is a major methodological constraint when trying to collect reliable strength data in children.[1628] Test–retest reliability of muscular strength measures with young people is not well researched but values in the range of 5–10% have been reported with both isometric[95, 198] and isokinetic[198, 1050] methods, although young children below the age of about 6 years tend to be somewhat unco-ordinated and unreliable in their efforts.[768] Reliability also appears to vary with joint complex and movement, for example, shoulder flexion movements have been observed to be less reproducible than knee flexion and extension, elbow flexion and extension, and shoulder extension movements in pre-pubertal boys.[1632]

Subject motivation does not appear to be a major problem with the assessment of children's and adolescents' muscular strength using either isometric[1133] or isokinetic contractions.[1628] Field tests of muscular fitness are, however, notorious for their reliance on motivation[41, 1348] and as they rely predominantly on muscular endurance rather than muscular strength they will not be considered further in this chapter.

Development of muscular strength

Studies of muscular strength development through childhood and adolescence have been extensively reviewed.[183, 198, 950, 967] Cross-sectional data are more abundant than longitudinal data and several studies rely on isolated muscle groups (e.g. grip strength), however, despite the nuances of testing procedures and variation in the nature of strength measures, the extant literature is remarkably consistent.

Muscular strength and chronological age

In boys, muscular strength increases linearly with chronological age from early childhood until about 13 or 14 years of age when there is a marked increase in strength through the pubertal years, followed by a slower increase into the early or mid twenties.[183, 198] Girls experience an almost linear increase in muscular strength with chronological age until about 15 years of age with no clear evidence of an adolescent spurt.[92, 957] Grip strength appears to reflect composite strength[198] and its variation with age and sex is illustrated in Fig. 8.1.

Sex-related differences in strength have been reported in children as early as 3 years of age but gender differences are small prior to puberty and there is a considerable overlap of male and female scores. The small prepubertal strength difference between boys and girls is greatly magnified during adolescence and by this time few girls outscore boys on strength measures.[541, 957] The sex-related difference is more marked in the upper extremity and in the trunk than in the lower extremity, even after adjusting for body size differences.[92] There are clear physiological reasons for the sex-associated differences in muscular strength but the contention that the augmented difference in upper extremity strength may be influenced by sociocultural factors cannot easily be dismissed.[76]

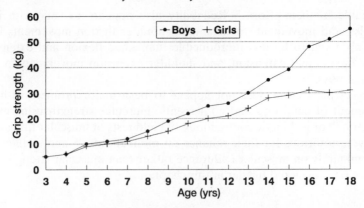

Fig. 8.1. Variations in grip strength with age and sex. Adapted from data reviewed in Blimkie, C.J.R. (1989). Age and sex associated variation in strength during childhood. In C.V. Gisolfi and D.R. Lamb (Eds.), Perspectives in Exercise Science and Sports Medicine, Vol 2, *Youth, Exercise, and Sport*. Indianapolis, IN, Benchmark Press, pp. 99–161.

Muscular strength and body size

In common with other performance measures, muscular strength is highly correlated with body size. For males aged 9–18 years, correlation co-efficients between stature and mass, and isometric strength characteristics range from $r = 0.77$ to $r = 0.93$.[198] Based upon conventional expression of strength in simple ratio with either stature or mass, grip strength increases steadily until around 13 years of age in boys. The rate of increase then accelerates during the pubertal years tapering in late adolescence.[198] In girls, a similar pattern of mass-related grip strength occurs although the growth curve is substantially flatter. The pubertal spurt in strength is also much less accentuated and values reach a plateau by the age of 15 years. Throughout the age range (7–18 years) boys are consistently stronger than girls, with absolute grip strength scores normalized for stature, the sex difference is minimal around the age of 13 years. Subsequently, boys' values accelerate rapidly whereas values in girls remain relatively static, reflecting their earlier attainment of PHV.

Concerns with the use of ratio standards to normalize data (see Chapter 3) also apply to the interpretation of strength data. Although early studies incorporated dimensional analyses into their interpretation of the growth of strength,[93, 95] few subsequent studies have investigated the applicability of alternative scaling techniques.

In boys aged 10–16 years, an average 10.1% yearly increase in composite (combined upper and lower body) mass-related strength has been observed[311] compared to a value of 18.3% when expressed relative to stature. Based upon previous work[93, 95] these authors applied dimensional theory to examine the extent to which the observed strength gains in 10–16-year-old boys could be predicted by the increase in the linear dimension (stature) alone. Their results indicated that the observed increase in composite strength across the age range was almost twice the value predicted for the changes in stature^2 (7.9% vs. 3.9%). These findings may suggest that qualitative changes in the muscular contribution to strength occur during maturation or may simply reflect the disproportionate increases in muscle cross-sectional area relative to stature^2 observed during male adolescence.[128] Alternatively, it has been suggested that neural maturation enables a more co-ordinated recruitment of muscle fibres.[93, 311]

A recent study[1249] examined longitudinal changes in the isometric strength of the knee extensors and elbow flexors in 8–13-year-old boys and girls using multilevel modelling (see Chapter 3). The results showed that knee extensor strength in girls increased in proportion to the increase in stature and mass over this age range. In contrast, in boys, the increase in the strength of these muscles was disproportionately larger than the increase in body size but was explained when testosterone was incorporated into the analysis. Hormonal differences could not, however, explain the observed sex difference in elbow flexor strength, suggesting that other factors influence the strength of these muscles during the adolescent period.

Although the data were generated from late adolescents and young adults, the study by Vanderburgh *et al.*[1564] using allometric modelling to examine sex-related differences in grip strength merits attention. Measured absolute grip strength was 64% higher in the males than the females and this difference reduced to 22% when values were expressed relative to body mass. With data scaled allometrically a common *b* exponent of 0.51 was derived and, with body mass partitioned out in this way, the sex difference increased to 42%.

Muscular strength and muscle

The maximal force that can be generated by an adult skeletal muscle is primarily a function of muscle size. Growth of muscle tissue during childhood and adolescence is characterized by constancy in number of fibres, an increase in fibre size and number of nuclei, and an increase in overall muscle mass.[967] There is no precise method of measuring total muscle mass in a living person and the amount of creatinine excreted in the urine is normally used as an indirect indicator of total muscle mass in the body. According to creatinine excretion rates muscle mass increases in boys from about 42–54% of body mass over the age range 5–17 years.[949, 967] Girls' muscle mass increases from about 40–45% of body mass between 5 and 13 years and then declines in relation to body mass due to fat accumulation during adolescence.[949, 967] At all ages beyond 7 years males have a larger

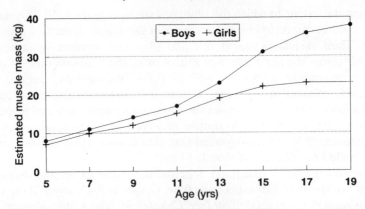

Fig. 8.2. Variation in muscle mass with age and sex. Adapted from data reviewed in Malina, R.M. and Bouchard, C. (1991). *Growth, Maturation, and Physical Activity*. Champaign, IL, Human Kinetics, pp. 115–32.

absolute and relative (to body mass) amount of muscle compared to females. Both boys and girls experience peak gains in muscle strength after peak gains in muscle cross-sectional area although there are individual variations.[311, 541, 1466] The pubertal spurt in muscle mass is substantially greater in boys. As muscle strength is highly dependent upon muscle size the gender differences in the development of muscle mass may account for much of the observed age- and sex-related differences in muscle strength although factors other than muscle size also contribute.[950] (Figure 8.2.)

Ethical constraints limit our understanding of young people's muscle structure and function. Few experimenters have been willing to use the needle biopsy technique for muscle sampling with children and there is therefore a paucity of data on muscle fibre type differentiation, distribution, and size during childhood and adolescence. Muscle fibre size (diameter) increases with age and although there are no obvious sex-related differences until about 16 years of age fibre areas increase into the mid twenties in males.[9, 344, 957] The percentage distribution of type II fibres increases during childhood and adolescence to reach adult levels during late adolescence.[165, 344, 562] There is, however, no reliable evidence of the influence of muscle fibre diameter or fibre type distribution on young people's muscular strength, although the recent development of magnetic resonance imaging (MRI) techniques of estimating fibre type distribution open up intriguing avenues of research.[735]

Some data are available on measurements of contraction time (elapsed time from the onset of force deflection following an electrical stimulation

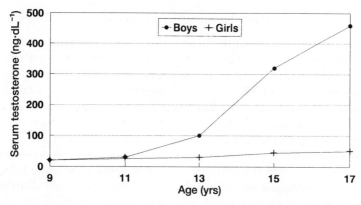

Fig. 8.3. Variation in serum testosterone with age and sex. Adapted from data reviewed in Sale, D.G. (1989). Strength training in children. In C.V. Gisolfi and D.R. Lamb (Eds.), Perspectives in Exercise Science and Sports Medicine, Vol 2, *Youth, Exercise, and Sport*. Indianapolis, IN, Benchmark Press, pp. 165–216.

to attainment of peak force) and half-relaxation time (elapsed time from peak force to half the peak force during recovery) during evoked isometric contractions.[400, 609, 610, 992] It appears that for the muscles studied there is little change in contraction time from childhood through adolescence into adulthood for males, whereas for females contraction time increases with advancing age. Half-relaxation time shortens slightly during childhood, with no further change during adolescence in girls, but decreases progressively in males from early childhood through to adult life.

Neuroendocrine factors may influence the relationship between muscle and muscular strength during growth and maturation. During childhood, circulating levels of testosterone are not significantly different between the sexes but, in comparison to girls, there is a dramatic increase in serum testosterone concentration in boys during adolescence.[1675] However, although muscle growth is clearly influenced by hormonal regulation[555, 556] well-controlled paediatric studies of concomitant changes in sex steroids, muscle size, and muscular strength are currently not available and any causal relationship remains to be determined. Nevertheless, comparison of Figs 8.1, 8.2, and 8.3 reveal that causal relationships are an intuitively appealing hypothesis.

The ability to activate motor units is fundamental to the expression of muscular strength. Little information is available on young people and whether there is a sex-associated variation in motor unit activation is unknown. It has been suggested that the ability to activate voluntarily muscle during isometric effort may vary across muscle groups[198] but this requires further substantiation.

Muscular strength and genetics

The few available studies of the heritability of muscular strength are difficult to interpret and they have produced widely different results for the same muscle groups as well as for different muscles.[956] Moderate degrees of heritability of composite isometric strength have been reported.[227, 505] Some studies have suggested a low to moderate amount of heritability for selected isometric strength measures whereas other studies have observed little or no significant genetic effect for the expression of isometric strength.[227]

If muscular strength is inheritable the effect could be mediated through the genetic determination of muscle fibre composition and distribution within a muscle. High heritability estimates for percentage of type I fibre distribution in the vastus lateralis have been recorded[844] but a more recent and comprehensive study reported no significant genetic effect for either the distribution of muscle fibre types or for muscle fibre areas for the vastus lateralis in either sex.[230]

Studies of a genetic influence on muscular strength have produced equivocal findings and although there are some indications of strength heritability the case remains to be proven.

Exercise (resistance) training and muscular strength

The factors affecting the interpretation of exercise training studies identified in Chapter 7 also apply to resistance training programmes and little credence can be given to studies which do not attempt to control for young people's growth and maturation.

It is well documented that adolescents can achieve significant increases in muscular strength through isometric, isotonic, or isokinetic resistance training programmes[199, 200, 1029, 1035, 1296, 1606, 1628] although girls may experience a less dramatic response to that seen in boys.[197] However, there is a popular view that resistance training programmes are ineffective with prepubescent children. A study by Vrijens[1586] has been widely cited to support this contention.

Vrijens[1586] trained 16 prepubescent boys (mean age 10.4 years) and 12 adolescent boys (mean age 16.7 years) three times per week for 8 weeks. The boys performed isotonic exercises involving the arms, legs, back, and abdomen, and the isometric contraction strength of arm flexors and extensors, leg extensors and flexors, and abdominal and back muscles was tested before and after the training programme. Muscular development was studied by soft-tissue radiology. Vrijens[1586] observed an increase in strength in all tested muscle groups in the adolescent group but no consistent pattern of strength improvement in the prepubescent group. Abdominal and back strength increased proportionally more in the prepubescent boys than in the adolescents but no significant increases in arm or leg strength were noted in the prepubescent group. The mean cross-sectional area of muscles in the arm and thigh remained unchanged in the prepubescent boys whereas a significant increase of muscle mass in both arm and thigh was observed in the adolescent group. Vrijens[1586] concluded that,

In childhood the absolute strength of the extremities is not changed by specific exercises. The absolute trunk muscle strength of prepubescent boys surprisingly increased significantly by strength training.[1586, p. 156]

However, Vrijens'[1586] study had several flaws. No control groups were included in the design, the exercise itself may not have been sufficient to induce strength changes in prepubescent boys, and although the subjects trained isotonically they were tested using isometric muscular contractions. Subsequent better controlled resistance training studies with prepubescents have clearly demonstrated that appropriate training programmes can induce increases in muscular strength during childhood.[199] Studies which have failed to induce strength increases with prepubescents have used low training loads,[1586] failed to provide progressive resistance loading as strength improved,[1391] or were of short duration.[452]

Blimkie[199] has suggested that the effectiveness of strength training seems to be more dependent on the intensity of loading than on either training duration or mode. Strength increases have been reported in as few as 3–6 weeks of high-intensity isotonic,[1125] maximal isokinetic[692] and maximal isometric[1030] training. When training intensity and volume are high significant improvements in muscular strength can be achieved with as few as two isotonic,[531] three isometric,[1105] and three isokinetic[1629] training sessions per week. Table 8.2 describes well-controlled studies which have involved prepubescent subjects, employed a control group, and used a training programme of at least three sessions per week for 9 weeks.

The most comprehensive study to date of prepubescents' responses to resistance training involved progressive isotonic resistance training for three sessions per week for 20 weeks.[1194] Emphasis was placed on overloading the elbow flexor and knee extensor muscle groups. Criterion tests included training mode-specific tests and non-specific isometric and isokinetic tests. The effects of learning were controlled by performing interim testing[204] and measures of muscle strength which were independent of learning (evoked twitch responses). The training mode-specific test was the one repetition maximum (1 RM), the maximal load that a muscle group can move through a range of motion. Significant improvements in 1 RM bench press, 1 RM arm curl, and maximal voluntary isometric elbow flexion strength were observed after 10 weeks of training.[204] By the end of the study significant increases were reported in 1 RM double leg press (22%), 1 RM bench press (35%), maximal voluntary isometric knee extension (25%), and elbow

Table 8.2.   Resistance training studies with children

Study	Subjects' age (yrs)	Sex	Training programme		Strength increase
			Type	Duration (wks)	
Blimkie et al.[205]	9–11*	M	Isotonic	10	Yes
Ramsay et al.[1194]	9–11*	M	Isotonic	20	Yes
Fukunaga et al.[592]	9.2	M & F	Isometric	12	Yes
Sewall & Micheli[1367]	10–11*	M & F	Isotonic & accommodating resistance	9	Yes
Pfeiffer & Francis[1166]	10.3*	M	Isotonic	9	Yes
Rians et al.[1203]	8.3*	M	Isotonic	14	Yes
Weltman et al.[1629]	8.2*	M	Concentric accommodating resistance	14	Yes

* Classified as prepubescent by authors.

flexion (37%) strength, and maximal voluntary isokinetic knee extension (21%), and elbow flexion (26%) strength.[1194] These results unequivocally demonstrate that progressive resistance training can increase the muscular strength of prepubescents.

Results from early European studies which observed at least some improvement in prepubescents' strength through training indicated that they were less susceptible to improvement than adolescents or adult subjects.[712, 823] More recent findings, from generally better controlled studies, have challenged this view in both girls[1105, 1636] and boys.[1167, 1293, 1296] However, it is difficult to make a fair comparison between strength gains made by prepubescents, adolescents, and adults. Older subjects tend to demonstrate more significant changes in absolute strength but prepubescents demonstrate similar relative strength gains compared to adolescents and adults in response to similar resistance training programmes. More research is required before the question of relative trainability of children and adolescents is resolved but it is readily apparent that children can benefit from an appropriate resistance training programme.

Adaptations to resistance training

As the expression of muscular strength is a function of the cross-sectional area and specific tension (force per unit cross-sectional area) of the involved muscles and the ability of the central nervous system to fully activate the muscles, it follows that increases in muscular strength after resistance training could be due to a combination of neural and muscular adaptations.[1296] In adults, it appears that neural adaptation predominates in the early stages of resistance training and then after several weeks muscle hypertrophy occurs. With long-term resistance training programmes muscular adaptation predominates and further strength development is dependent upon muscle hypertrophy.[843, 1085, 1295]

Increases in muscle size with resistance training in adolescents are well documented[411, 867, 1586] but there is little evidence to suggest resistance training-induced muscle hypertrophy during prepubescence even in studies that reported significant increases in muscular strength.[204, 692, 1125, 1293, 1391, 1629] The lack of muscle hypertrophy in most studies can be partially explained by short duration training programmes and imprecise measures of muscle size. However, a recent study using computerized axial tomography (CAT) also failed to demonstrate a significant increase in muscle size following 20 weeks of resistance training, despite significant and substantial increases in muscular strength.[1194]

The only study to seriously challenge the assertion that resistance training during prepubescence induces increases in muscular strength without significant changes in muscle size is Mersch and Stoboy's[1030] report on the effects of 10 weeks of maximal isometric knee extension training on one boy from each of two pairs of monozygotic twins. The other twin acted as control. Magnetic resonance imaging revealed a 4–9% increase in quadriceps cross-section complemented with a 38% increase in isometric knee extension strength in the trained boys. These results leave open the possibility of muscle hypertrophy through resistance training in prepubescents, but the weight of evidence suggest that strength gains are largely independent of changes in muscle size with prepubescent children.

Several authors have attributed muscular strength gains in prepubescent children to neurological adaptations[591, 692, 1629] but only two studies have effectively addressed the problem.[204, 1125, 1194] One study reported a significant 16.8% increase in integrated electromyographic amplitude during maximal isokinetic elbow flexion, and a corresponding increase of 27.8% in maximal isokinetic strength following an 8 week resistance training programme.[1125]

Ramsay and her colleagues[1194] used the twitch interpolation technique[163] to assess the contribution of changes in motor unit activation to training-induced strength increases in 13 prepubertal boys. Following a 10 week resistance training programme motor unit activation of the elbow flexors and knee extensors increased by 9% and 12%, respectively.[204] A further 10 weeks of training resulted in additional increases of only 3% and 2%, respectively.[1194] The changes in motor unit activation were, however, much less than the changes in muscular strength. Maximal voluntary isometric strength increased by 40% for the elbow flexors and 25% for the knee extensors over the 20 week training period. Ramsay *et al.*[1194] concluded that the observed increases in muscular strength could be attributed only partially to an increase in motor unit activation. They noted an increase in evoked twitch torque (a measure of intrinsic muscle strength) and suggested that intrinsic muscular adaptations may also contribute to resistance training-induced strength increases during prepubescence. It is likely, however, that improved motor co-ordination (learning) also plays an important role in strength gains following training during childhood.[199, 200]

Adaptations to de-training

As described in Chapter 7 it is difficult to determine the effects of a period of de-training on children and adolescents because of their continued growth and maturation during the de-training period. Nevertheless, the limited evidence available suggests that training-induced strength gains will not persist through a period of de-training.[203, 1367] De-training in adults results in a relatively rapid reduction in neuromuscular activation and a more gradual and smaller reduction in muscle size.[1085] As resistance training has a less dramatic effect on muscle size, especially with children, the reduction in training-induced strength gains with young people is attributable predominantly to changes in the level of neuromuscular activation and motor co-ordination.

It has been demonstrated that, with 9–11-year-old boys, a maintenance programme consisting of 8 weeks of once per week high-intensity weight training is not sufficient to conserve strength gains achieved after 20 weeks of training three times per week.[203] It appears that long-term benefits of resistance training depend upon the maintenance of the programme into adult life.

Risks of resistance training

The American Academy of Pediatrics[19] recommends that children and adolescents should avoid the practice of weight lifting, power lifting, and body building, as well as the repetitive use of maximal amounts of weight during strength training programmes, until they have reached Tanner stage 5 of sexual maturity. There are numerous reports of injuries sustained during power lifting[238, 258] and anabolic steroid misuse has been reported in strength-reliant sports.[271, 1518] In the present context, however, we are concerned with appropriate resistance training for children and adolescents and not with the sports of weight lifting and power lifting, or other competitive sports in which strength training may be advantageous.

Reports of epiphyseal fractures resulting from weight training during childhood and adolescence are common[169, 663, 1252, 1285] but in most cases they have been attributed to improper lifting technique, excessive loading, or the performance of ballistic movements that result in high sheer forces and a greater potential for fracture.[200, 1034, 1035] Micheli[1035] has claimed that acute growth plate injuries are actually rare in adolescents and even less likely in prepubescents as the growth plate is much stronger and more resistant to sheer stress in children than in adolescents. Blimkie[200] has commented that, as in prospective resistance training studies with young people there have been no reported incidences of epiphyseal fractures, the concern over potential epiphyseal fractures during supervised resistance training may be overstated.

Resistance training is associated with a risk of injury due to repetitive microtrauma to musculoskeletal structures.[238, 258] Soft tissue injury appears to be the most prevalent, and the lower back seems the most susceptible site.[200] Nevertheless, there is little evidence to suggest that closely supervised resistance training is more likely to induce musculoskeletal injury than participation in many popular sports.[679, 1034, 1203, 1468]

Cardiovascular responses to resistance exercise are well documented in adults[554, 1163] and concern exists over the possibility of syncope (blackout) following changes in blood pressure during and after resistance exercise. Rare cases of blackout during weight lifting have been reported in adults[1200] but not in children or adolescents.[200] Data on young people's blood pressure responses to resistance exercise are sparse[138, 1089, 1481] but it appears that both systolic and diastolic blood pressure responses to resistance exercise are comparable to those reported in studies of adult subjects performing similar lifts. The effects (if any) of long-term resistance training on children's and adolescents' cardiac dimensions and function are unknown.[200]

Exercise prescription

Adults working with children and adolescents must stress the importance of taking sensible precautions before, during, and after exercise sessions. When external resistances, as in weight training, are used adult supervisors carry additional responsibility when working with young people and close supervision and monitoring are required. Supervisors should be suitably qualified and cognizant of all relevant safety regulations. All young participants should be taught proper lifting and appropriate breathing techniques and emphasis should be placed upon the safety and well-being of the young people involved in the training programme.[577, 847, 1606]

Resistance training programmes should be introduced sensitively and neither adult programmes nor unmodified adult equipment should be imposed on children. Ideally, individualized programmes should be developed and the young person actively involved in the exercise prescription process.[847, 1606] Each session should include a warm-up and cool-down phase incorporating a series of stretching exercises (see Chapter 14).

Effective resistance training programmes can be designed around isometric, isotonic, or isokinetic contractions. They should adhere to the principles of training (Table III.1) and appropriate overload and rate of progression should be carefully considered. Maximal or near maximal repetitions should be avoided with children[1088, 1538] and training should be advanced with small increments with respect to both the amount of resistance used and the motor skills required.[1606] Training programmes should include exercises for all major muscle groups, and there should be a good balance between exercises for agonist and antagonist muscle groups.[847, 1606] It is usual to exercise large muscle groups first and then to progress to smaller ones.[79, 847]

To illustrate guidelines to be followed in the development of an appropriate resistance training programme we will focus upon weight training (isotonic contractions) and the concept of a repetition maximum (RM). RM is the maximal load that a muscle group can lift over a given number of repetitions before fatiguing. Recommendations for an appropriate overload for young people vary (e.g. 7–11 RM,[1035] 6–15 RM,[465, 1088] 8–12 RM,[1428] 12–15 RM[1538]) but there is a general consensus that not more than a 6 RM load should be used. Sale[1296] suggested 8–12 RM for use in upper limb exercises and 15–20 RM for use in lower limb exercises. The greater number of repetitions in lower limb exercises was recommended because more repetitions can be executed with a given percentage of the 1 RM. We concur with Sale's[1296] recommendations for both children and adolescents and in addition to increases in muscular strength this protocol should also enhance muscular endurance.

Initially, young people will need to determine, for upper limb exercise, their 8 RM load by trial and error and then implement the training programme. As training progresses the overload will be increased first by increasing the number of repetitions until, in this case, 12 repetitions are achieved. At this point a new 8 RM load will need to be determined and the process repeated over time (progressive overload).

Progressive overload can also be increased through the volume of exercise. The young subject should begin with a single set of approximately 6–10 different exercises and gradually progress to 3 sets in a workout which

Table 8.3. Resistance exercise prescription

Frequency	2–3 times per week
Intensity	8–12 RM per set for upper limb exercises
	15–20 RM per set for lower limb exercises
Time	30–60 min (1–3 sets)
Type	Weight training

From recommendations in Sale, D.G. (1989). Strength training in children. In C.V. Gisolfi and D.R. Lamb (Eds.), Perspectives in Exercise Science and Sports Medicine, Vol 2, *Youth, Exercise, and Sport*, Indianapolis, IN, Benchmark Press, pp. 165–216, and Kraemer, W.J., Fry, A.C., Frykman, P.N., Conroy, B. and Hoffman, J. (1989). Resistance training and youth. *Pediatric Exercise Science*, **1**, 336–50.

should last perhaps 40 min.[847, 1296] There should be at least 1 day of rest between each workout and a minimum training period of 8–12 weeks should be programmed. Our recommended programme is outlined in Table 8.3.

A well-structured, progressive resistance training programme can be recommended for enhancing both children's and adolescents' muscular strength but muscular fitness is only one component of health-related fitness and other components, particularly aerobic fitness, should not be ignored. In our view, young people should be encouraged to engage in a wide range of physical activities throughout childhood and adolescence as early specialization in one aspect of health-related physical activity is unlikely to promote a lifetime commitment to a balanced programme of physical activities.

Summary

The assessment of young people's muscular strength can be problematic but despite the nuances of testing procedures the data are consistent. Both boys and girls experience an increase in muscular strength with increases in chronological age, body size, and muscle mass. Sex-related differences in strength have been reported as early as three years of age but gender differences are relatively small prior to puberty. Boys experience a significant increase in strength through the pubertal years and the small prepubertal strength difference between boys and girls is much more pronounced during adolescence. Ethical considerations restrict our understanding of young people's muscle structure and function but increases with growth and maturation of muscle size and, in boys, serum testosterone concentration reflect changes in muscular strength.

Resistance training with young people must be closely supervised and carried out cautiously but a well-designed programme will induce increases in the muscular strength of both children and adolescents, although girls may experience a less dramatic response to that seen in boys. Children are less likely to demonstrate muscle hypertrophy than adolescents. Training-induced strength gains will not persist through a period of de-training and long-term benefits depend upon the maintenance of a resistance training programme into adult life.

Appropriate resistance training can be recommended for young people but they should be encouraged to participate in a variety of other sports and active recreations and not exclusively focus upon enhancing muscular strength.

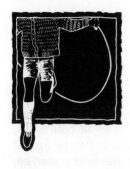

9
Physical activity and coronary artery disease

Coronary heart disease

Despite recent evidence of a decline, coronary heart disease (CHD) remains the leading cause of death in most Western countries, accounting for 26% of deaths in England and 23% in the United States.[417, 1666] In England, CHD is responsible for 2.5% of total National Health Service expenditure and results in 35 million lost working days per year.[417] In the United States, the cost of CHD is estimated at $50 billion per annum.[570, 1602]

Atherosclerosis refers to the progressive build-up of fibrotic, lipid-filled plaques in the walls of the arteries. Atherosclerotic CHD involves the development of plaques in the coronary arteries leading to a reduced blood flow to the myocardium. The effect on the heart depends on the degree of ischaemia. If blood flow is reduced and insufficient to satisfy the myocardial oxygen demand it results in angina. A poorly perfused myocardium is also prone to arrhythmias. If blood flow is totally cut off the portion of the myocardium fed by the occluded artery will suffer major damage: a heart attack. In general, the severity of the heart attack depends on the amount of tissue destroyed.

Paediatric origins of coronary artery disease

The clinical manifestations of atherosclerotic CHD normally occur in adult life but there is evidence that the origins lie in childhood.[25, 368, 395, 1686] Saltykov,[1318] in his study of the degenerative changes of the aorta, first called attention to the paediatric origin of atherosclerosis when he stated,

the so-called fatty changes in the arteries of childhood and youth, especially in the aorta, are nothing less than the beginning of atherosclerosis.[1583, p. 812]

Many investigators have since described these lesions and documented their presence in childhood.[731, 1583, 1712]

One of the earliest recognizable lesions is the fatty streak. Fatty streaks are lipid-containing intimal lesions with no significant underlying vascular changes. They are flat or only slightly elevated and do not significantly narrow the lumen of the artery. Fatty streaks are clinically harmless and potentially reversible, whereas the progression of fatty streaks to fibrous, calcified, and complicated plaques may be the critical event in atherosclerosis.[1478]

Holman *et al*.'s[731] autopsy studies documented the presence of fatty streaks in the aortas of many children less than three years of age. The paediatric aspects of coronary and aortic lesions were further investigated by Strong and McGill[1477] who used a subsample of autopsy results from the International Atherosclerosis Project.[996] Autopsies of 4737 cases of both sexes, aged 10–39 years from six location groups were studied. By the age of 10 years, fatty streaks were present in almost all of the aortas studied. Coronary artery fatty streaks were less common than aortic fatty streaks but they were found even in the 10–14-year-old age group.[1511] In the sample located in New Orleans fatty streaks were present in the coronary arteries of all persons over 20 years of age.[1477]

Fibrous plaques are firm, elevated lesions with a potential for narrowing the arterial lumen and causing the complications of progressive atherosclerotic CHD. Whether fatty streaks advance to fibrous plaques is controversial and may depend upon the location and type of fatty streak under consideration.[572] Examination of the aorta has often led to the conclusion that fatty streaks do not progress into fibrous plaques but histological studies have clearly indicated that coronary artery fatty streaks can progress to fibrous plaques and more advanced lesions.[611, 1454, 1455]

Fatty streaks have been observed in the same sites of the arterial wall as are fibrous plaques later in life[1051] and transitional lesions having the gross and microscopic characteristics of both fatty streaks and fibrous plaques are relatively common in the coronary arteries of young adult males.[997] McGill[998] comprehensively reviewed the available evidence and concluded that,

in a highly vulnerable site in the coronary arteries, we can trace the evolution of clusters of monocyte and macrophage foam cells at about age 20.[998, pp. 445-6]

and, in his Duff Memorial lecture, he asserted that,

I believe that we can say with certainty that coronary atherosclerosis has its origins in childhood, at least by age 10 and possibly earlier.[998, p. 450]

Further support for the hypothesis that coronary atherosclerosis begins early in life was provided by autopsy studies of United States soldiers killed in Korea[506, 507] and in Vietnam.[1018] These studies confirmed the presence of severe occlusive lesions in late adolescence and early adulthood. Lesions involving one or more of the coronary arteries were identified in 77% of 300 soldiers, mean age 22 years, killed in action in Korea. In 12%, the occlusion was 50% or more of the arterial lumen. In the Vietnam series, using more stringent criteria, 45% of 105 fatal casualties of a similar age were shown to exhibit atherosclerotic lesions. These findings substantiate the

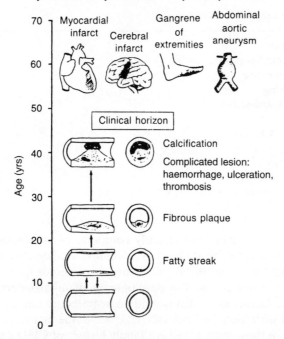

Fig. 9.1. The natural history of the atherosclerotic process. From McGill, H.L., Geer, J.C. and Strong, J.P. Natural history of human atherosclerotic lesions. In M. Sandler and G.H. Bourne (Eds.), *Atherosclerosis and Its Origins*. New York, Academic Press, p. 42. Reprinted with permission.

view that the process leading to coronary atherosclerosis has its origins in childhood and adolescence. (Figure 9.1)

Coronary risk factors

A risk factor is an identifiable characteristic which, when present, is associated with a higher than expected incidence of a disease. Coronary risk factors may therefore be defined as,

those abnormalities demonstrable in persons free of clinical coronary heart disease and known to be associated with significantly increased risk of developing the disease in subsequent years.[1452, p. 230]

The concept of coronary risk factors evolved from prospective epidemiological studies relating personal characteristics of participants to subsequent incidence of CHD.[780, 816] Risk factors are based on associations, therefore they may be directly causative, secondary manifestations of more

Table 9.1.   Coronary risk factors

Major risk factors
Adverse lipid and lipoprotein profile
Raised blood pressure
Cigarette smoking
Inadequate physical activity

Contributory risk factors
Obesity
Diabetes mellitus
Some psychological traits

---

basic underlying abnormalities or early symptoms of the disease.[778] Nevertheless, several prospective studies have demonstrated definite associations between certain environmental, biochemical, physiological, genetic, and pathological conditions and the development of atherosclerosis.[779, 815, 1451] Some of these factors have also been demonstrated, in autopsy studies, to be associated with increased risk of CHD.[731, 996] Some factors are fixed; the risk is higher in those with a positive family history of CHD and mortality from CHD is higher in men than in women. Other factors can be altered through changes in behaviour (see Table 9.1).

Extrapolation of the risk factor concept to children may be speculative but there is a growing conviction that the identification of adult coronary risk factors at an early age may identify some potential coronary candidates in childhood.[66, 171, 782, 883, 1479, 1602] Fundamental to the concept of coronary risk factors in children is the phenomenon of 'tracking' or examining trends over time. Several longitudinal investigations have addressed the incidence of risk factors in children[170, 171, 886, 1119] and they have demonstrated that initial levels of risk factors are predictive of follow-up levels over four,[880] five,[1607, 1608] six,[339, 1192] and even 10–12 years later.[119, 884, 1609] Furthermore, studies in Bogalusa, Louisiana have documented the importance of risk factor levels in childhood to early anatomical changes in both the aorta and the coronary arteries[572, 1110] and these studies lend strong support to the concept that atherosclerotic CHD begins in childhood.

The relationship between most risk factor levels and coronary atherosclerosis is continuous, linear, or curvilinear, and there is no evidence to support the view that threshold levels of risk factors are biologically plausible. The assignment of practical cut-off points at which continuous variables are to be considered risk factors does, however, facilitate the identification of coronary-prone individuals.[527] This concept has been extended to young people on many occasions[59, 220, 617, 1667, 1668, 1691] but it is difficult to compare directly studies due to the range of subject age, the

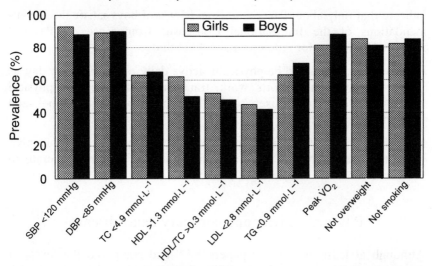

Fig. 9.2. Prevalence of health indicators for cardiovascular disease in young people aged 11–16 years. DBP, diastolic blood pressure; SBP, systolic blood pressure. Peak $\dot{V}O_2$ criteria: boys >40 mL·kg⁻¹·min⁻¹; girls >35 mL·kg⁻¹·min⁻¹. Figure drawn from data reported by Armstrong, N. *et al.* (1990–94).[59, 85, 612]

variety of proposed threshold levels, methodology, data analysis, and sample size.

The American Health Foundation (AHF)[1691] proposed thresholds for coronary risk in children of 4.65 mmol·L⁻¹ serum cholesterol, 130 mmHg for systolic blood pressure, and 85 mmHg for diastolic blood pressure. Application of these thresholds to young people (aged 11–16 years) examined in our laboratories[59] reveals 47.5% of the girls and 41.3% of the boys exceeding the AHF serum cholesterol threshold and 6.9% of girls and 8.5% of the boys exceeding at least one of the blood pressure thresholds.

Members of the European Pediatric Work Physiology Group[164] have proposed both 'health and risk indicators for cardiovascular disease in children'. Figure 9.2 illustrates data collected in our laboratory[59, 85] in relation to the proposed health indicators. As the assessment of young people's body fatness is problematic (see Chapter 10) we have chosen to use the Royal College of Physicians'[1275] criterion of 'overweight'.

Although the majority of children and adolescents exceed the cardiovascular health thresholds significant numbers of young people do not, and adverse lipid and lipoprotein profiles appear to be quite common. As peak $\dot{V}O_2$ is only weakly related to habitual physical activity (see Chapter 7) its use as a surrogate for activity is problematic. Data on the same subjects[57] indicate that only about 0.6% of girls and 3.9% of boys satisfy the recommendations of the International Consensus Conference on Physical Activity Guidelines for Adolescents[1309, pp. 307–8] that:

- All adolescents should be physically active daily, or nearly every day, as part of play, games, sports, work, transportation, recreation, physical education, or planned exercise, in the context of family, school, and community activities.

- Adolescents should engage in three or more sessions per week of activities that last 20 min or more at a time and that require moderate to vigorous levels of exertion.

Physical activity and coronary heart disease

Although at least two earlier papers[1152, 1287] had compared the levels of energy expenditure of workers in different jobs with their cardiac health Morris and his co-workers[1069] were the first group to attract serious attention to the hypothesis that physical activity may be inversely related to CHD. Morris' group[1069] studied CHD in 31 000 London Transport workers, comparing the drivers with the more active conductors on double-decker buses. They reported that the conductors had 50% fewer heart attacks (both fatal and non-fatal) when compared with the drivers. The findings of the study were, however, subsequently criticized on the basis of self-selection of occupation and further weakened by Morris' own analysis,[1068] which confirmed that the conductors were more lightly built than the drivers and that this difference was present from the time of taking up employment with London Transport. Nevertheless, Morris' pioneering work stimulated numerous epidemiological investigations into the effects of physical activity on CHD.

Subsequent studies which provide sufficient data to calculate a relative risk or odds ratio for CHD at different levels of physical activity have been comprehensively reviewed by Powell *et al.*[1177] who concluded that,

The inverse association between physical activity and incidence of CHD is consistently observed, especially in the better designed studies; this association is appropriately sequenced, biologically graded, plausible, and coherent with existing knowledge. Therefore, the observations reported in the literature support the inference that physical activity is inversely and causally related to the incidence of CHD.[1177, p. 283]

More recent meta-analyses have reinforced Powell *et al.*'s[1177] conclusions and confirmed that there is a cause-and-effect relation between physical activity and CHD.[181, 486] Potential mechanisms by which physical activity may reduce the incidence of CHD are illustrated in Table 9.2

Table 9.2. How physical activity may reduce the incidence of coronary heart disease in adult life

---

- Improves blood lipid and lipoprotein profile

- Reduces arterial blood pressure

- Reduces cigarette smoking

- Decreases adiposity

- Increases psychological well-being

- Retards atherosclerosis

- Lowers circulating catecholamines

- Decreases platelet adhesiveness

- Increases fibrinolysis

- Increases plasma volume

- Increases coronary artery diameter

- Increases coronary collateral vascularization

- Improves aerobic fitness

Several of these mechanisms are speculative and some beneficial adaptations have yet to be demonstrated convincingly in human subjects.[234, 343, 1151, 1405] Similarly, the appropriate volume (intensity, duration, and frequency) of physical activity for heart health benefits has yet to be established. Current research suggests that adults should engage in a minimum of 15–20 min physical activity, of at least brisk walking intensity (7.5 kJ·min^{-1}), three times a week as a contribution towards the prevention of CHD.[6, 24, 702]

The following sections review the effects of physical activity on blood lipids, blood pressure, and cigarette smoking during childhood and adolescence. Subsequent chapters address the relationship between physical activity and body fatness, diabetes mellitus, and psychological well-being. The effects of exercise training on aerobic fitness are examined in Chapter 7.

Blood lipids

Initial concern about total blood cholesterol as a coronary risk factor has generated major advances in the understanding of the metabolism, transport, and regulation of lipids. It is now generally accepted that lipoproteins and apolipoproteins fill important roles in the association between blood lipids and coronary artery disease.

Composition of blood lipoproteins

Chylomicrons circulate freely in plasma but other lipids form complexes with proteins (apolipoproteins) and are carried in macromolecular complexes called lipoproteins. Lipoproteins may be classified according to their size, floating densities in an ultracentrifugal field, electrophoretic mobilities, or protein composition. Current practice is to classify by density and, in general, the larger the lipoprotein particle, the greater its lipid content and the lower its density (see Table 9.3). Chylomicrons, which are predominantly triglyceride, are the largest and least dense. The next largest is the very low-density lipoprotein (VLDL) whose principal lipid is also triglyceride. The primary carrier of cholesterol is the low-density lipoprotein (LDL), which transports about one-half to two-thirds of the cholesterol in the blood. The smallest of the lipoproteins is high-density lipoprotein (HDL) which is about one-half lipid and one-half protein by weight, and together with LDL, contributes to the blood cholesterol level. The HDL family can be divided into several subfractions of which the two most extensively studied are the lighter, lipid-rich HDL_2 and the heavier, lipid-poor HDL_3. Other lipoprotein subfractions, such as intermediate-density lipoprotein and lipoprotein (a), exist and comprehensive analyses are available elsewhere.[97, 1382, 1498]

Table 9.3. Lipoprotein composition

Lipoprotein	Source	Density (g·mL⁻¹)	Protein (%)	Lipid (%)
Chylomicrons	Intestine	<0.96	1–2	98–99
VLDL	Liver and intestine	0.96–1.006	7–10	90–93
LDL	VLDL and chylomicron	1.019–1.063	21	79
HDL_2	Intestine and liver	1.063–1.125	33	67
HDL_3	Intestine and liver	1.125–1.210	57	43

Lipids have several important biological functions. Cholesterol is used in the synthesis of steroid hormones and as a component, in conjunction with phospholipids, of cell membranes. Triglycerides are stored as fat in adipose tissue and used for energy production. It is, however, the apolipoprotein portion of the particle that regulates the interaction of the lipoprotein complexes with tissue receptors and lipolytic enzymes. Specific apolipoproteins are associated with certain lipids. Apolipoprotein A-1 is primarily associated with HDL and is distributed among both HDL_2 and HDL_3 subfractions. Apolipoprotein A-11 is also mainly found with HDL, predominantly HDL_3, whereas apolipoprotein B makes up over 90% of the apolipoprotein content of LDL. Durstine and Haskell[478] provide a detailed description of apolipoproteins and their functions.

Blood lipids and coronary heart disease

Many patients with CHD have high levels of blood triglyceride, but the role of blood triglycerides in CHD remains a controversial issue.[527, 643] Increased triglyceride levels are inversely related to HDL concentration,[398] and a graded and direct relationship between blood triglycerides and the development of CHD, independent of blood cholesterol, has been noted.[309] The severity of CHD has been positively correlated with blood triglyceride levels[246] but several population studies have not found blood triglyceride to be an independent risk factor for CHD.[743, 780, 1682] The Study Group of the European Atherosclerosis Society[527, p.82] concluded that,

elevated triglyceride has yet to be shown to be a cause of atherosclerosis [although], there is reason to suspect that among the triglyceride-rich lipoproteins certain subclass [remnant particles] play a causal role in atherogenesis.

The evidence incriminating the blood total cholesterol in the evolution of CHD is extensive and unequivocal.[636, 779, 1451] In adults, cholesterol levels rising above 4.7 $mmol \cdot L^{-1}$ demonstrate a direct and graded risk for development of CHD[1452] and a cholesterol level of 5.7 $mmol \cdot L^{-1}$ represents a twofold increase in the incidence of CHD when compared with a level of 4.7 $mmol \cdot L^{-1}$.[780] The atherogenicity of the blood cholesterol is dependent upon the relative proportion associated with HDL and LDL. LDL-cholesterol is directly associated with CHD[87, 639] and the available evidence suggests that LDL-cholesterol may act through causing direct damage to the arterial endothelium with subsequent proliferation of arterial smooth muscle cells resulting in an accumulation of lipids and progression to atherosclerotic plaque formation.[1338, 1351]

HDL-cholesterol concentrations, particularly HDL_2, appear to have an inverse relationship with CHD.[779, 1038] Potential mechanisms by which HDL may reduce or retard development of atherosclerosis include the facilitation of the transport of cholesterol from peripheral tissues to the liver for subsequent degradation and the inhibition of LDL-cholesterol uptake by peripheral cells by affecting the LDL receptor site.[303, 1039, 1040, 1333]

Apolipoproteins A-1 and B have been associated with coronary artery disease.[478] Angiographic evidence suggests that elevated levels of apolipo-protein A-1 are associated with a low incidence of coronary artery disease,[944] whereas apolipoprotein B has been positively identified with increased risk for coronary artery disease.[681]

Blood lipids and lipoproteins during childhood and adolescence

Analytical variation in the estimation of blood lipids makes data collected in different studies difficult to interpret and comparative analyses must therefore be viewed with caution. Wynder and his associates[1691] attempted to standardize total cholesterol measurements for 5331 13-year-olds from 15 countries and although it was not possible to standardize methodology, their results clearly demonstrated wide geographical variations in young people's blood cholesterol level. The highest mean values were found in Finland followed by other Northern European countries. Southern European children, from countries such as Greece and Italy, had relatively low mean total cholesterol levels.

At birth, blood cholesterol, LDL, and triglyceride levels are very low and they increase rapidly during the first year of life.[865] Despite some conflicting evidence the consensus of opinion is that during childhood and adolescence lipid and lipoprotein levels generally remain relatively stable with few sex differences.[11, 59, 1500] The exception is HDL, which, following an often marked decline in boys during adolescence,[157, 1517, 1568, 1577] is significantly lower in boys than in girls.[59, 1024, 1116, 1569] There are, however, wide individual differences and Fig. 9.3 illustrates data collected in our laboratory from 11–16-year-olds.[59]

Physical activity and blood lipids

Studies with adults

In adults, physical activity has often been demonstrated to elicit a beneficial effect on blood lipid and lipoprotein profiles,[1661, 1679, 1680] but some contrasting results have been reported.[595, 690, 1155] In the most systematic reviews of the literature to date, Tran and his colleagues[922, 1540] carried out meta-analyses of 66 studies on males and 27 studies on females. These analyses demonstrated that conflicting findings could be due to the effect or influence of confound-ing variables known to interact with blood lipid levels (e.g. age of subjects, body mass, body fatness, aerobic fitness, cigarette smoking, alcohol con-sumption, diet, oral contraceptive use, menstrual cycle phase, and intensity, duration, frequency, and mode of physical activity), being neither controlled nor reported in many studies. Nevertheless, Tran's meta-analyses indicated that physical activity results in desirable changes in blood lipids and lipoproteins, although women seem to respond with significantly smaller changes than men. The precise changes in blood lipid profile induced by physical activity are not fully understood but following an excellent review of the literature Durstine and Haskell[478] concluded that, the important changes in lipoprotein composition associated with physical activity are increased HDL-cholesterol, HDL_2-cholesterol, and apolipoprotein A-1 concentrations.

Although no investigation of blood lipids and lipoproteins in relation to physical activity has addressed the issue in a dose–response design[1495] it appears that dynamic, continuous aerobic physical activity with large muscle groups is the most effective moderator of lipid and lipoprotein profiles.[717, 798, 1677] Resistive exercise has been shown to be beneficial in some studies[632, 746, 762] but a comprehensive review of the literature concluded that,

the issue of whether strength training can favourably alter blood concentrations of lipids and lipoproteins has not been adequately addressed.[842, p. 270]

There is no clear answer to how long or how intense physical activity needs to be and both vigorous[173] and low-intensity physical activity[352] have produced favourable results. It is probable that the optimum amount of physical activity varies with the blood lipid-lipoprotein profile of the individual. Superko[1495] reviewed available studies and came to the conclusion that physical activity equivalent to jogging 10 miles (16 km) per week for 6 months would be likely to result in an increase of HDL-cholesterol, HDL_2 mass, and often a reduction in triglyceride. (Table 9.4.)

Physical activity exerts both acute and chronic effects on blood lipids and lipoproteins. The precise mechanisms are not fully understood but it appears that factors such as diet, adiposity, body mass loss, and hormone and enzyme activity interact with physical activity to alter the rates of synthesis, transport, and clearance of lipid and lipoproteins from the blood.[478, 631] Potential mechanisms are summarized in Table 9.5.

Studies with children and adolescents

The literature concerned with the response of young people's blood lipid and lipoprotein levels to physical activity is relatively scarce when compared to the number of adult studies, but increasing interest in this area can be mapped through a series of published reviews.[68, 78, 140, 278, 425, 906, 1260, 1555] Armstrong and Simons-Morton[78] have provided a detailed, tabulated analysis of all relevant studies to 1994.

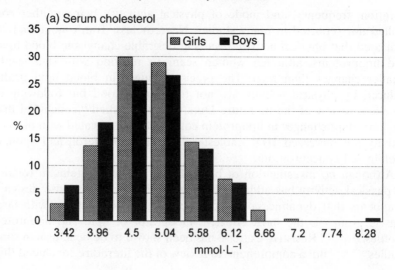

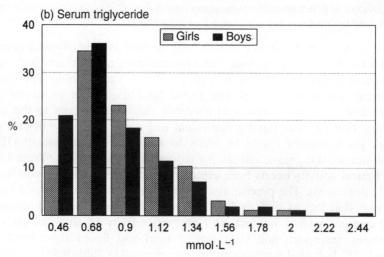

Fig. 9.3. Serum lipids in young people aged 11–16 years: (a) serum cholesterol; (b) serum triglyceride; (c) HDL cholesterol; (d) LDL cholesterol. Figures drawn from data reported by Armstrong, N., Balding, J., Gentle, P. and Kirby, B. (1992). Serum lipids and blood pressure in relation to age and sexual maturity. *Annals of Human Biology*, **19**, 477–87.

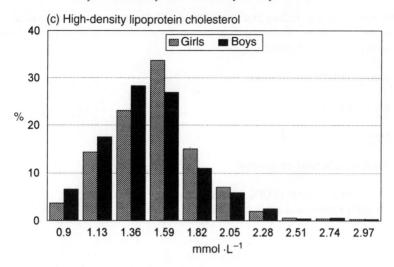

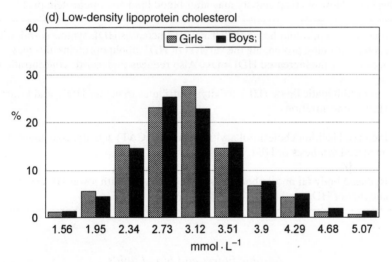

Fig. 9.3. *Cont'd.*

Table 9.4. Physical activity and blood lipid and lipoprotein changes in adults

---

- Increased HDL-cholesterol

- Increased HDL$_2$-cholesterol

- Increased apolipoprotein A-1

- Decreased triglyceride

- No change in total cholesterol

- Only minor changes in LDL-cholesterol,
  its subfractions, and apolipoproteins

Table 9.5. How physical activity may alter blood lipid and lipoprotein profile

---

- Increased lipoprotein lipase (LPL) activity: increases HDL synthesis and, with exercise training prolonging the survival of HDL apolipoproteins, this may account for the increased HDL mass. Also reduces triglyceride concentration

- Reduced hepatic lipase (HL) activity: contributes to higher HDL$_2$ and lower HDL$_3$ concentrations

- Increased lecithin cholesterol acyltransferase (LCAT) activity: contributes to increased synthesis of HDL$_2$-cholesterol

- Reduced body fat and/or body mass loss: associated with lower HL activity and higher HDL and HDL$_2$ concentrations.

Aerobic fitness and blood lipids

A number of studies have investigated the relationship between measures of aerobic fitness and blood lipids during childhood and adolescence. Peak $\dot{V}O_2$ (or $\dot{V}O_{2\,max}$) has been found to be unrelated to total cholesterol,[15, 58, 107, 582, 617, 869, 1423, 1575, 1667] to HDL-cholesterol,[15, 58, 86, 582, 869] to LDL-cholesterol,[15, 869, 939] to triglyceride,[15, 582, 617, 939] and to apolipoproteins.[821, 939] One study reported aerobic fitness to be significantly correlated with HDL and HDL$_2$ in boys but not in girls,[107] whereas another study found girls in a high fitness group to have higher HDL-cholesterol than girls in a low fitness group. No differences were detected in boys.[1575] Male and female data were combined in one study[1423] and negative correlations between aerobic fitness and triglyceride and LDL-cholesterol and a positive relationship between aerobic fitness and HDL-cholesterol were reported. Kwee and Wilmore[869] observed a negative correlation between aerobic fitness and triglyceride in boys. Armstrong *et al.*[86] found a negative relationship between peak $\dot{V}O_2$ and cholesterol in boys but not in girls. When the common effects of body fatness were statistically partialled out the relationship was no longer significant.

Other studies that have used less direct measures of aerobic fitness or estimates of exercise tolerance as independent measures have reported similar findings,[468, 471, 716, 1055, 1496] although a positive relationship with HDL-cholesterol has been more consistently suggested in both boys[1349, 1557, 1591] and girls.[1349, 1516]

Habitual physical activity and blood lipids
Several investigators have studied the relationship between young people's habitual physical activity and their blood lipid and lipoprotein profile. However, on the basis of studies to date, it must be concluded that significant differences in blood lipids and lipoproteins between active and sedentary young people remain to be proven. There are some indications that active children and adolescents may have higher HDL-cholesterol[470, 471, 1496, 1575, 1578] and perhaps lower triglyceride[1496, 1516, 1578] than do sedentary youngsters, but the evidence is not compelling. Most studies have reported no significant relationship between physical activity patterns and blood lipids.[15, 58, 86, 468, 821, 892, 939, 1349, 1464]

Any relationship between blood lipids and habitual physical activity may be confounded by the difficulty in estimating young people's physical activity patterns (see Chapter 6) and by a possible interaction between physical activity, body fatness, and blood lipid and lipoprotein profile. In addition, because there is a smaller variance in both levels of physical activity and levels of blood lipids and lipoproteins in children and adolescents than there is in adults, blood lipids may be less likely to vary with physical activity.[1053]

Exercise training and blood lipids
Cross-sectional analyses of 'trained' versus 'untrained' young people have consistently demonstrated higher levels of HDL-cholesterol in the trained subjects, with no difference between trained and untrained subjects in levels of total cholesterol.[107, 194, 938, 1107, 1423, 1557, 1591] Some studies have reported lower triglyceride levels and/or lower LDL-cholesterol levels in trained subjects.[938, 1107, 1423, 1557, 1591] Macek *et al.*[938] observed favourable apolipoprotein profiles in trained subjects, and Atomi *et al.*[107] reported trained subjects to have higher HDL_2-cholesterol levels than untrained controls.

These data need to be interpreted with caution as few studies defined their criteria of 'trained', 'control/normal', or 'inactive' subjects and little indication was given of selection procedures. This is compounded by small sample sizes, and no control of training intensity, frequency, duration of session, or length of programme. Pre-training blood lipid and lipoprotein profiles are generally not reported and in several studies male and female data have been pooled. Furthermore, it is often impossible to ascertain whether changes in blood lipid profile have been accompanied or influenced by changes in body composition, aerobic fitness, or diet.

Several prospective training studies have been carried out with young children. Some studies have reported no significant changes in blood lipids and lipoproteins following exercise training[167, 481, 615] whereas others have found favourable, but often transitory, changes.[550, 614, 1336, 1530] Studies with older children and adolescents have also been generally unimpressive[267, 268, 430, 744, 908] although several studies have lacked rigour in both design and execution.

In a well-controlled study Linder et al.[907] randomly assigned 50 male volunteers, aged 11–17 years, to either a control or a physical conditioning group. Each subject in the physical conditioning group was required to participate in an exercise training programme which consisted of three days of an alternating walk–jog protocol. Each walking segment was completed in 60 sec. The jogging segments were run at a speed that increased the subject's pulse rate to 80% of maximum. In addition, competitive soccer or rugby was played 1 day per week for a minimum of 60 min. The programme continued for 8 weeks and 21 experimental and 18 control subjects underwent post-training examination. No significant differences between the two groups in levels of triglyceride, total cholesterol, HDL-cholesterol, or LDL-cholesterol were detected. The investigators expressed surprise at this 'unexpected' result and speculated that either a longer period of training was necessary to alter the lipid and lipoprotein profile of adolescents, or that a critical level of blood lipoproteins may exist in young people below which alterations with physical activity are difficult.

Two studies have evaluated the influence of resistance training on blood lipid and lipoprotein profile. Weltman et al.[1630] demonstrated a 15.7% reduction in total cholesterol but no change in triglyceride in prepubertal boys following 14 weeks of hydraulic resistance strength training, but their results are confounded by the initial elevated total cholesterol of the boys and the training-induced increase in $\dot{V}O_{2\,max}$. Fripp and Hodgson[581] evaluated 14 adolescent boys following a 9 week resistance exercise programme and observed no change in total cholesterol, apolipoprotein B or $\dot{V}O_{2\,max}$ but significant favourable changes in HDL-cholesterol and LDL-cholesterol.

The evidence from these short-term prospective studies is not encouraging, although Bar-Or[140, p. 325] has suggested that,

the findings leave open the possible usefulness of conditioning as a means of altering the lipid and lipoprotein profiles in non-obese children and adolescents.

Table 9.6.   Summary of findings relating physical activity to blood lipids and lipoproteins during childhood and adolescence

---

Prospective exercise training studies
No strong evidence of changes in blood lipid and lipoprotein profile

Comparison of trained and untrained subjects
Evidence of an association with favourable changes in HDL, LDL, and triglyceride

Relationship with aerobic fitness
Evidence of an association with favourable change in HDL

Relationship with habitual physical activity
Evidence of a weak association with favourable change in HDL

In the light of adult data,[1495] it may be that physical activity intervention programmes of much longer duration are necessary to induce favourable changes in young people's blood lipids and lipoproteins.

The findings of studies relating physical activity to blood lipid and lipoprotein profiles in young people are summarized in Table 9.6. Observational studies indicate that exercise training, aerobic fitness, and high levels of habitual physical activity may be associated with favourable changes in blood lipids. Prospective studies do not provide any significant support of a relationship. It must be concluded, therefore, that the case for physical activity positively influencing blood lipids and lipoproteins during childhood and adolescence remains to be proven.

Blood pressure

Elevations in diastolic or systolic blood pressure are predictive of CHD.[781, 783] A plausible explanation for the effect of elevated blood pressure on the atherosclerotic process is through the distending pressure of the blood within the vessel exerting shearing forces that damage the intima. This may be followed by intimal smooth muscle proliferation, production of a connective tissue matrix by the smooth muscle cells, and deposition of lipid within and among the cells.[1602] Regardless of the mechanism there does not appear to be a single critical level of blood pressure beyond which risk is markedly increased. The risk is continuous: the higher the blood pressure the greater the risk of CHD. The importance of elevated blood pressure as a risk factor for CHD becomes apparent when one considers that 15–25% of adults in Western societies may have hypertension.[784, 785, 1117]

Blood pressure during childhood and adolescence

Despite many years of experience with the non-invasive measurement of children's blood pressure, through sphygmomanometry, discussion continues concerning its reliability, the wide variation observed in individual subjects, and the uncertain validity of comparisons between persons or groups over time.[1162, 1687] A well-controlled evaluation of the measurement of children's blood pressure in a single epidemiological multicentre study concluded that,

comparisons of blood pressure values in different areas should be done cautiously.[1550, p. 79]

Nevertheless, even when interpreted cautiously, Wynder *et al.*'s[1691] comparative study of 13-year-old children in 15 countries illustrates geographical variations. Wynder reported that the highest mean systolic blood pressures were found in Finland (117 mmHg for both boys and girls) and France (117 mmHg for boys and 114 mmHg for girls). Low values in boys were found in Yugoslavia and Thailand (103 mmHg) and the lowest mean values in girls were present in Yugoslavia and Nigeria (102 mmHg). Geographical comparisons are complicated by the finding that black children tend to have higher blood pressures than white children.[170] When black youngsters are compared with white, they exhibit an increased blood pressure response,[538] and a greater hypertensive response on a high-salt diet when given a noradrenaline challenge.[439] Other factors related to young people's blood pressure include obesity and dietary salt.[885] (and see Chapter 10)

The wide range of blood pressures recorded in different studies partially reflects methodological differences but remarkable inconsistencies have emerged from within studies relating blood pressure to age, sex, and sexual maturity. Figure 9.4 illustrates the variation in the blood pressures of 11–16-year-olds in a single study.

Girls have been reported to have higher diastolic blood pressures (DBP) than boys in some studies[1120, 1188, 1568, 1570] whereas other studies have reported no sex differences in DBP.[59, 332, 1503, 1655] Some experimenters have observed that girls under the age of 14 years have higher DBP than similarly aged boys[448, 856] but others have reported girls' DBP to be higher than boys' DBP only at 14 years and above.[909]

Systolic blood pressure (SBP) has been reported to be higher in boys,[59, 332, 1120, 1568] although some studies have found no sex differences.[448, 1187, 1569] Two studies reported no sex differences in SBP until the age of 14 years when boys experienced marked increases in SBP.[909, 1655] The association of higher SBP with increasing sexual maturity appears to be well established,[59, 390, 1188, 1568, 1570] although some investigators have only observed the association in boys.[1120, 1569]

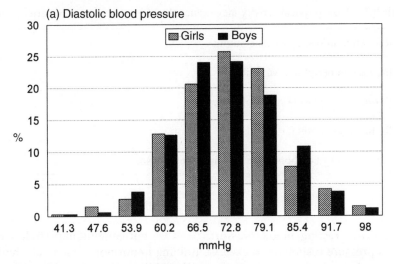

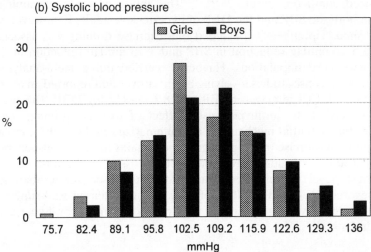

Fig. 9.4. Blood pressure of young people aged 11–16 years: (a) diastolic; (b) systolic. Figures drawn from data reported by Armstrong, N., Balding, J., Gentle, P. and Kirby, B. (1992). Serum lipids and blood pressure in relation to age and sexual maturity. *Annals of Human Biology*, **19**, 477–87.

Physical activity and blood pressure

Studies with adults

The relationship between physical activity and resting blood pressure in adults has been well researched and several reviews are available.[88, 668 1057, 1352, 1532, 1533] Cross-sectional studies indicate that physically active or fit adults

Table 9.7. How physical activity may reduce the blood pressure of hypertensives

---

• Reduction in resting cardiac output

• Increase in peripheral vasodilation

• Reduction in plasma catecholamines

• Reduction in body fat

• Adaptations to carbohydrate and lipid metabolism

---

have lower resting blood pressures[360, 1057, 1532] but longitudinal studies of blood pressure responses to exercise training in normotensive adults have produced conflicting results.[215, 630, 1352] The ability of exercise training to reduce both the SBP and the DBP of hypertensive adults is, however, well established. Tipton[1532, 1533] concluded that exercise training was associated with a 5–25 mmHg reduction in SBP and 3–15 mmHg reduction in DBP in hypertensive populations. Hagberg[668] carried out a meta-analysis of 25 chronic exercise studies involving hypertensives and reported an average reduction of 10.8 mmHg for SBP and 8.2 mmHg for DBP. The precise mechanisms of the antihypertensive effect of exercise training remain unclear but potential mechanisms are summarized in Table 9.7. Similarly, the optimum exercise training programme remains to be established, probably because few studies have addressed the issue of the dose–response relationship.[987, 1091] Tipton[1533] lends support to both prescribing aerobic endurance exercise between 40–70% of $\dot{V}O_{2\,max}$ and initiating well-supervised and monitored weight or circuit training programmes for hypertensive populations.

Studies with children and adolescents

Relatively few studies have addressed the effect of physical activity on blood pressure in either normotensive[16] or hypertensive[16, 37] children and adolescents. Controlled, prospective studies with young people are sparse.

Aerobic fitness, habitual physical activity, and blood pressure
Several studies have reported significant relationships between peak $\dot{V}O_2$ (or $\dot{V}O_{2\,max}$) and blood pressure[86, 412, 582, 869] but only one study appears to have observed a favourable relationship, with DBP in girls, robust enough to withstand the removal of the common effects of body fatness.[412] The findings from studies employing less rigorous measures of aerobic fitness

are mixed. Most studies have reported some favourable relationships between aerobic fitness and blood pressure[156, 233, 482, 571, 1053, 1128, 1311, 1516] but in those studies where statistical adjustments were made for body fatness the strength of these relationships generally was substantially reduced, often to levels that did not achieve statistical significance.

Habitual physical activity does not appear to be related to blood pressure[86, 553, 830, 980, 1311, 1516] although one study demonstrated an association of lower levels of leisure time activity with higher SBP.[1475]

Exercise training and blood pressure

Normotensives   Eight week,[8, 907] 12 week[268] and 14 week[481] aerobic exercise programmes have failed to elicit any effect on the blood pressure of normotensive young people. Although one 12 week, 30 min per day, 5 days per week programme resulted in no change in SBP but a significant reduction in DBP.[550]

Two longer-term studies have, however, reported relatively small but significant reductions in both DBP and SBP following an exercise training programme.[522, 682] Eriksson and Koch[522] trained 9 boys, for 1 h per day, 3 days per week, for 4 months using high-speed running and demonstrated significant reductions in SBP and DBP and a significant increase in $\dot{V}O_{2\,max}$. As part of the Odense schoolchildren study, 18 boys and 17 girls, aged 9–11 years, experienced three extra physical education lessons a week for 8 months in which, on average, heart rates for each child exceeded 70% of maximum for 35 min of each 50 min lesson.[682] After 3 months neither aerobic fitness nor blood pressure had changed significantly. After adjustment for values in body mass, stature, heart rate, and the variable in question before training, aerobic fitness rose significantly and both SBP and DBP fell significantly by the end of the training programme.

Other studies with obese adolescents have demonstrated reductions in DBP and SBP with combined dietary and exercise programmes.[1005, 1221]

Hypertensives   Several studies have demonstrated reductions in both DPB and SBP of hypertensive young people following exercise training programmes.[393, 569, 682] The only study which appears to have exclusively employed a weight training programme with hypertensives did not induce any significant changes in either DBP or SBP.[872] However, repeated episodes of intense resistance training did not increase SBP or DBP at rest which indicates that it may not be necessary to restrict hypertensive youth from resistance training.

It is, however, the work of Hagberg and his colleagues[670–672] which has provided the most valuable insights into the effect of both endurance and resistance exercise training on the blood pressure of hypertensive adolescents. Hagberg[671, 672] evaluated the effects of six months of endurance running on 25 adolescents whose blood pressure was persistently above the

Table 9.8. Summary of findings relating physical activity to blood pressure during childhood and adolescence

---

Prospective exercise training studies
Weak evidence of changes in the blood pressure of normotensives
Aerobic exercise training is related to a reduction in both DBP and SBP in hypertensives

Relationship with aerobic fitness and/or habitual physical activity
No clear association established after adjustment for differences in body mass/fatness

---

95th percentile for their age and sex. They exercised three times per week, for 40 min, at an intensity of 60–65% of peak $\dot{V}O_2$. Both DBP and SBP decreased significantly although no significant change in either body mass or skinfold thickness was detected. When the subjects were reassessed 9 months after the cessation of the training programme, SBP had returned to pre-training levels but DBP was still significantly below pre-training levels in the subjects who had diastolic hypertension initially. Five of the subjects continued with a 5 month weight training programme immediately following the endurance training programme.[670] SBP of the weight training group remained significantly lower than when measured at the beginning of the project. The two subjects who initially had diastolic hypertension maintained the reduction in DBP achieved by endurance training. Hagberg concluded that,

weight training in hypertensive adolescents appears to maintain the reductions in blood pressure achieved by endurance training and may even elicit further reductions in blood pressure.[670, p. 147]

The findings of studies relating physical activity to blood pressure are summarized in Table 9.8. With normotensive young people the evidence that exercise training will induce significant reductions in either SBP or DBP is not convincing. Aerobic exercise training appears to be effective in reducing both DBP and SBP of hypertensive children and adolescents. Resistance training may be effective in maintaining reductions in blood pressure induced by a previous aerobic exercise training programme.

Most studies have been of relatively short duration, few have been adequately controlled, and individual variations in response to exercise training have not been addressed. No dose–response relationship has been established between physical activity and blood pressure in young people.

Smoking

The prevalence of cigarette smoking in English adults has fallen from 51% of men and 40% of women in 1974 to 29% of men and 27% of women in 1992.[418] Smoking among English adolescents has, however, remained virtually unchanged at 10% during the period 1982–1993.[418] A WHO study[820] surveyed young people, aged 11, 13, and 15 years, in nine countries and Fig. 9.5 illustrates the percentages of respondents (total

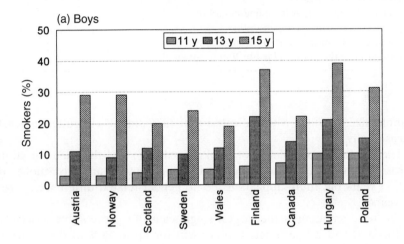

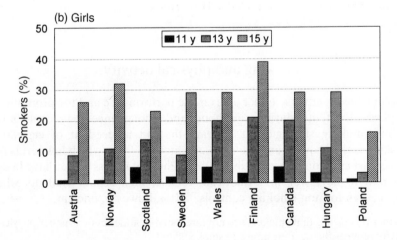

Fig. 9.5. Percentage of young people who smoke at least occasionally: (a) boys; (b) girls. Figures drawn from data reported by King, A.C. and Coles, B. (1992). *The Health of Canada's Youth*. Canada, Minister of Supply Services.

Table 9.9. How cigarette smoking may promote coronary heart disease

Nicotine causes

An increase in resting heart rate

An increase in resting DBP and SBP

An increase in myocardial oxygen demand

An increase in platelet adhesiveness and aggregation

An increase in free fatty acids

A reduction of the ventricular fibrillation threshold

Carbon monoxide causes

Displacement of oxygen from haemoglobin

Reduction of maximal oxygen uptake

Adverse effects on the electron transport system

A reduction of the ventricular fibrillation threshold

---

sample size, 41 904), who indicated that they smoke cigarettes at least occasionally.

The increasing prevalence of smoking with age and the wide variation across countries are readily apparent. More boys than girls smoke at age 11 years but there appears to be no gender-related difference at age 15 years.

Cigarette smoking is the largest single cause of preventable mortality in England and it is estimated to account for up to 18% of deaths from CHD.[417] for those who smoke, stopping smoking is the single most effective means of reducing risk for CHD. How smoking may promote CHD is summarized in Table 9.9.

Smoking and physical activity

Smoking has an adverse effect on exercise performance and the promotion of physical activity during childhood and adolescence may contribute to anti-smoking strategies. It appears that an antecedent of cigarette smoking is the acquisition of a 'smoker's lifestyle'[1705] to which low levels of sports participation may contribute.[1244, 1294] Physical fitness scores have been reported to be lower for American, female, high school students who smoke, than for non-smoking controls.[1373] It is, however, unclear,

whether this means that smokers are not interested in athletics or whether physical activity reduces the need or desire to smoke.[1258, p. 126]

Questionnaire studies of 2831 Finnish children and 13 181 British adolescents have indicated that more active children smoked significantly less than those who are inactive.[124, 870, 1539] In our laboratory we have detected a weak negative relationship between smoking habits and level of physical activity in boys but not in girls.[612] A six year longitudinal study of young people aged 12 years, 15 years, and 18 years at the outset observed that subjects leading a sedentary lifestyle were more likely to take up smoking. Those subjects who remained physically active throughout the study 'hardly ever started to smoke during the follow-up'.[1193, p. 203]

There are few studies which have been able to associate young people's physical activity with a low incidence of cigarette smoking and no cause and effect relationship has been established. The argument that physical activity has a significant role to play in reducing the prevalence of young smokers is intuitively appealing but unproven.

Exercise prescription

Dose–response data relating the effects of physical activity to blood lipids, blood pressure, and cigarette smoking in young people appear to be non-existent. Prescribing a specific exercise training programme is therefore speculative. Current evidence and extrapolation from adult data suggest that a minimum exercise training period of 6 months would be required before beneficial effects could be expected. Extending Superko's[1495] recommendation of jogging 10 miles (16 km) per week to a population of children and adolescents would involve the young person in approximately 2 h per week of jogging (e.g. at a rate of 8 km·h^{-1}). In our experience this intensity of exercise is equivalent to about 80% of maximal heart rate with children and perhaps 75% of maximal heart rate in adolescents. Four 30 minute sessions of large-muscle group exercise per week, at an intensity equivalent to 75–80% of maximal heart rate, may therefore be an effective exercise prescription. It is likely that young people with adverse lipid profiles and hypertensive individuals whose physicians allow strenuous physical activity would benefit most from this type of programme.

We do not recommend that asymptomatic young people are encouraged to follow the above exercise prescription for the purpose of reducing coronary risk factors during childhood and adolescence. We believe that youngsters likely to benefit the most in terms of protection against chronic disease are those who adopt active lifestyles that are sustained through adult life. We support the idea of exposing young people to exercise training programmes in which they may develop understanding of fitness concepts, fitness skills, and self-efficacy for maintaining regular participation in lifetime fitness activities. However, we recommend emphasis be placed upon promoting an increase in enjoyable physical activities involving large-muscle groups. Appropriate activities in the present context include walking, jogging, cycling, dancing, swimming, skating, and cycling.

Summary

Coronary atherosclerosis has its origins in childhood and adolescence and there is a growing conviction that the identification of adult coronary risk factors at an early age may identify some potential coronary candidates in childhood. The effect of regular physical activity in lowering blood lipids and reducing high blood pressure during adult life is well established but the case for physical activity positively influencing cigarette smoking, blood lipids, lipoproteins, or blood pressure during childhood and adolescence remains to be proven.

Cross-sectional comparisons of trained and untrained, active and sedentary, fit and unfit children and adolescents include the combined effects of fitness, leanness, and physical activity and may be further contaminated by self-selection of subjects. This may explain why convincing evidence for a beneficial effect of regular activity on levels of blood pressure and HDL-cholesterol is more apparent in cross-sectional studies than in short-term longitudinal investigations. The results of longitudinal studies are unimpressive but with the exception of Linder *et al.*'s[907] investigation, which demonstrated no significant changes in blood lipids, lipoproteins, or blood pressure, the studies are generally lacking in rigour in both design and execution. Controlled, prospective studies of at least 6 months duration need to be carried out before firm recommendations on appropriate physical activity can be established. In the meantime the best advice to young people in this context may be to encourage them to adopt more active lifestyles and to give up or not to take up cigarette smoking.

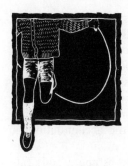

10
Physical activity and body fatness

Body fatness and health

Fat is an essential component of the human body and is necessary for normal physiological function. Fat is stored in the bone marrow, in vital organs including the heart, lungs, liver and kidneys, and in the lipid-rich tissues of the nervous system. The majority of body fat, however, is deposited as storage fat in adipose tissue, primarily in subcutaneous sites but also around the organs. Some of the visceral fat serves a role in protecting the vital organs from trauma but an over-accumulation of fat (obesity) is undesirable.[162] Obesity is incrementally associated with increased morbidity and mortality from causes such as non-insulin dependent diabetes mellitus (NIDDM), stroke, coronary heart disease (CHD), some cancers, and arthritis.[136, 607, 1079, 1087, 1275]

Estimation of body fat

The estimation of body fat as a percentage of body composition is complex. The methods available for body composition assessment have been extensively reviewed in relation to both adults[249, 250] and young people.[918, 920] Numerous techniques are available including measurement of skinfolds, stature–mass indices, bioelectrical impedance, near infrared interactance, densitometry (underwater weighing), computed tomography (CT), and magnetic resonance imaging (MRI).

In the laboratory, densitometry with correction for pulmonary residual volume[281] is recognized as the 'gold-standard' method for determining body density.[214, 918, 1663] Body density is subsequently converted to percentage fat using standard equations.[264, 1406] Although densitometry has been used with children[1161] the limitations of this method with young subjects are well documented. The method assumes chemical maturity,[920] but changes in body composition during growth and maturation affect the conceptual basis for estimating fatness and leanness; in particular changes in bone density and hydration of the fat-free body which occur with maturation make the application of adult-derived equations to young people untenable.[914–917]

The simple, inexpensive, and non-invasive nature of anthropometric body composition assessment methods have popularized their use with children and adolescents. Stature–mass indices such as the Quetelet index, more usually referred to as the body mass index (BMI)[1] have been widely used.[803, 909] However, although the BMI may be useful to monitor adolescent growth[1233] the inability of the index to differentiate between lean and fat components of body composition proscribe its use as a measure of body fatness[1602] unless other methods are either unavailable or not practicable.[918] For example, during adolescence an increase in BMI in boys may reflect a rapid development of muscle and bone rather than the accumulation of fat.[920]

Skinfolds are easily measured and routinely used to estimate body fatness.[688, 1129, 1223] However, the change in the relationship between anthropometric dimensions and body fatness during maturation, as estimated from body density, precludes the accurate prediction of young people's total body fatness from skinfold data.[920] Multicomponent, criterion-referenced skinfold prediction equations which account for age, gender, and maturational stage have been developed[1414] and received support[759, 919] but further research is required to explore their validity. Nevertheless, skinfold thicknesses provide a useful indicator of children's and adolescents' subcutaneous fatness and inter-study comparisons can be based upon raw scores without attempting to convert to percentage body fat.[86, 300, 1239] However, consideration must be given to the large inter-observer variability typically associated with skinfold measurements.

Although electrical conductivity was first used in body composition research in the early 1960s[1527, 1528] bioelectrical impedance has only recently become an accepted assessment technique in adults.[866, 1357, 1559] The few studies which have examined the usefulness of bioelectrical impedance for the estimation of body fatness in children have produced promising relationships between resistive index and total body water[405] and resistive index and fat-free mass determined from underwater weighing.[366, 736, 737] However, the validity of the method is dependent upon stringent preparatory measures including standardization of fasting state, phase of menstrual cycle, prior physical activity, and electrode placement.[426, 902]

Near infrared interactance has been promoted as a tool for body composition assessment[349] but attempts to validate the technique with adults have not been encouraging.[734, 1008] The methodology has not been widely used with children and adolescents[251, 318] and results indicate that it offers either no or minimal advantage over multiple-component reference skinfold or BMI methods.[916]

With the recognition that body fat distribution, rather than body fat excess *per se*, is related to increased morbidity, methods that can differentiate and quantify internal or visceral fat from subcutaneous fat stores are of particular value. The waist–hip ratio (WHR) has been widely used

---

[1] Body mass index (BMI) = mass divided by stature squared (kg·m^{-2}).

in adults to indicate central fat deposition. Relationships have been observed between visceral fat and WHR[91, 1361] but others have concluded that although WHR is an independent predictor of numerous metabolic aberrations, its correlative power is not explained by an ability to predict visceral fat deposition.[1245] Similarly, research with both obese and non-obese children has shown WHR to be a poor predictor of intra-abdominal fat deposition determined from MRI.[240, 567]

Computed tomography has frequently been used to assess abdominal fat deposition in adults[91, 868, 1359, 1360] but the radiation exposure entailed precludes its use with children. MRI is a non-invasive, harmless alternative[1153, 1456] which produces results similar to CT[1361] and has been used to quantify abdominal fat deposition in young people.[240, 422, 567] The prohibitive cost of MRI has led several investigators to research for anthropometric correlates of MRI-determined fatness. In girls of normal body mass, waist, hip, and trochanter circumferences have been shown to be highly correlated to fat surface area at the same sites computed from MRI scans.[422] In both boys and girls we have observed that abdominal skinfolds and thigh circumference correlate strongly with MRI-determined total fat.[1161] Data from the same population of children indicated that intra-abdominal fat deposition in the boys was best reflected by the subscapular/triceps skinfold ratio with the subscapular skinfold alone the best correlate in girls.[567] In contrast, only in the obese children studied by Brambilla *et al.*[240] was MRI-determined intra-abdominal fat positively correlated with trunk/extremity circumference ratios. Despite these relationships, it has been concluded that even the best anthropometric correlates are not sufficiently sensitive for the clinical determination of visceral fat in individual children.[567] The main advantages and disadvantages of body composition assessment techniques are summarized in Table 10.1.

Obesity

In the Western world and those countries more recently 'industrialized' over-fatness is an increasing problem. A recent survey of English adults reported that the prevalence of 'serious' obesity, defined as a BMI greater than 30, doubled between the years of 1980–1991 with 13% of men and 16% of women now falling into this category.[420, 1180] These data are reflective of a general trend towards a population increase in levels of body fat, with significant shifts in the number of individuals falling into all BMI bands associated with overweight.[420, 1180]

In the United States, it is estimated that 31% of adult males and 35% of adult females are obese,[1086] with the prevalence of clinical obesity rising to 50% of females in some ethnic groups.[861] If the increase in obesity in the United Kingdom continues at its current rate it has been estimated that by the year 2005 over 18% of men and 24% of women will be obese.[420]

Table 10.1.   Methods of assessing body fatness: advantages and disadvantages

Method	Advantages	Disadvantages
Skinfold thickness	Inexpensive and simple to administer	Large inter-observer error Regression equations for conversion to percentage body fat not well validated for young people
Body mass index (BMI)	Simple, non-invasive technique Useful to indicate adolescent growth	Unable to quantify body fatness
Waist/hip ratio	Correlates with metabolic diseases	Does not accurately predict internal fat deposition
Bioelectrical impedance	Non-invasive Validity demonstrated in adults	Validity not well established in young people Requires careful standardization of nutritional and activity status
Near infrared reactance	Non-invasive	Poor validity demonstrated with adults and young people
Densitometry (underwater weighing)	Considered the 'gold-standard' measure in adults	Adequate submersion in water may be difficult in some young subjects Changes in chemical maturity with growth make it difficult to estimate accurately body density
Computed tomography (CT)	Measures visceral fat deposition	Radiation exposure limits use of CT with young people
Magnetic resonance imaging (MRI)	Non-invasive Measures visceral fat deposition	Prohibitively expensive for routine use

Given the potential health consequences of obesity, it is not surprising that overweight and obesity are recognized as a major public health problem and targeted for significant public health initiatives. For example, in the United Kingdom the Department of Health has set targets to reduce obesity by 25% in men and by 33% in females by the year 2005.[420]

The growing problem of adult obesity is reflected by an increase in childhood and adolescent overweight and obesity. Japanese authors have reported a doubling in childhood obesity in the 10 years to 1987 with the highest frequency of cases observed in early pubescence.[1334] Obesity has been described as the most common childhood metabolic disorder in developed nations[1378] and moderate levels of obesity appear characteristic of North American teenagers.[633]

The precise quantification of body fatness during growth is confounded by many factors and as a result, obesity is difficult to define clinically as a fat percentage of total body composition. In adults, over-fatness is more often classified according to the BMI with indices greater than 25 and 30 constituting 'overweight' and 'obesity', respectively.[420] Other studies with both adults[326] and young people[358, 1334, 1706] have used criteria based upon the percentage above normative data for body mass, stature, and age with 10% greater than predicted mass defined as overweight and 20% greater as obese.

Some investigators have attempted to circumvent the problems associated with a simple mass for stature criterion by defining overweight as a body mass greater than the 75th percentile of normative data; reported to correspond to an approximate BMI of 22–24 in 13–18-year-olds.[1079] The inclusion of a measure of body fatness is perhaps more meaningful with subjects defined as overweight if displaying both body mass and triceps skinfold thickness greater than the 75th percentile.[160] Other national surveys have used a triceps skinfold equal to or greater than the 85th percentile for children of the same age and sex to denote obesity.[437] These discrepancies in the definitions of obesity make it difficult to determine accurately the exact prevalence of obesity in child and adolescent populations and have confounded the interpretation of studies attempting to modify body fat levels through physical activity.

Studies investigating the prevalence of obesity in youth have reported percentages ranging from 9[766]–40%.[1121] Data generated in our laboratory[83] from 685 11–16-year-old subjects, from communities whose demographic data demonstrate them to be representative of Southern England, revealed that 12.4% of boys and 9.7% of girls were at least 20% above the Royal College of Physicians'[1275] recommended mass for stature and age. A similar survey of over 250 10–11-year-olds found 21% of boys and 14% of girls exceeded the 75th percentile for both body mass and triceps skinfold thickness.[74] As many as 20% of 14-year-old girls have been reported to exceed by 10% their recommended body mass.[1706] American National Health surveys conducted 10–15 years apart noted that the prevalence of obesity increased by 54% in children aged 6–11 years and by 39% in adolescents aged 12–17 years over the time period studied.[640] When data were split into various age, sex, and ethnic groups the increase in prevalence ranged from 18% in 12–17-year-old boys to 91% in 6–11-year-old black boys and girls. Despite some reservations[684] the volume of evidence supports the view that the body fatness of children and adolescents is increasing.[1243, 1551]

Over-fatness in young people

Some authors have commented that it is uncertain whether or not childhood obesity represents an immediate hazard to health[633] but more recent evidence has associated childhood obesity with both immediate health consequences and adverse metabolic complications in adulthood. Childhood and adolescent obesity is associated with depressed growth hormone (GH) release, hyperinsulinaemia, carbohydrate intolerance, and elevated blood pressure.[341] Lipid disorders and left-ventricular hypertrophy have also been observed in obese young people.[666, 1100]

In over 4800 children involved in the Muscatine study, the presence of increased body mass and triceps skinfold was moderately associated with elevated blood pressure and lipoprotein levels.[883] In addition, children with an adverse lipid profile were reported to have a higher than average risk of these problems persisting into adulthood.[885]

Similar results have been reported in British children.[59] Here, body fatness, as indicated by sum of triceps and subscapular skinfold thicknesses, was significantly correlated with systolic blood pressure (SBP), diastolic blood pressure (DBP), serum triglycerides, and high-density lipoproteins (HDL) in 11–16-year-old boys and girls. In boys a similar significant relationship was observed between sum of skinfold thicknesses and serum total cholesterol.

Becque and associates,[160, p. 610] found that 97% of a group of 36 obese 13-year-olds had four or more risk factors leading them to state, '...obese adolescents have an alarmingly high incidence of multiple coronary heart disease risk factors'. Over 30% of the subjects had elevated total cholesterol levels, 92% had depressed HDL levels, and 23% had a SBP which exceeded by at least two standard deviations the mean normative values for children of comparable age and sex.

In addition to these immediate health complications, overweight and obesity during late adolescence appear to be strongly associated with adult mortality from CHD.[2, 728, 1126, 1436] The 55 year follow-up of the Harvard growth study which originally ran from 1922–1935 has provided unique data indicating that adolescent overweight is predictive of both increased risk of all-cause mortality and disease-specific mortality among men, although this relationship was not found in women. The risk of morbidity from atherosclerotic disease was increased in both men and women who had been overweight in adolescence. Sex-specific morbidity was also evident with colorectal cancer and gout prevalent in men and arthritis common in women who had been overweight in adolescence. Interestingly, overweight in *adulthood* was less predictive of morbidity. This was suggested to reflect the fact that central deposition of fat is characteristic of adolescents[428, 1074] but recent evidence from MRI does not support this hypothesis.[422, 567] Nevertheless, these data provide further evidence that juvenile obesity warrants early intervention.

Fat patterning

Although the adverse health outcomes associated with obesity are well established, there is a growing conviction that it is the distribution of fat within the body (fat patterning), independent of the level of obesity, which is particularly predictive of metabolic disease.[91, 786, 1153]

Obese individuals can be categorized into those who predominantly accumulate adipose tissue centrally (i.e. around the abdomen and upper body) and those whose fat is distributed more peripherally particularly around the thighs and buttocks. Central or android fat deposition is characteristic of males whilst a peripheral or gynoid distribution is typical of females.[857, 868, 1412] Increased CHD risk is associated with trunk–abdominal obesity and is highest in those with deep abdominal fat.[195, 425] Furthermore, trunk skinfolds in adults have been shown to have stronger correlations with the metabolic complications of obesity than arm skinfolds.[1232]

As fat patterning is closely associated with various pathologies, the identification of a predictive correlate of adult pathology-associated adiposity in children is important for targeting appropriate prevention strategies. Anthropometric indices (BMI, skinfolds, and WHR) may be used to indicate the predominance of body fat[1321] but such measures are unable to differentiate between intra-abdominal and subcutaneous fat depots.[240, 422] Several studies have used MRI scans to obtain a non-invasive measure of visceral fat deposition in young people.[240, 422, 567] The results have indicated that, in girls[422, 567] and boys[567] the deposition of visceral fat is lower than in adults of normal body mass and there appears to be no interpretable relationship between intra-abdominal fat and maturational age in either normal or obese boys or girls.[240, 567] Furthermore, excess adipose tissue accumulation at the waist site is predominantly subcutaneous in children[567] and increased maturity in girls is associated with gluteal rather than abdominal fat deposition.[422]

Brambilla *et al.*[240] used MRI to examine differences in peripheral and abdominal adiposity in normal and obese youngsters aged 10–15 years. Their data confirmed a predominance of subcutaneous fat deposition in both obese and control subjects and there was a wide overlap in the area of intra-abdominal fat between the two groups.

The lack of documentation in this area places constraints upon the conclusions which may be drawn, but these data provide strong indications that neither boys nor girls, whether of normal body mass or obese, display the characteristic over-accumulation of visceral fat deposition associated with increased morbidity in adults. Further studies are indicated to monitor the development of visceral fat deposition with progression to full maturity and adulthood.

Tracking of body fatness

There is compelling evidence to associate over-fatness during the formative years with over-fatness in later life. Strong links have been observed between overweight during infancy and childhood[699] and between childhood, adolescence, and adulthood.[833, 1211, 1234] It has been suggested that over 80% of overweight children become overweight adults[2] whilst others have estimated that the odds of an *overweight* adolescent becoming an *average* weight adult are 28 to 1.[1483]

Charney et al.[326] tested the hypothesis that a substantial correlation would be observed between body mass attained in the first six months of life and adult weight status in the third decade of life. Their results demonstrated that infants equal to or above the 90th percentile for body mass at least once in the first six months of life were 2.6 times more liable to be overweight or obese adults than infants of average and light body mass. Other factors which correlated significantly with an individual's adult weight status included the child's educational level, parental social class, and current weight status. A marked interactive effect was noted in that 51% of individuals overweight during infancy and having one parent overweight were obese as adults. Furthermore, youngsters who exceeded the 75th, and even more so, the 95th percentile had a significantly higher chance of becoming overweight adults than infants of low body mass.

These findings are consistent with data reported from the Harvard growth study[1079] which indicated that 52% of overweight adolescents remained overweight at follow-up 55 years later. The authors concluded that the BMI appears to be programmed early in life thus indicating intervention during childhood as necessary to reduce adult morbidity.

Physical activity and body fatness

Aerobic fitness of over-fat and overweight young people

Párizková[1131, p. 64] stated that, 'The functional capacity and cardiorespiratory efficiency is deteriorated in the obese as compared to adolescents of normal weight'. Although when expressed in absolute terms (L·min⁻¹) the peak aerobic fitness of obese subjects is similar to or higher than that of non-obese individuals[74, 945] support for Párizková's statement becomes apparent when aerobic fitness is expressed relative to total body mass. Significantly lower values of mass-related peak $\dot{V}O_2$ (mL·kg⁻¹·min⁻¹) have been consistently reported in overweight juveniles with typical values of 29–36 mL·kg⁻¹·min⁻¹.[86, 160, 403]

Because the expression of peak $\dot{V}O_2$ in mass-related terms penalizes heavy individuals,[1502] particularly where the high body mass results from an accumulation of body fat, simple division by body mass makes it impossible to determine whether a true functional deficiency of the cardiopulmonary system is characteristic of obesity. In a sample of 220 11–16-year-olds we observed mass-related peak $\dot{V}O_2$ to be significantly lower in overweight boys and girls than in those of normal body mass. Scaling the data using a log-linear model (see Chapter 3) reduced the discrepancy between overweight and normal subjects but the difference remained statistically significant.[74]

An innovative study by Cooper *et al.*[358] investigated the ability of obese and non-obese subjects to increase metabolic rate above the unloaded steady-state during incremental cycle ergometer exercise, enabling the oxygen cost of exercise (change in oxygen uptake/change in exercise intensity) to be determined. At maximal exercise levels the oxygen uptake observed was defined as 'delta $\dot{V}O_{2\,max}$'. In addition, breath-by-breath $\dot{V}O_2$, $\dot{V}CO_2$, and $\dot{V}E$ were measured during a 6 min period of submaximal exercise. The results indicated that the majority of exercise responses were within the normal range. However, the normal age-related increase in delta $\dot{V}O_{2\,max}$ was not observed in the obese subjects and one-third of the subjects had markedly abnormal responses on both size-dependent and size-independent measures. Despite these findings the authors pointed out that neither deficient aerobic fitness nor impaired cardiopulmonary responses to exercise are inevitable in obese children and many have normal aerobic fitness for their developmental stage.

A similar conclusion has been drawn by studies which have reported no significant differences in the aerobic fitness of obese young people and those of normal body mass when values are expressed in relation to lean body mass.[493, 945] It therefore appears that although overweight and obese youngsters are disadvantaged in activities which require their body mass to be supported (e.g. walking, running) their cardiopulmonary function and peak $\dot{V}O_2$ (L·min⁻¹) may be in the normal range.

Habitual physical activity of over-fat and overweight young people

If energy intake consistently exceeds energy requirements there will be a progressive accumulation of body fat. Obesity may therefore result from either high energy intake or low energy expenditure, or a combination of both factors. A regulated reduction in energy intake will promote significant loss of body mass in the obese.[511, 560, 1334] However, this strategy alone may result in a marked loss of lean tissue[560, 1704] and a reduction in metabolic rate thus attenuating the rate of body mass loss and increasing the likelihood of subsequent reversion to pre-intervention levels. Physical activity has the greatest potential for increasing an individual's energy expenditure. The advantages of increasing physical activity derive not just from the immediate increase in metabolic rate with activity but also from the potential for a persistent increase during the post-activity period[1529] and the ensuing maintenance or increase in muscle mass.[146, 1334] Low levels of physical activity are therefore implicated in the development of childhood obesity.[138, 652, 1585]

Several studies have reported lower levels of physical activity among obese or overweight youngsters than their non-obese or non-overweight peers.[273, 476, 766, 1234] One study reported that the children of obese parents were less active than those of lean parents, despite no significant difference in body composition between the two groups of children.[657] In contrast, other investigators have observed no relationship between body fatness or overweight and habitual physical activity[60, 74, 237, 1459] or energy expenditure.[410]

Bar-Or and Baranowski[146] reviewed comprehensively the extant literature and concluded that, on balance, obese young people tend to be less physically active than their leaner peers. However, because of their greater body mass obese or overweight youngsters may well expend more energy than those of normal body mass despite being less physically active.

Exercise training and body fatness

Many studies with young people have employed a multicomponent approach where increased physical activity is combined with dietary modification and/or lifestyle and nutrition education. Several of these programmes have failed to elicit significant changes in body fatness. For example, a 10 month programme of nutrition education, exercise, and psychological support in 350 obese young subjects failed to induce changes in either body mass or triceps skinfold.[988, 1363] In 10–17-year-old obese males and females, a 20 week programme of diet and behaviour modification reduced body fat by 4%. A parallel group who also participated in three sessions of aerobic activities per week lost an additional 2% body fat.[1221]

Other obesity management studies incorporating physical activity have elicited significant reduction in body mass or body fat. Seven week summer camps for obese children which promote body mass loss through an intensive programme of dietary modification through education, restricted diet, and increased aerobic exercise have proved particularly successful. Typical decreases in body mass of 10% with concomitant increases in lean tissue of 4–9% have been reported.[1131] These observations are consistent with the 10.9% reduction in percentage overweight, which accrued with a daily exercise and nutritional education programme in 90 obese children.[334]

Despite no changes in some studies,[436] others where the intervention has focused upon exercise training with no direct dietary modification have proved successful. A school-based study[1061] involved 28 obese girls and 12 normal girls in a 15 week programme of daily walking, jogging, and running. Although actual body mass loss was only minimal, 1.0 kg and 0.54 kg in obese and normal groups, respectively, skinfold thickness decreased markedly in the obese group. These positive effects were enhanced when the programme was extended to 29 weeks. In a study of similarly aged males, two 45 min lacrosse sessions per week produced a 10.9% decrease in body fat compared with a 2.3% reduction in the control group.[762]

More recently, an intensive programme of aerobic exercise in obese 11-year-old children incorporating daily 20 min running sessions decreased body fat by 40% in boys and 31% in girls after the first year of training. Concomitant decreases in body mass of 29% in boys and 37% in girls were observed.[1334]

These data clearly support the inclusion of exercise training in programmes designed to produce favourable changes in body composition in obese children and adolescents. Unfortunately, it is also evident that the majority of young people remain overweight at the end of exercise programmes and data on the permanency of positive changes are not encouraging. The changes in body composition reported by Párizková[1131] were reversed once subjects returned home. Furthermore, a cycle of improvement and deterioration was noted over a four year longitudinal period of attendance at summer camps indicating that lifestyle modification had not been established. They younger and less obese the child at the onset of treatment, the more marked and longer lasting were the results of intervention.[1131] These findings emphasize the need to identify and treat obese children from an early age.[341]

Other beneficial effects of exercise training in obese young people

Over and above the direct effects upon energy expenditure and body fat reduction, exercise training confers other metabolic and health benefits upon the obese individual. These include improvements in blood lipid profile, glucose metabolism, and overall coronary risk profile. Increased levels of sustained physical activity induce changes in lipid metabolism which promote the utilization of fat, rather than carbohydrate, during exercise[1131] thus enhancing the reduction of adipose tissue. Several studies have reported notable improvements in the blood lipid profiles of obese children. In their 2 year programme, Sasaki *et al.*[1334] found 16–19% increases in the HDL levels of boys and girls after the first year. By the end of the second year triglyceride concentrations had decreased by 33% in the girls only.

A 2 year intervention programme[1694] combining caloric restriction and 30–60 min aerobic training three times a week resulted in positive changes in HDL, HDL/total cholesterol ratio, and decreased triglycerides in the 10 subjects who achieved normal or near normal body mass during the study. However, 27 subjects did not achieve similar health-related benefits. Although in this study no suggestions were offered as to why some subjects failed to improve, it is documented that some obese subjects remain refractory to any interventions to reduce body mass[146] suggesting a genetic component to the response or non-response of obese subjects to exercise training.[228]

Elevated resting and exercise blood pressure are common in obese children.[1132] The addition of five 60 min exercise sessions to a 20 week intervention programme of dietary restriction and behaviour modification has been shown to produce greater decreases in resting and submaximal exercise SBP and DBP in obese subjects compared with those whose programme did not include exercise. This beneficial effect occurred despite no significant changes in body composition.[1221]

Other cardiovascular improvements include an increase in left-ventricular end-diastolic volume observed in 10–11-year-old obese children following a one year programme of jogging five times per week.[697] The authors suggested that this reflected augmented diastolic filling consequent to brady-cardia rather than a volume overload hypertrophy as there was no accompanying increase in the thickness of the left ventricular posterior wall.

Becque and associates[160] reported that diet, behaviour modification counselling plus exercise for a 20 week period elicited significantly greater improvements in overall coronary risk in obese adolescents compared with control or diet and behaviour groups. This again was despite only minor differences in the magnitude of changes in fat and body mass between the two experimental groups.

Exercise may also control insulin resistance and reduce insulin levels in obese subjects[136, 425] particularly if combined with a low-fat, high-complex carbohydrate diet, which has similar independent effects upon insulin sensitivity. Such a decrease has been indicated by the findings of Ylitalo[1694] in obese children and adolescents following a two year conditioning programme.

Exercise prescription

As the functional aerobic fitness of many obese subjects does not appear to be impaired,[74, 358, 945] prescriptions which primarily focus upon increasing total daily energy expenditure rather than improving cardiopulmonary fitness are recommended.[145, 1132] This is best achieved by activities which use large muscle groups as recommended in Chapter 7. Body mass-bearing activities are particularly valuable to promote optimal bone mineral deposition during periods of body mass loss and dietary restriction (see Chapter 12). The activity programme should effect a 10–15% increase in daily energy expenditure which may be achieved during approximately 30–45 min of mild to moderate intensity exercise.[145, 1132] The inclusion of a resistance training component may be a beneficial aid to preserving muscle mass in obese children undergoing dietary restriction.

Individual adherence to any exercise programme is essential for a successful outcome. In this respect, programmes that are regimented and monotonous or include vigorous activity are unlikely to foster adherence.[145, 509–511] Similarly, it is essential that young people participate in activities they enjoy and do not perceive as threatening or embarrassing.[145]

By advocating moderate intensity physical activities adherence is encouraged in addition to producing favourable changes in body composition, regulating the complications of abdominal obesity, and enhancing other health indicators.[425]

Finally, an increase in general lifestyle activities such as walking to school, undertaking household chores, using stairs, and more active play should be emphasized. Not only does this significantly increase daily energy expenditure, but lifestyle modification appears essential to the prolonged success of obesity management strategies.[508, 510] The general characteristics of an exercise programme suitable for obese young people are outlined in Table 10.2.

Table 10.2. Characteristics of an optimal activity programme for the management of juvenile obesity

---

- Emphasizes use of large muscle groups

- Moves the whole body over distance

- Emphasizes duration rather than intensity

- Raises daily energy expenditure by 10–15%

- Includes activities to promote muscle strength

- Includes daily physical activity

- Volume of physical activity is increased gradually

- Incorporates the child's preferred activities

Adapted from Bar-Or, O. (1995). Obesity. In B. Goldberg (Ed.), *Sports and Exercise for Children with Chronic Health Conditions*. Champaign, IL, Human Kinetics, pp. 335–54.

Summary

Some body fat is essential for normal physiological function but an over-accumulation is associated with increased morbidity and mortality from a variety of metabolic diseases. Recent years have seen major advances in methodologies for estimating body fatness but assessment during childhood and adolescence remains problematic. Adult-derived equations for converting body density determined during underwater weighing, or skinfolds to percentage body fat are inappropriate with young people and youth-generated equations require further validation. Stature–mass indices provide some useful information regarding changes in body composition with growth but are unable to distinguish between fat and lean components of body composition. MRI is an ethical, non-invasive means of quantifying subcutaneous and internal fat deposition in young subjects, but it is too expensive for routine use.

Adult over-fatness and obesity are an increasing problem in the Western world and there is evidence of a corresponding rise in childhood and adolescent overweight. Juvenile obesity is associated with various immediate health problems and appears predictive of adult obesity and CHD. In adults, abdominal fat deposition is highly related to increased risk of CHD. Young people appear to deposit less fat intra-abdominally than adults and no reliable anthropometric correlates of abdominal fat have been identified for this population.

The aerobic fitness of obese children and adolescents is not well documented but the available data indicate that cardiopulmonary function and aerobic fitness are not necessarily impaired in obese youngsters. Although the data are equivocal they suggest that obese young people are less physically active than their non-obese peers. However, because of their greater body mass obese youngsters may well have higher energy expenditures than young people of normal body mass. Exercise training may elicit reductions in body fatness, particularly with concurrent dietary modification, although follow-up studies indicate high recidivism. Increased physical activity may also have positive effects on blood lipid profile, blood pressure, and glucose metabolism. Exercise prescription for obese youth should emphasize increasing daily energy expenditure rather than aerobic fitness. Lifestyle modification is likely to be essential to long-term success in obesity management.

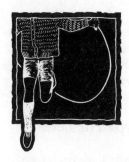

11
Physical activity and diabetes

Diabetes mellitus results from the failure of the mechanisms which regulate blood glucose levels.[1101] In diabetic individuals, the ability to secrete insulin is absent or grossly impaired resulting in elevated blood glucose levels and tissue starvation of carbohydrate. Muscle cells are forced to rely upon fat and protein predominantly mobilized from muscle and adipose tissue stores, causing the progressive wasting characteristic of untreated diabetes. In untreated diabetic patients the high levels of fatty acid mobilization lead to the production of ketone bodies which accumulate in the blood. If diabetes continues untreated the accumulation of ketones causes metabolic acidosis, coma, and eventually death will ensue. The excess glucose in the blood of diabetics exceeds the kidney's capacities for dealing with it and glucose 'spills over' into the urine (glycosuria). The presence of glucose in the urine is thus one of the simplest diagnostic tests for diabetes.

Young people who spontaneously develop diabetes most frequently suffer from type I or insulin-dependent diabetes mellitus (IDDM) which is one of the most common chronic disorders among children and adolescents. The condition may also develop later in adult life, usually after the age of 40 years, and is then termed maturity onset, type II or non-insulin dependent diabetes mellitus (NIDDM). Type I diabetes is characterized by such a severe deficiency or even absence of insulin production that exogenous administration of the hormone is essential to control blood glucose levels and prevent death. IDDM appears in genetically predisposed individuals due to either an autoimmune reaction or damage to pancreatic cells resulting from an environmental factor such as a viral infection.[1101] Aside from the immediate problems associated with the disturbance to glucose homeostasis, diabetics are at increased risk of numerous long-term medical complications, including non-atherosclerotic and atherosclerotic heart disease, neuropathy, nephropathy, and retinopathy.[732]

Adult onset, type II diabetes is frequently associated with obesity and has strong familial links.[801] Frank insulin deficiency is not necessarily involved, but rather there is a reduction in the cell receptor sites for insulin. This reduces the uptake of the hormone and attenuates its regulatory effects. Although symptoms of insulin deficiency develop, a programme of weight loss, dietary modification, and hypoglycaemic drugs will often adequately control the diabetes without the need for exogenous insulin.[1101] However, poorly controlled type II diabetics are at high risk of developing vascular diseases such as atherosclerosis, kidney disease, and coronary disease.[599, 801] Both IDDM and NIDDM damage the microcirculation leading to major vascular damage in organs such as kidneys, eyes, and peripheral nerves.

Physical activity in the management of type I diabetes

The blood glucose lowering properties of physical activity have been recognized for many centuries and even after the discovery of insulin the incorporation of an exercise programme into the diabetes management of juveniles has been strongly advocated.[772] With the addition of diet, this triad (insulin, activity, and diet) underpins the management of type I diabetes[732, 801]. However, the research evidence documenting the precise nature and extent of both immediate and long-term benefits of regular physical activity upon diabetes in young people is relatively scarce and the results equivocal.

Glucose homeostasis during exercise

In normal individuals, insulin levels progressively fall during exercise whilst glucagon levels are maintained (at moderate exercise intensities) or increased (during high-intensity or prolonged exercise). The falling insulin levels also affect other aspects of energy metabolism, facilitating lipid oxidation, and providing amino acid precursors for hepatic gluconeogenesis. These hormonal changes ensure that blood glucose levels remain relatively constant through balancing rates of peripheral utilization of glucose with hepatic gluconeogenesis. Exercise in the diabetic individual does not produce declining insulin levels and this carefully matched regulatory mechanism fails. If exercise is undertaken within a short time of insulin administration, plasma levels of the hormone may actually increase subsequent to an enhanced absorption of insulin from the subcutaneous injection site[177, 178, 802] as a result of mechanical stimulation of the site.[548] This effect is pronounced if the injection site is close to the exercising muscles.[841] By avoiding exercise within 60–90 min of an insulin injection this effect can be minimized.[732] Although a residual level of insulin is required during exercise to optimize muscular glucose uptake[801] the sustained elevation seen in exercising diabetics has serious metabolic consequences. The major effect is an inhibition of hepatic glycogenolysis and gluconeogenesis[1714] such that glucose utilization is not matched with hepatic glucose production and blood glucose levels fall eventually resulting in hypoglycaemia. This effect is accentuated in diabetic individuals whose glucagon response to hypoglycaemia is deficient[732] and may occur more frequently in individuals undergoing intensive insulin therapy or where the diabetes is very tightly controlled.[313, 888] The risk of developing hypoglycaemia during prolonged exercise may be minimized by decreasing insulin dosage prior to exercise and consuming supplementary carbohydrate throughout the exercise bout.

Post-exercise hypoglycaemia is a problem for diabetics. Insulin sensitivity may be increased for several hours after exercise increasing the risk of hypoglycaemia occurring during this period or even the following day. It has been shown in a prospective study of 300 young diabetics followed for two years that 16% experienced late-onset post-exercise hypoglycaemia, frequently occurring at night, some 6–15 h post-exercise.[934] The causes of this delayed hypoglycaemia are not well understood but most likely result from continuous glucose uptake and replenishment of energy stores within the exercised muscles.[212, 413]

During high-intensity exercise (exceeding 80% peak $\dot{V}O_2$) blood glucose levels in normal individuals increase transiently in response to the hormonal changes which produce a marked stimulation of hepatic glucose production.[732] Glucose levels reach a peak 5–15 min post-exercise and return to pre-exercise levels within an hour.[1046] On cessation of exercise, insulin levels rise rapidly to counteract glucose production, enhance glucose uptake and return blood levels to normal. In undiagnosed and poorly controlled diabetics with elevated glucose levels and inadequate insulin these regulatory mechanisms fail and hyperglycaemia worsens. In individuals treated with continuous, subcutaneous infusions of insulin the magnitude of post-exercise hyperglycaemia has been shown to be related to pre-exercise glucose levels.[1046] The explanation for this phenomenon may be the absence of the post-exercise 'rebound' insulin response during the recovery periods.[180] Due to these effects, management of glucose is more complicated for the diabetic participating in sports which require short, intense bursts of activity than for moderate, sustained activity. Careful, frequent monitoring of blood glucose levels during such activities is essential to minimize the risk of hyper- or hypoglycaemic states. Small doses of insulin following exercise may be necessary if hyperglycaemia develops.[733] In cases of severe insulin deficiency and hyperglycaemia, failure of the glucose regulatory changes during exercise may precipitate the development of ketosis as a result of increased lipolysis in response to hypoinsulinaemia.[732, 801]

Despite the metabolic hazards faced by the diabetic individual, there are good reasons for promoting physical activity in this population. Accelerated atherosclerotic disease is a common long-term outcome of diabetes with many diabetics dying prematurely from stroke or coronorary heart disease (CHD).[801, 1101, 1581] Physical activity may therefore be beneficial in ameliorating adverse lipid profiles, reducing hypertension, increasing aerobic fitness and increasing insulin sensitivity in the same way as in normal individuals,[1335] (see also Chapters 7 and 9).

Aerobic fitness of diabetic children and adolescents

Non-atherosclerotic CHD (cardiomyopathy) leading to congestive heart disease and heart failure is a complication of adult diabetes[542] and pre-clinical signs of myocardial dysfunction during exercise testing in adolescents have been observed in some studies[977, 1571] leading authors to suggest that this might be the explanation for the lower levels of aerobic fitness observed in these same individuals. Other studies have failed to identify incipient cardiomyopathy in adolescents.[1270] Furthermore, it has been suggested that diabetic individuals may be reluctant to participate in vigorous physical activity fearing a severe hypoglycaemic reaction.[754, 1589] Documentation of the physical activity patterns of diabetic children is extremely scarce, however, an indirect measure of physical activity as reflected by participation in athletic activities within and outside school concluded that diabetic children participated as often as their non-diabetic counterparts.[1646] Given these findings it is of interest whether or not impaired aerobic fitness is intrinsic to diabetes.

Investigations into the aerobic fitness of diabetic children and adolescents have produced equivocal findings. Many studies have included small sample sizes, sometimes of mixed sex or with the control or non-diabetic group not adequately matched for age, anthropometric characteristics, and sex making it difficult to draw definitive conclusions.

Several studies of aerobic fitness in young diabetics have reported peak $\dot{V}O_2$ values not significantly different from those observed in non-diabetic individuals of comparable age.[297, 391, 667, 1158, 1270] However, conflicting results have also been obtained with reports of lower aerobic fitness in diabetic individuals.[109, 298] One of the earliest studies to investigate aerobic fitness in diabetic youth used a submaximal cycle ergometer test[497] and indicated an age and size-related effect in 6–16-year-old subjects, with young diabetic boys having lower aerobic fitness than non-diabetic boys with no significant differences apparent in the older subjects. In the female subjects, the reverse was observed with significantly lower aerobic fitness being demonstrated only in the older diabetic girls.

In several of the studies indicating lower peak $\dot{V}O_2$ in diabetic youngsters, a programme of regular aerobic training has significantly enhanced their fitness, raising peak $\dot{V}O_2$ to a level comparable with the non-diabetic controls.[298, 874] Where pre-training fitness levels have been the same in diabetic and control groups, peak $\dot{V}O_2$ has been shown to both increase[297] or fail to change[391] although the training stimulus in the latter study may have been inadequate in view of recent recommendations.[1309] Surprisingly, improved peak $\dot{V}O_2$ has been noted with only one training session per week for either 3 months in 16 8–17-year-olds[746] or 5 months in 6 diabetic adolescent boys.[878]

Despite some conflicting results, recent studies indicate that aerobic fitness levels in diabetic young people are comparable with the non-diabetic population and diabetic children appear to be as trainable as non-diabetics. The disparate findings may be due more to methodological inconsistencies than to physiological or metabolic effects.

Physical activity and diabetic control

The level of glycosylated haemoglobin (Hb A_1) in the blood is an important gauge of diabetic control. Haemoglobin (Hb) has a high affinity for glucose which attaches to the haemoglobin molecule when blood glucose levels are elevated. The higher the blood glucose, the more Hb A_1 is formed. The attachment of the glucose molecule displaces 2,3-diphosphoglycerate (2,3-DPG), interfering with the oxygen affinity of the Hb molecules. This reduces oxygen delivery to tissues, a situation which is exacerbated by the already low level of 2,3-DPG observed in diabetic individuals.[1101] As red blood cells have an average life-span of 120 days, Hb A_1 levels provide a sensitive index of glycaemic control over the previous 6–8 weeks. Levels of Hb A_1 around 8.5–10% are typical in diabetics with lower levels indicative of good control.[211]

Several studies have investigated the effect of a prolonged period of structured physical activity upon diabetic control as reflected by Hb A_1 but the findings are inconclusive. Some studies have observed improved control after a period of regular physical training in diabetic children and adolescents[391] whilst others have noted an absence of change.[746, 1473] Although the divergent results from these studies might, in part, be attributed to an insufficient training stimulus, other well-controlled studies whose training programmes satisfy current guidelines[1309] have shown disparate findings in both supporting[297] and refuting[298, 874, 1272] improved glycaemic control.

The results of these studies must be interpreted cautiously in view of the small, often mixed sex, samples involved which inevitably preclude firm conclusions. In addition, it is apparent that in those studies eliciting improvements, pre-training glycaemic control was often poor[297, 391] whereas those showing no change demonstrated better control prior to the training programme.[746, 874] These findings suggest that the extent of amelioration of diabetic control is directly related to the degree of control pre-training.[1589] In addition, the metabolic importance of the small (e.g. 1.2%), but statistically significant, improvements in control is questionable.[297] Furthermore, many factors other than physical activity affect glycaemic control particularly management of glucose levels prior to the training sessions, for example, reductions in insulin dosage and increases in carbohydrate consumption both influence long-term glycaemic control. The extent to which these variables have been controlled for in the various studies is not always evident further confounding interpretation of the results. However, on the basis of the studies presented here it would appear that regular physical activity *per se*, has a minor role in the daily management of glycaemic control.

Despite these inconclusive findings, several studies have noted relationships between aerobic fitness and glycaemic control (Hb A$_1$) in diabetic adolescents[109, 1175] indicating that for this specific measure of diabetic control, optimizing aerobic fitness may be a more significant factor than regular physical activity.

Physical activity and insulin sensitivity

Vigorous exercise enhances glucose tolerance for a period of several days and induces increased insulin sensitivity for a considerable period post-exercise.[801, 1589] Muscular activity and insulin act synergistically to increase glucose uptake over and above the rates produced by each factor independently.[138, 1589] Regular physical activity thus enables diabetic individuals to increase carbohydrate consumption without a concomitant increase in injected insulin requirement.[138] This effect has frequently been reported to occur seasonally where increased reported physical activity during summer vacations can permit a more than halving of daily insulin requirements.[754, 763] Similar effects have been noted in children participating in special camps which focus on raising physical activity levels.[280]

Physical activity, diabetes, and blood lipids

Of the many complications associated with diabetes, CHD occurs frequently, at an earlier age, and is the most common cause of death in diabetics.[603, 1101] This risk is enhanced by the hypertension, hyperglycaemia, and dyslipidaemia frequently observed in diabetics.[603]

Until recently, dyslipidaemia, notably increased levels of low-density lipoproteins (LDL), very low-density lipoproteins (VLDL), and triglycerides, has received little attention as an independent risk factor in diabetics as high cholesterol levels are apparently no more prevalent in diabetic than non-diabetic adults.[603] However, abnormalities in the composition and metabolism of lipoproteins unique to diabetes are a concern and it as been suggested that cholesterol levels in diabetics should be reduced to levels lower than recommended for normal individuals, with even lower targets set for children.[603]

As in normal adults, training appears to ameliorate the blood lipid profile of IDDM adults as evidenced by an increase in the ratio of HDL to LDL, and decreased LDL.[1589] Limited evidence suggests that triglycerides may be reduced in diabetic children subsequent to a 5 month programme of 'hard physical activity of increasing intensity'.[879]

Several studies have examined the relationships between diabetic control, physical activity and lipid levels. In adults with poor control, increased levels of the ratios total cholesterol/HDL and free fatty acid (FFA)/albumin have been observed[153] with physical activity serving to reduce the ratio of total cholesterol to HDL. Improved diabetic control alone has been shown to evoke a rise in HDL levels[976] although in young people with adequate control, a sedentary lifestyle is associated with increased ratios of total cholesterol to HDL, and FFA to albumin.[153] Therefore, although both physical activity and improved glycaemic control appear to improve the blood lipid profile of diabetics, each acts independently. A 12 week aerobic training programme incorporating three exercise sessions per week resulted in a reduction in LDL levels in young diabetics.[298] However, there were no relationships detected between any of the blood lipids measured and Hb A_1 either before or after training despite a significant improvement in glycaemic control. Whereas in non-diabetic children and adolescents, peak aerobic fitness is unrelated to lipid levels,[78] (and see Chapter 9), as for glycaemic control, fitness may be an important correlate of lipid levels in diabetic adolescents.[109]

Physical activity guidelines for diabetic young people

Despite the potential hazards, increased physical activity may confer significant benefits to diabetic young people. Aerobic fitness appears to correlate with indices of diabetic control and blood lipid levels and there appear to be no intrinsic reasons why diabetic children and adolescents should not attain normal levels of aerobic fitness. Increased physical activity also has much to offer young diabetics in terms of increased psychological well-being, particularly as these individuals are learning to take responsibility for a serious, chronic disease.[733]

Practical guidelines for the management of diabetes within exercise, particularly strategies for avoiding hypo- or hyperglycaemic responses are widely available.[454, 732, 733, 1589] A synopsis of the key recommendations relating to pre-exercise blood glucose levels and strategies to counter hypo- and hyperglycaemia are presented in Tables 11.1 and 11.2.

Planned, regular physical activity of moderate intensity is preferable to sporadic periods of high-intensity exercise[454] and the guidelines presented in Table 7.6 may be considered equally suitable for diabetic individuals. Where exercise sessions are planned, the individual is able to more accurately anticipate and adjust carbohydrate and insulin requirements. The need for the young person to be in good glycaemic control cannot be overemphasized and medical evaluation of diabetic status, with particular reference to glycaemic control and other contraindications to exercise, such as autonomic neuropathy or cardiomyopathy, is essential prior to

Table 11.1. Recommendations for physical activity based upon pre-exercise blood glucose levels

Blood glucose level	Action
Lower than 5.5 mmol·L⁻¹	Consume extra carbohydrates
Between 5.5 and 14 mmol·L⁻¹	Safe range for exercise
Higher than 14 mmol·L⁻¹	Check urinary ketones. If negative exercise is usually safe. If positive administer insulin and delay exercise until ketones are negative and blood glucose is less than 14 mmol·L⁻¹

Adapted from Wallberg-Henriksson, H. (1992). Exercise and diabetes mellitus. *Exercise and Sport Sciences Reviews*, **20**, 339–68, and Horton, E.S. (1995). Diabetes mellitus. In B. Goldberg (Ed.), *Sports and Exercise for Children with Chronic Health Conditions*. Champaign, IL, Human Kinetics, pp. 355–73.

Table 11.2. Strategies to avoid hypo- or hyperglycaemia during or post-exercise

Adjustments to insulin regime

Administer insulin at least 1 h prior to exercise. If less than this, use a site away from the exercising muscles

Reduce the dose of both short- and intermediate-acting insulin before exercise

Where exercise is regular (>3 times per week) total insulin dose may be reduced

Adjustments to diet

Eat a meal 1–3 h before exercise

If exercise continues longer than 30 min consume an extra 15–30 g of carbohydrate every 30 min

Following prolonged, vigorous activity increase food intake for up to 24 h post-exercise to avoid late-onset hypoglycaemia

Monitoring glucose and ketones

Check blood glucose before, during, and after exercise and adjust insulin and food intake accordingly

Postpone exercise if blood glucose is <5.5 mmol·L⁻¹ or >14 mmol·L⁻¹, or if ketones are present. Correct metabolic control prior to exercise

Note individual metabolic responses to exercise of different types and intensities at different times of day

Note individual metabolic responses to training and competition

Adapted from Wallberg-Henriksson, H. (1992). Exercise and diabetes mellitus. *Exercise and Sport Sciences Reviews*, **20**, 339–68, and Horton, E.S. (1995). Diabetes mellitus. In B. Goldberg (Ed.), *Sports and Exercise for Children with Chronic Health Conditions*. Champaign, IL, Human Kinetics, pp. 355–73.

increasing physical activity. Certainly, in the presence of excessive hyper-glycaemic or ketotic states exercise is absolutely contraindicated until glycaemic control has been restored through appropriate insulin therapy.

Summary

Diabetes mellitus arises from the failure of the normal blood glucose regulatory mechanisms, specifically insufficient or absent insulin produc-tion. Diabetic individuals are at risk of developing long-term medical complications including heart disease, neuropathy, nephropathy, and ret-inopathy. The recognized blood glucose lowering properties of exercise has led to its incorporation into diabetes treatment strategies in conjunction with dietary modification and insulin administration. Exercise in diabetic individuals does not initiate the normal hormonal changes which ensure stable blood glucose levels and steps must be taken to reduce likelihood of the development of hypo- or hyperglycaemia. Although some studies have indicated impaired aerobic fitness in diabetics others have failed to identify differences compared with normal subjects. Diabetic children and adoles-cents appear as trainable as their non-diabetic counterparts. Increased physical activity has not been shown to consistently improve diabetic con-trol as reflected by glycolysated haemoglobin but insulin sensitivity may be enhanced allowing exogenous insulin administration to be reduced. Exer-cise training has beneficial effects upon the unfavourable blood lipid pro-files observed in diabetic young people and in contrast to non-diabetics, aerobic fitness may be correlated with blood lipid levels. Although in-creased physical activity and exercise training do not appear to improve directly the diabetic state, planned, regular physical activity plays an im-portant role in the management of the many medical complications associ-ated with the condition.

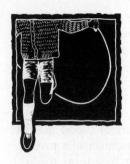

12
Physical activity and skeletal health

Skeletal health

Bone is a dynamic living tissue which is continually being remodelled. From childhood through adolescence and into early adult life bone is deposited faster than it is broken down, and bones become larger and more dense. The remodelling process then reverses its direction, bone mineral is resorbed and excreted faster than it is deposited and bone mineral content falls progressively from its peak value.[537, 990] This process continues into old age and, through an accelerated decline of bone mass following the menopause, women have a fracture prevalence six times greater than in men in most populations.[687, 777, 1209]

Osteoporosis is characterized by low bone mass and microarchitectural deterioration of bony tissue, leading to enhanced bone fragility and a consequent increase in fracture risk.[346] It is widely recognized as a major public health problem[1276, 1688] and current evidence indicates that the incidence of osteoporosis is likely to increase in the future for both men and women.[881, 1023]

Bone mineral density (BMD) in the elderly is dependent upon peak BMD attained during growth and maturation, maintenance of BMD during mid life and loss of BMD in later years.[329, 741] Failure to attain a sufficient level of BMD during growth and maturation may contribute significantly to low BMD in older populations.[740, 741, 1198] As no current treatment can significantly restore the amount of bone lost in severe osteoporosis emphasis should be placed upon maximizing peak BMD and reducing subsequent bone loss.[537] Promotion of skeletal health and the prevention of osteoporosis should therefore begin in childhood and adolescence.[491, 537, 926]

Skeletal maturation

The continual remodelling of bone is controlled by the action of osteoblasts and osteoclasts which cause bone formation and bone resorption, respectively. The rate of remodelling is governed by hormones and factors, such as skeletal loading (e.g. through physical activity) and nutrition. BMD progressively increases from birth through childhood and adolescence into early adult life but adolescence appears to be a very important period for the development of bone mass in both boys[1210] and girls.[1521] Studies of adolescents have consistently reported marked increases in BMD during

Table 12.1.   Factors affecting bone mineral density (BMD) and risk of osteoporosis

---

• Peak BMD attained during childhood,
  adolescence, and early adult life

• Maintenance of BMD during mid life

• Loss of BMD in later years

---

puberty although the size of increase varies according to skeletal site.[1421] Increases in BMD ranging between 15 and 75% of total adult value in girls[218, 620, 808] and between 5 and 70% of total adult value in boys[218, 808] have been reported.

The wide variation in the data reported can be attributed in part to confounding factors such as hormonal milieu,[1421] genetics,[984] the anti-osteogenic effects of cigarette smoking,[1419] inadequate nutrition,[152] and physical inactivity.[118] However, data generated using different techniques must be interpreted cautiously and methodological differences cannot be ignored.[1181] For example, projectional methods of determining BMD such as dual X-ray absorptiometry (DEXA) provide areal densities which are confounded by size changes accompanying growth.[115] Larger bones resulting from growth will yield a higher areal BMD measurement than smaller bones of a similar density because volumetric change resulting from increasing bone depth is not considered. Quantified computerized tomography (QTC) is therefore a superior method of assessing BMD as it provides real volumetric values. As the DEXA method can overestimate values of BMD and the values recorded by QTC indicate about a 15% volume BMD increase in adolescent girls[621] it has been suggested that increases of this order during puberty are a more realistic expectation.[808]

The age at which peak BMD is achieved is unclear. Cross-sectional studies suggest an age period of reaching peak BMD in males between 16 and 25 years and in females between 16 and 23 years.[269, 620, 624] Recent longitudinal studies indicate that in females the age of peak BMD is reached around 30 years of age[404, 1199] but few data appear to be available for males.[537] The differences reported are probably due to methodological factors including the skeletal site assessed[1421] but it is safe to conclude that overall peak BMD is not achieved before about 30 years of age.[537]

Assessment of skeletal maturity

All children progress from a skeleton of cartilage prenatally to a fully developed adult skeleton of bone. As both the beginning and endpoints of maturation are known and the ossification process of bones occurs in a reasonably consistent pattern, skeletal age provides a convenient indicator of maturity status. In association with chronological age skeletal age can be used to determine whether a child is biologically advanced or delayed. In the exercise sciences skeletal age has been used to examine the relationship between biological maturity and variables, such as peak $\dot{V}O_2$.[809, 849, 1387]

Because calcified cartilage and bone are radiopaque the progress of the skeleton to maturity can be monitored through a series of radiographs. The hand–wrist is reasonably typical of the whole skeleton and it is these bones which are normally evaluated[655, 1222, 1505] although other joints such as the knee[1224] have also been used. The initial appearance of specific bone centres is noted and the characterization of each bone by gradual shape differentiation as it progresses to the adult form is examined.

For the evaluation of skeletal age two principal techniques have been used. In the atlas method popularized by Greulich and Pyle,[655] a given radiograph plate is compared with a set of standard radiographs taken at ages ranging from birth to maturity. The bone-specific method of Tanner *et al.*,[1505] after Acheson,[4] relies on a series of written criteria for stages through which each bone passes. Both methods are limited by their reference population but provide useful markers of maturity which are related to both somatic and sexual maturity indicators (see Chapter 1). Girls are more advanced in skeletal maturity than boys and reach full skeletal maturity earlier, but neither physical activity nor exercise training have any apparent effect on skeletal maturity of the hand and wrist in either sex during the period 11–16 years.[960]

Hormonal milieu and skeletal health

The protective effect of oestrogen on bone has been well documented in women and during the years following the cessation of menses there is a rapid loss of bone associated with the decrease in endogenous oestrogen levels.[458, 926, 1432] There is no evidence that calcium supplementation or physical activity or a combination of the two can prevent this loss although the effectiveness of hormone replacement has been consistently demonstrated.[458] Similarly, the skeletal hazards associated with amenorrhoea in adults are well known[433, 913] but few studies have been carried out with adolescents despite the frequent observation of eating disorders, delayed menarche and/or amenorrhoea in girls who train intensively (see Chapter 14).

It has been demonstrated that amenorrhoeic adolescents have lumbar BMDs below that of normally menstruating girls.[1644] A later onset of menarche and reduced total oestrogen exposure have been associated with lower peak vertebral bone mass.[39] The lumbar and whole body BMD of anorexic girls, aged 12–20 years, have been shown to be significantly lower (18–26%) than that of healthy girls.[111] Physical activity does not protect against this type of osteopenia. Regardless of its origin, prolonged amenorrhoea in young females has adverse effects on skeletal health and the bone loss may not be reversible.[118, 926, 928]

Few studies have involved young males but a marked increase in serum testosterone has been observed to be followed by a rapid rise in forearm bone mineral content[846] and, in a retrospective study, delayed onset of puberty was associated with reduced BMD in men.[549] The effects of physical activity on hormonal status in boys are not well understood but studies carried out with adult males indicate that intensive exercise is associated with low levels of serum total and free testosterone[35] although this may not be the case with boys.[1267]

Nutrition and skeletal health

Although much of the variability in bone growth and mineral density may be attributed to hormonal status and to genetics[1172, 1420, 1424] peak BMD is also dependent upon environmental factors, particularly nutrition and physical activity. Adequate nutrition during childhood and adolescence is vital for optimal growth and maturation and sufficient calcium appears to be a prerequisite for skeletal health.[330, 537, 656] Low dietary phosphate levels are unusual in the Western world as almost all foods contain phosphates in organic or inorganic form. However, there is some concern that excessive phosphate intake may have a detrimental effect on BMD because diets high in phosphates and low in calcium have been shown to increase serum parathyroid hormone levels and therefore influence calcium regulation.[30, 294]

The amount of calcium required to allow bone to be mineralized is quite low and only severe restrictions in calcium intake lead to rickets and delayed growth[152, 894] but the potential benefits of calcium intakes above the minimum requirement are not well understood. The relationship between physical activity, calcium intake, and bone accretion in young people remains to be unravelled. Calcium appears to act as a threshold nutrient, where the threshold represents the level of nutrient intake below which some aspect of nutrient status is influenced by intake of the nutrient, and above which is independent of intake.[985] This may account for much of the inconsistency in the findings of both observational and prospective studies. The effect of calcium supplementation on the BMD of young people with dietary calcium intakes above the threshold level may not be appreciable.[658] It is, therefore, possible that some subjects in studies that did not detect a relationship between calcium and BMD may have had calcium intakes that met or exceeded the threshold, making detection of an association difficult.[152] It has been suggested that an optimal level of peak bone mass cannot be achieved by young people with average daily intakes of calcium below 1000 mg per day in males and 850 mg per day in females.[1150] Others have suggested higher thresholds of 1500 mg per day[700] and 1800 mg per day[984] but what constitutes the threshold level of calcium intake, if it exists, remains open to debate.

Matkovic and his colleagues[986] were among the first to draw attention to the importance of calcium intake to BMD. They examined the bone mass and fracture incidence of adults, aged 30–90 years, living in two regions in Croatia, one with a relatively high calcium intake (approaching 1000 mg per day) and the other with a low calcium intake (about 500 mg per day). The residents of the high calcium intake region had significantly higher BMD from the age of 30 years and a reduced incidence of fracture. It was suggested that the greater BMD in the high calcium region was due to a larger bone mass formed in childhood. The study was not well controlled and the results could have been confounded by other differences in diet such as protein and energy intake. It appears that the residents of the high calcium intake region were also more physically active than the population of the other region. Nevertheless, this study focused attention on the potential benefits of high calcium intakes to bone accretion.

Two more recent studies have retrospectively investigated the relationship between BMD and calcium intake during the early portion of the life cycle in pre-menopausal[676] and post-menopausal[1392] women. Both studies emphasized the apparent importance of adequate calcium nutrition during adolescence and early adulthood for the attainment of optimal bone mass.

The results of cross-sectional studies of BMD and calcium intake in healthy young people have been inconsistent. Some studies have reported a positive relationship between dietary calcium and BMD[323, 1365, 1547] whereas others have reported no association.[797, 1563, 1644] The equivocal findings can be attributed to a number of potentially confounding factors. For example, a wide age range of children and adolescents have been used as subjects[e.g. 323] and both BMD and calcium intakes are difficult to assess.[152] Reliable estimates of calcium intake require several days of monitoring[1037] and some studies have only assessed calcium intake over a short period,[e.g. 1644] whereas others have not provided sufficient detail of how calcium intake was assessed.[e.g. 797]

Prospective data on calcium intake and BMD during youth are sparse. Matkovic *et al.*[984] supplemented the diet of a small cohort of 14-year-old girls with milk or calcium carbonate but over a 2 year period they were unable to demonstrate a statistically significant difference in BMD between the experimental group and the control group. The authors suggested that their small sample size ($n = 28$) was inadequate, in terms of statistical power, to detect any differences between the two groups.

In an 18 month supplementation trial of 500 mg per day of calcium versus placebo, in 94 girls initially aged 11.9 years, significantly greater increases in lumbar spine BMD and whole body BMD were detected in the supplemented group.[912]

A three year study of supplementation with 1000 mg per day of calcium versus placebo was conducted with 45 pairs of identical twins.[764] Among the 22 pairs of twins who were prepubertal throughout the study the calcium supplemented twins demonstrated significantly greater increases in BMD at the radius and lumbar spine than the placebo groups. No benefit from calcium supplementation was observed among the 23 twin pairs who were either pubertal at the onset of the study or entered puberty during the study. The 22 prepubertal twin pairs were re-examined in a follow-up study one year after the cessation of calcium supplementation.[1422] The dietary calcium intake of the twins averaged 1020 mg per day and at the follow-up examination the significant differences between the previous supplemented and unsupplemented twins disappeared. It therefore seems likely that high calcium intakes need to be maintained for differences in BMD to persist.[152]

The Amsterdam Growth Study[805] provided a 15 year longitudinal analysis of the effect of daily calcium intake during adolescence and young adulthood on the development of peak bone mass at age 27 years. Dietary calcium intake was assessed longitudinally six times and a high calcium intake by boys during their teen years was related to high lumbar BMD at age 27 years. The association between BMD and calcium intake was not found in females.[1627] However, when the influence of body mass and mass-bearing physical activity was accounted for statistically calcium intake was found to be no longer a significant predictor of BMD in males.[1626]

Physical activity and skeletal health

Skeletal loading

In the nineteenth century, Julius Wolff noted that bone tissue reorganizes itself when mechanical forces change[972] and Wolff's law states,

the general form of bone being given, alterations to the internal architecture and external form occur as a consequence of primary changes in mechanical stress.[115, p. 97]

Bone mass adapts to the mechanical strain placed upon it by skeletal loading. Changes in internal strain in bone (i.e. the deformation that occurs in response to loading), seems to activate osteocytes which subsequently alter the sensitive balance between bone resorption and bone formation. Because of the highly invasive nature of measuring loads on bone surfaces *in vivo* data on young people are virtually non-existent and much of our knowledge is based on studies with animals. Nevertheless, the results are remarkably consistent and can be applied to humans with confidence.

Repeated application of skeletal loads which produce strain above a threshold level stimulate an increase in bone mass and enhanced structural and mechanical properties in proportion to the induced level of strain;[1278] an application of the principle of overload. This increased bone mass will have the effect of reducing the internal strain from a given load. The stimulus to further bone formation will therefore be reduced until an equilibrium is reached at which strain is normalized and a new balance between bone resorption and bone formation is achieved, but at an increased level of bone mass.[588, 589] This state continues until there are further increases in skeletal loading and the cycle repeats itself (i.e. progressive overload). At a fixed level of load per unit area (skeletal stress) more compliant immature bone experiences greater increases in bone formation than mature bone.[389, 1191]

Changes in bone mass are localized to the induced strain and there may be net bone formation and net bone loss occurring simultaneously in different parts of the skeleton.[118, 1432] Static stress (continuous applied loading) does not appear to be osteogenic and for optimal effect cyclic stress (intermittent loading) is required.[115, 331] However, if strains are intermittent, high in magnitude, and high in rate, few repetitions appear to be necessary to produce a substantial osteogenic effect.[1277]

Skeletal loading studies suggest that physical activity designed to increase BMD and bone strength should involve loads of high magnitude and high rate, should be intermittent in nature, and should involve varied and diverse patterns of stress. Relatively few loading cycles are required, so physical activity would not need to be sustained.[331] Traditionally, dynamic (intermittent), body mass-supporting physical activities such as walking, jogging, and running have been recommended for the promotion of skeletal health. Peak strain magnitudes during this type of physical activity are, however, not particularly high and strain distribution is not altered to a great degree.[331] Weight (resistance) training offers skeletal loading of high magnitude and varied patterns of stress, through lifting exercises with strain distributions which are different from those encountered in normal daily activities.[331] For example, the forces produced at the lumbar vertebrae during jogging are about 1.75 times body weight[302] compared with the five to six times body weight forces which have been reported during weight lifting activity.[646] In weight lifting, however, loading is more static in nature and is applied at lower rates than in activities such as running.

The role of physical activity during adult life in the prevention of osteoporosis has been extensively researched and a number of comprehensive reviews are available.[331, 457, 458, 665, 1432] The mode of physical activity that best promotes BMD is yet to be determined. Most studies have used body mass-supporting activities such as walking, running, and dancing as the activity intervention but when resistance exercise has been used a better osteogenic stimulus has often been observed.[1432] However, several of the studies which have employed resistance training have used highly selective groups and/or not screened for steroid use.[331]

Habitual physical activity and skeletal health

The problems associated with the assessment of habitual physical activity were discussed in Chapter 6 and studies relating habitual physical activity to skeletal health need to be viewed in this context. Several recent studies have used questionnaires to estimate current physical activity levels and all have reported positive associations with BMD.[206, 855, 1420, 1421, 1564] The relationships observed between physical activity and BMD have, however, been modest and site-specific. One study observed a positive relationship in boys but not in girls.[1564]

Studies employing retrospective questionnaires with adults and examining relationships between estimated physical activity during childhood and adolescence and adult BMD have reported equivocal findings. Significant relationships have been reported[353, 993, 1499, 1549] but one study failed to demonstrate a relationship[852] and another reported a relationship between childhood physical activity and adult BMD in girls but not in boys.[541]

A Dutch study[1626] focused on body mass-supporting activities estimated from six interviews during a 15 year longitudinal study. A significant association was observed between body mass-supporting activity and BMD in males but not in females and the effect of physical activity on BMD appeared to be dependent upon the amount of physical activity.

In a unique study Faulkner *et al.*[539] compared the BMD of dominant and non-dominant limbs in 124 girls and 110 boys, aged 8–16 years. The BMD of the dominant arm was significantly greater in both boys and girls but no significant differences in BMD were detected between dominant and non-dominant legs. The authors conclude that the greater BMD of the dominant arm was likely to be a result of increased tensile loading compared to the non-dominant arm. The similarity in BMD of the legs was probably due to a lack of biased stress in the legs as body mass support is generally an evenly distributed stress. The finding that the overall mean BMD of the arms was 0.62 g·cm^{-2} compared to an overall mean BMD of 0.94 g·cm^{-2} for the legs reinforces the importance of body mass-supporting activity on bone mineralization. (Table 12.2.)

Exercise training and skeletal health

Factors affecting the interpretation of exercise training studies have been discussed in Chapter 7 and the following discussion needs to be viewed in this context.

Little league baseball players have been shown to have significantly higher bone mineral content in their dominant humerus at all ages from 8–19 years.[1604] The high impact activity of gymnastics has often been suggested to be beneficial for bone health and BMD has consistently been

Table 12.2. Factors influencing the attainment of peak bone mineral density

- Genetics

- Early or late onset of puberty

- Menstrual dysfunction

- Hormonal status

- Cigarette smoking

- Nutrition

- Physical activity

demonstrated to be higher in young gymnasts than in swimmers or control subjects.[319, 659, 1104] Soccer may also promote skeletal health.[994] A study of élite male junior weightlifters found them to have 13–30% greater spine and femoral neck BMD than age-matched non-weightlifters.[345] Swimming does not appear to be as beneficial to skeletal health as body mass-supporting activities.[319, 659, 994, 1104]

In what appears to be the only controlled, prospective study of exercise training on the skeletal health of adolescents Blimkie *et al*.[205] studied the effects of resistance training on the BMD of healthy girls after the onset of menstruation. Thirty five girls between 14 and 18 years of age, matched for age, body mass, and sports participation were randomized into either a training ($n = 17$) or a control ($n = 18$) group. A 26 week training programme consisted of four sets of 13 exercises of varying and progressive resistance performed three times weekly on hydraulic resistance machines. Despite significant increases in strength no significant changes in whole body BMD or lumbar spine BMD were detected in the training group at the end of the 26 week period. A significant mid point increase (4.6%) in lumbar spine BMD had been observed but it proved to be transient. (Table 12.3.)

Adaptations to de-training

Observations of de-training effects with children and adolescents are not available but adult studies have demonstrated that following a period of de-training BMD regresses towards its pre-training value.[e.g. 392] De-training effects, however, may be reflected by periods of immobilization and studies with children have clearly demonstrated the detrimental effects of immobility and inactivity on the skeleton.[116, 706]

Table 12.3. Summary of findings relating physical activity to skeletal health during childhood and adolescence

---

Prospective exercise training studies
No evidence of changes in BMD

Comparison of trained and untrained subjects
Evidence of a positive association between
body mass-supporting sport participation and BMD

Relationship with habitual physical activity
Evidence of a modest, positive association between
body mass-supporting physical activity and BMD

Comparison of dominant and non-dominant limbs
Evidence of a positive association between
limb dominance and BMD

Risks of exercise training

Several studies with adults have demonstrated that extremely high training loads may have a detrimental effect on bone.[331, 1432] It has been suggested that there may be a threshold level of exercise that stimulates bone formation, with higher levels of exercise having less effect as altered hormone responses override the load-induced stimulus for bone formation.[331] Data on children and adolescents are not available.

Exercise prescription

The development of optimum BMD is complex and, on the basis of the available scientific evidence, it is not possible to confidently prescribe a specific exercise programme for the promotion of skeletal health. However, some prudent recommendations can be offered.

The maintenance of skeletal integrity is a lifetime task and young people should be encouraged to make a lifelong commitment to a balanced programme of physical activity. Emphasis should be placed upon body mass-supporting (e.g. running, skipping) rather than body mass-supported (e.g. cycling, swimming) activities. Short, intense bouts of regular physical activity are likely to be more beneficial than infrequent, prolonged activity, some resistance training may be beneficial, and immobilization should be avoided whenever possible. If bedrest is inevitable (e.g. during sickness) even brief daily body mass-supporting or resistance activity may help to prevent a reduction in BMD.

Physical activity is only one of the factors which influence skeletal health and young people should avoid cigarette smoking and disordered eating patterns. A well-balanced diet which provides adequate protein and energy is important and sufficient calcium is vital for the development of BMD. Adolescence appears to be a period, at least with girls, where calcium intake may fall substantially as the consumption of low calorie soft drinks increases.[416, 926]

Diets designed to maintain calcium levels are available elsewhere.[e.g. 656] The importance of adequate calcium intake cannot be overemphasized and physical activity may be ineffectual in promoting skeletal health if calcium level falls below its threshold value.

Summary

Bone is continually being modelled and remodelled and BMD in mid- and late-adult life is dependent upon peak BMD which is probably attained by the age of 30 years. Appropriate hormonal status and adequate phosphate and calcium intake appear to be prerequisites for optimal bone mineralization. The optimal level of calcium intake during growth and maturation remains to be determined and whether physical activity influences the threshold for calcium intake has not been systematically studied.[152] The positive effects of calcium intake and physical activity on bone accretion may be independent[1199, 1549] but it is likely that adequate calcium is an important enabling factor in physical activity-related effects on BMD.[776] The interaction between hormonal milieu and physical activity appears to be dependent upon the intensity of the activity. Physical activity, however, is unlikely to compensate for the osteopenic effects of low levels of oestrogen or testosterone.[118]

Mechanical loading of bone increases BMD. For optimum effects intermittent skeletal loads of high magnitude and high rate are necessary. Body mass-supporting activities, such as walking and running, have been recommended but resistance training may provide a better osteogenic stimulus. Studies investigating the effects of physical activity on young people's skeletal health are sparse and generally not well controlled. Nevertheless, there are indications that body mass-supporting physical activities induce increases in BMD although the case for resistance training during childhood and adolescence remains to be proven. A period of immobilization has detrimental effects on skeletal health.

A specific exercise prescription for the promotion of young people's skeletal health cannot be recommended on the basis of current data. However, children and adolescents should be encouraged to avoid cigarette smoking, to maintain an adequate calcium intake, and to engage in a range of body mass-supporting physical activities.

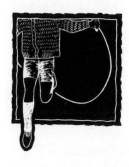

13

Physical activity and mental health

Mental health

Mental illness is a serious and often underestimated cause of distress and disability. Approximately 30–40% of adults in the Western world experience psychiatrically significant mental problems during their lifetime[1218, 1258] although only about 20% of those who suffer seek professional help.[1369] Mental illness accounts for an estimated 14% of certificated sickness absence, 14% of National Health Service (NHS) inpatient costs, and 4% of NHS pharmaceutical costs in the United Kingdom.[417] In the United States mental illness is estimated to account for 8–15% of the nation's health budget.[1258] Although mental illness is not normally associated with young people the UK Department of Health[417] suggests that,

The mental health of children and adolescents is a particularly important area as many are vulnerable to physical, intellectual, emotional, social or behavioural developmental disorders which, if not treated, may have serious implications for adult life.[417, p. 83]

In Western society, mental health problems among young people have been reported to have an incidence of 5–20%, depending on the population surveyed and the severity threshold employed.[1258, 1283, 1579] The incidence of depression rises in adolescence and major depression is found in 2–8% of young people, particularly among females.[418] Boys are much more likely than girls to show disorders of anxiety and sleep[444] whereas eating disorders are 8–11 times more common in girls.[419, 1115] Bulimia nervosa and anorexia nervosa are the principal eating disorders and their onset peaks in adolescence[418] (and see Chapter 14).

Girls are more likely to attempt self-harm than boys[418, 602] but suicide is more common in young males.[698] Against national trends in other age groups suicide rates among adolescent males in England have risen in recent years.[418] This presents a particular challenge to the Health of the Nation initiative[417] which has identified prevention of suicide as one of its key targets.

Children and adolescents themselves are not immune to mental health problems, and it has been suggested that adult mental health problems may have a childhood onset or origin.[444, 1258] *Mens sana in corpore sano*, a healthy mind in a healthy body, is a concept to which we subscribe and although

Physical activity and health

Table 13.1. Exercise and mental health

• Physical fitness is positively associated with mental health and well-being

• Exercise is associated with reduced state anxiety

• Exercise is associated with a decreased level of mild to moderate depression and anxiety

• Long-term exercise is usually associated with reductions in traits such as neurosis and anxiety

• Exercise results in reductions in various stress indices

• Severe depression usually requires professional treatment but exercise may act as an adjunct

• Exercise has beneficial emotional effects across all ages in both sexes

---

Consensus statement of the National Institute of Mental Health, adapted from Morgan, W.P. and Goldston, S.E. (1987). *Exercise and Mental Health.* Washington, DC, Hemisphere Publishing, p. 156.

Part III is primarily focused on physical health and well-being it would be remiss of us not to address briefly the role of physical activity in the promotion of mental health and well-being.

Physical activity and mental health

The use of physical activity to promote mental health is not a new concept and Hippocrates is known to have prescribed exercise for patients suffering from mental illness.[1283] In recent years there has been a surge of interest in the possible benefits of physical activity to mental health in the adult population[257, 442, 1111, 1393, 1509] and the National Institute of Mental Health in the United States has published a consensus statement on the topic (Table 13.1).

At the time the statement was agreed in 1984, the comment, 'exercise has beneficial emotional effects across all ages in both sexes' was largely conjecture as little was known of the effect of physical activity on young people's mental health.[see 261] Although data from children and adolescents are now less sparse very few well-designed studies possessing good external and internal validity have been conducted. In general, the extant literature on physical activity and mental health consists primarily of descriptive, correlational, and cross-sectional studies in which association may be indicated but causality is not resolved. Common methodological problems include the use of inadequate sample sizes, the failure to assign subjects

Table 13.2. Potential mechanisms for an association between physical activity and mental health

---

- **Biochemical hypothesis** physical activity induces chemical changes (perhaps involving amines and/or endorphins) known to improve mood

- **Thermogenic hypothesis** physical activity causes an elevation of body temperature which reduces anxiety and induces a sensation of well-being

- **Distraction hypothesis** physical activity diverts attention away from environmental stressors

- **Self-significance hypothesis** participation in physical activity fosters feelings of mastery and competence

- **Control hypothesis** stresses created by physical activity are seen as stable and improvements can be clearly seen and achieved

---

randomly to experimental conditions, the absence of a placebo or control group, the failure to utilize double-or-total blind designs, and the use of different criterion measures.[257, 1434] The Hawthorn Effect (i.e. any treatment may induce an effect because the subjects are aware of it), which is problematic in studies in which psychological and behavioural responses serve as the dependent variable,[350] has often been ignored.[257, 444] Additional issues which have arisen in paediatric studies include the challenge of accurately assessing physical activity in this population (see Chapter 6), high attrition rates, and the use of measures which have been developed with adults and not validated with children and adolescents. Most studies have used white, middle, or upper-middle class, urban subjects, making generalizations to other socioeconomic and ethnic groups problematic.[293]

The casual mechanism or mechanism of any relationship between physical activity and mental health are unknown but a number of hypotheses have been proposed (see refs. 982, 1064, 1066, 1164, 1435, for detailed discussion). Potential mechanisms are unlikely to be totally independent of one another and there is still much to be learned about the relationship between physical activity and mental health (Table 13.2).

Physical activity: self-concept and self-esteem

According to Gruber[661, p. 30] 'self-concept is our perception of self and self-esteem is a value we place on our self-image'. Self-esteem is non-existent at birth and forms during childhood and adolescence. Its source is the interaction between the person and environmental/social experiences.[444]

Gruber[661] evaluated the relationship between physical activity and self-esteem through a meta-analysis[623, 1525] of 84 studies involving primarily prepubescent children. He concluded that physical activity enhances self-esteem. The effect was much greater in children with special needs (e.g. emotionally disturbed, trainable mentally retarded, economically disadvantaged, educable mentally retarded, or perceptually handicapped) than in normal children (effect sizes 0.57 and 0.34, respectively). This is probably an illustration of the principle that those in most need are likely to demonstrate the greatest gains. The other interesting point to emerge from Gruber's[661] review was that participants in physical fitness or aerobic activities showed a much greater improvement in self-esteem than participants in creative movement, sports skills, or perceptual-motor skills programmes (effect sizes 0.89, 0.32, 0.40, and 0.29, respectively).

Some of the studies analysed by Gruber[661] included youngsters who were probably adolescent and positive effects of physical activity on self-esteem were still apparent.[694, 845, 1000, 1010] A study of 98 14–18-year-old, incarcerated, juvenile delinquents demonstrated improved self-concept following a 12 week, three times per week aerobic exercise training programme[1011] but the attrition rate was high (30%). Another study with a high attrition rate investigated the effect of a 16 week, three times per week resistance training programme on a sample of 59 16-year-old girls.[730] Although poor adherence to the study reduced the resistance training group from 13 to only six subjects and the length of the programme to 12 weeks improved self-esteem was reported.

Calfas and Taylor[293] published an excellent review of the effects of physical activity on psychological variables in adolescents and of the 10 studies they identified as addressing self-esteem or self-concept a positive relationship or experimental effect was demonstrated in nine.[262, 557, 694, 725, 730, 845, 1000, 1011, 1337] They calculated effect sizes for controlled trials where experimental and control group means and standard deviations were provided. Effect size was calculated by subtracting the control group mean from the experimental group mean and dividing the difference by the pooled estimate of the standard deviation. Calfas and Taylor[293] commented that effect sizes calculated using a small number of studies should be interpreted with caution and reported a low effect size of 0.12. They concluded, however, that physical activity can contribute to the promotion of both children's and adolescents' self-esteem and self-concept.

Physical activity: intelligence and academic achievement

Kirkendall[822] comprehensively reviewed research associating physical activity with intellectual development and commented that,

In the 1950s and 1960s, physical educators were grasping for ways to justify exercise and physical education programs. If it could be shown that activity programs contributed to intellectual development, then they would gain credibility and be justified. Many studies aimed at showing this were conducted during the 1970s. Now it has become increasingly evident and accepted that exercise and physical activity programs are justified and needed because of their physical benefits. There has been no real need recently to prove that physical activity programs contribute to mental performance.[822, p. 59]

Few studies on the topic therefore appear to have been carried out in recent years[293] and many of the earlier investigations were limited by the methodological issues discussed above. For example, athletes have been reported to have higher grade-point averages than non-athletes[489] but, of course, athletes may enrol in less demanding classes and/or receive preferential treatment from tutors.

Nevertheless, Kirkendall[822] concluded that there is a modest positive association between motor performance and intellectual performance, especially with motor performance involving cognitive processes such as co-ordination and balance tasks. It appears that the association between motor and intellectual performance is strongest during the early stages of development and gradually decays with age. There is no conclusive evidence regarding the effects of physical activity on intellectual development.[822] However, although evidence relating physical activity to academic achievement is sparse[293] at least one study has demonstrated improvements in academic performance following the inclusion of an additional 5 h per week of physical activity in the curriculum and the corresponding reduction in classroom time.[1388] Increased physical activity is unlikely to improve intelligence but it may have the potential to improve academic performance. No study has demonstrated an impairment of intellectual development through increases in physical activity.[822]

Physical activity: other psychological variables

Calfas and Taylor[293] identified 11 studies which focused upon anxiety/stress variables and found physical activity to be associated with reductions in anxiety and stress in eight [refs 113, 176, 259, 260, 483, 557, 725, 1110 (2 studies), 1337, 1371]. An effect size of 0.15 was calculated from those studies providing sufficient information for the determination.

The type of physical activity required to elicit positive effects is unclear. Petruzzello *et al.*[1164] reported that only aerobic physical activity reduced anxiety but this observation is in conflict with other studies. Brown and Seigel[260] investigated the effect of physical activity and life stress on the health of 212 adolescent girls. The negative impact of stressful life events on health declined as physical activity levels increased but both aerobic and anaerobic physical activity were equally effective in buffering stress. Hilyer *et al.*[725] employed an exercise programme which included flexibility exercises, resistance training, and aerobic exercise. Following a 20 week, three times per week regime with 30 randomly selected, adolescent male inmates of a school for young offenders they observed significant reductions in depression and anxiety, and enhanced self-esteem.

Evidence relating physical activity to hostility/anger is both sparse and inconsistent. One study demonstrated improvements in depression, anxiety, and hostility following an aerobic exercise training programme[176] whereas others have detected no significant association between exercise training and hostility/anger.[558, 1110]

Physical activity has been shown to exert an anti-depressant effect for mild to moderate forms of depression and a meta-analysis of studies on both children and adults reported exercise to be a better anti-depressant than relaxation and other enjoyable pursuits.[1111] Calfas and Taylor[293] reported a positive relationship or experimental effect in nine of the 11 studies they located which focused on physical activity and depressed mood [176, 259, 262, 483, 557, 725, 1011, 1110 (2 studies), 1195, 1371]. An effect size of 0.38 was determined from studies which provided sufficient information for the calculation. The studies which observed a positive effect on depression generally employed aerobic exercise training programmes as the independent variable.

Although there are potential negative outcomes of physical activity on mental health[1067, 1189] causal relationships between physical activity and impaired mental health have not been documented in children and adolescents.[293] The evidence suggests that physical activity is psychologically beneficial for young people and there are no data which suggest that physical activity may create psychological harm in this age group. Data on the effects of de-training on mental health appear to be non-existent.

Table 13.3. Physical activity and psychological health and well-being

- Improves self-esteem and self-concept

- No effect on intellectual development

- May improve academic performance

- Reduces anxiety and stress

- Reduces depression

- No effect on hostility or anger

Exercise prescription

Physical activity is positively associated with improvements in the mental health of children and adolescents. However, dose–response data from well-controlled studies are not available and the optimal frequency, intensity and duration of exercise needed to promote mental health are unknown. The effects of different types of physical activity on psychological health and well-being have not been well documented.

Most studies have focused on aerobic exercise training programmes and reviews of the literature have recommended exercise programmes for the promotion of mental health similar to the programme we outlined in Chapter 7.[261, 293] However, anaerobic training,[260] resistance training,[730] and mixed exercise programmes[725] have also been shown to be effective.

Further research is needed before an appropriate exercise programme can be confidently prescribed. In the meantime, a good behavioural goal is for young people to develop the skills necessary to enjoy a wide range of physical activities and to continue being active throughout their adult lives.[75, 293] If aerobic or resistance exercise training programmes are required the programmes described in Chapters 7 and 8 respectively will be appropriate but the optimum duration of exercise training programmes for improving psychological health and well-being is unknown.

Summary

Young people are not immune from psychological problems and disturbances in adult mental health may be initiated during childhood and adolescence. The mechanisms by which physical activity may influence mental health are not well understood but physical activity has been associated with improvements in self-esteem, and reductions in anxiety, stress, and depression. Physical activity may promote academic achievement although this remains to be proven. There is no evidence to suggest that physical activity may induce psychological harm in young people.

The specific effects of various types of physical activity on mental health have not been documented and dose–response data from well-controlled studies are non-existent. The exercise training programmes described in Chapters 7 and 8 may have positive effects on psychological health and well-being. However, a good behavioural goal would be for children and adolescents to adopt physically active lifestyles. As enjoyable early activity experiences are likely to foster future participation young people should be encouraged to develop a repertoire of motor skills, so that they may achieve success in a range of activities and feel confident enough in their own abilities to want to pursue more active lifestyles.

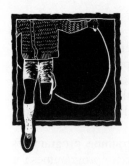

14

Intensive participation in sport and exercise

Intensive training and élite competition may start at a young age[947, 969] and even prepubertal children may be engaged in several hours per week of strenuous exercise.[691] Social and psychological concerns with intensive participation in exercise during childhood and adolescence have been reviewed elsewhere[287] but there are a number of physiological issues which need to be addressed. These include overuse injuries, temperature regulation during exercise, the use of performance-enhancing drugs, eating disorders, and, in girls, menstrual dysfunction.

Overuse injuries

Musculoskeletal damage

Young people involved in intensive exercise training are at risk of two major categories of musculoskeletal injury. The first of these, injury due to a single acute 'macrotrauma', is a risk of many sports regardless of age[1453] and is the predominant source of athletic injury.[601] In youth, soccer is the sport most frequently implicated.[757, 854, 1548] Acute fractures typify this type of injury but the characteristics of ossifying bone result in additional bony injuries typically observed in children.[1647] These include plastic deformation, torus fracture (compression of the metaphyseal cortex), greenstick fractures where the periosteum remains intact, acute ephiphyseal plate injury, and acute apophyseal avulsion.

During growth, particularly during the growth spurt, rates of bone matrix formation may exceed the rate of mineralization resulting in a temporary weakness in the bone.[1453] Consequently, patterns of bony injury in children differ from those in adults. Although the bone may be more resistant to impact during this phase, buckling or bowing rather than breaking, a sudden overload may cause serious damage and the peak rate of distal radius fractures coincides with the age of PHV.[121] It has been suggested that the epiphyseal area is some two to five times weaker than the structures (ligaments, tendons) supporting the bone[947] and is thus more vulnerable than the surrounding bone to shearing and tensile forces.[1647] Therefore, the type of injury that would cause damage to ligaments in adults may cause a serious fracture within the epiphyses of a growing child. Such injury may lead to bone deformity, chronic joint disease, or actually arrest limb growth.[1264]

The sequelae of unresolved, repeated microtrauma comprise the second type of injury characteristic of intensive exercise participation. Such overuse injuries have potential long-term consequences for the growth and health of the musculoskeletal system.

Epiphyseal plate injuries

Studies with animals demonstrating adverse effects of exercise stress upon skeletal health[38, 210, 1476] have led authors to express similar concerns regarding the possibility of epiphyseal damage as a result of intensive exercise in young people.[34, 210] There is clear evidence that epiphyseal overuse injuries do occur, particularly in gymnastics and baseball, where repetitive compressive loads produce the premature growth plate closure which has been observed in some young gymnasts.[12] Widening or 'beaking' of the distal radial epiphyses and shortening of the radius compared with the ulna have also been reported by several authors in this population.[312, 288, 1274] Injuries to the elbows of young baseball pitchers caused by the repetitive valgus stress of overhand throwing[499, 1546] occur frequently and are well documented. A variety of degenerative and inflammatory changes contribute to 'little league elbow' including damage to, and premature closure of the proximal radial epiphysis.[1264, 1535] Epiphyseal stress fractures are not common in other sports; even the repetitive stresses to the epiphyses of the long bones during distance running do not appear to regularly induce stress injuries at these sites in young athletes.[34]

Stress fractures

Runners in particular, and other athletes involved in repetitive training, are at increased risk of developing stress fractures. Although relatively rare in children, the incidence appears to be increasing in parallel with the increased participation rates.[1032] The femoral neck, fibula and tibia, and metatarsals are particularly vulnerable sites[336, 946] with individual sports associated with specific patterns of stress fractures. For example, competitive running involves the tibia and fibula,[742] jumping sports the pelvis and femur,[946] whilst all of the upper body is at risk in gymnastics.[1431] Stress fractures in adults usually involve cortical bone.[429] In contrast, cancellous bone with compressive stress applied to trabecular bone is implicated in young people, although very intensively trained young athletes may show the more adult pattern of fracture.[1032]

Stress fractures typically result from inappropriate training. In runners, abrupt increases in training volume, changes in running surface, or inappropriate shoes are common culprits.[580] Prompt identification and treatment of stress fractures in young athletes are essential. Progression from stress fracture to frank fracture is possible if training continues[239] and there is a risk of potential lifelong damage, for example, disabling degenerative arthritis where the hip joints are involved.

Osteochondritis and osteochondritis dissecans

The points at which the major tendons attach to bone, the apophyses, are particular areas at risk of overuse injury in the young athlete. In adults, stress to these points results in soft tissue damage (i.e. to the muscles and tendons themselves). In young athletes, however, training strengthens the soft tissues more quickly than the bone is developing. Furthermore, bone length increases relatively faster than muscle length during the growth spurt. This produces an exaggerated pull on the tendon–bone insertion. Overstress to these points can disrupt the process of ossification leading to chronic inflammation, avulsion of cartilage and bone from the developing area with tendinous microtears, and haemorrhages.[1647] This damage and fragmentation to bone is termed 'osteochondritis' or 'traction apophysitis'. In adolescents, damage to the insertion of the patellar tendon at the tibial tubercle (Osgood–Schlatter's 'disease') and the insertion of the Achilles tendon into the calcaneous (Sever's 'disease') are the two most commonly affected sites. The onset of these conditions is typically between the ages of 11–15 years, and usually coincides with the initiation of the growth spurt.[336] Osgood–Schlatter's disease is the most frequent adolescent overuse injury of the knee[1118] and this painful condition can persist for many months usually disrupting training for periods exceeding 7 months.[863]

Sever's disease is the comparable condition in the ankle and is the most common cause of heel pain in the adolescent athlete.[1032] Gymnasts are frequently affected, as are soccer players.[1036] This perhaps explains the predominance of the condition in boys. The duration of Sever's disease is usually somewhat shorter than for Osgood–Schlatter's disease and treatment by rest, physiotherapy, and orthotics allows the majority of sufferers to return to sport within 2 months.[1036]

Osteochondritis dessicans is a disorder of the joint surfaces which occurs when segments of subchondral bone and articular cartilage become avascular, die, and separate from the underlying bone forming a loose body. Caused by repetitive jarring of the joint, the injury occurs commonly in the knees but also in the ankle, hip, and elbow. This form of degeneration, although not frequently observed is one of the components of 'little league elbow'[7] which results from compression overuse injury of the lateral compartment of the elbow.[32] The worrying feature of osteochondritis dessicans is the potential for permanent disability if the condition is not recognized early and treated appropriately.[946]

Prevention and rehabilitation

Overuse injuries are provoked by a variety of factors including incorrect, overzealous training, the 'too much too soon' phenomenon,[1034, 1453] incorrect or inappropriate techniques in throwing or contact sports, poorly fitting footwear or protective gear, and inappropriate pressure from parents and coaches.[1453] It is particularly important to ensure that training is geared to the maturational stage of the child. The problems associated with decreased epiphyseal strength have been alluded to previously, but the relative inflexibility and diminished strength of young athletes during periods of rapid growth leave the athlete particularly vulnerable to overuse injury of the muscles or joints.[79, 1032, 1453] Intensive participation within a single sport characteristically produces muscle tightness in those muscles which are continually stressed. For example, adolescent tennis players demonstrate lower flexibility of the shoulder and lower back than other athletes[325] and a similar pattern of sport-specific inflexibility is noted in prepubescent tennis and soccer players.[817] Flexibility training should therefore be an integral part of the young athlete's training programme as a preventative measure.

Stretching exercises to improve flexibility can be either ballistic or static in nature. Ballistic stretching uses momentum to produce the stretch by 'bouncing' within a stretched position. This type of stretching, is therefore not recommended in young athletes as it carries a high risk of an excessive stretch damaging already taut muscles.[79] Static stretching exercise involves stretching a muscle comfortably beyond its normal length and produces fewer muscle tears and soreness. Table 14.1 provides an appropriate training schedule for flexibility training in this population. Assisted passive stretching and the use of proprioceptive neuromuscular facilitation are advanced stretching techniques[17, 1019] which must be used cautiously with young athletes.

Correct and complete rehabilitation of overuse injuries (the recovery of normal endurance and strength with full motion[1453]) is essential in children and adolescents given the serious long-term consequences to growth if the injury becomes chronic or prolonged.[336] In cases of epiphyseal and apophyseal injuries and stress fractures, complete rest is often the essential initial requirement[336, 1690] with a very gradual resumption of physical activity as symptoms recede. Premature return to full participation and competition is likely to perpetuate the injury or promote re-injury.[1453] Ensuring training programmes are appropriately geared to the young athlete's physiological maturity and progress in intensity by no more than 10% per week,[1034] combined with sufficient rest to allow restitution of any microtrauma, will contribute to the prevention of serious overuse injury.

Table 14.1. Guidelines for training flexibility in young people

Frequency	3–7 times per week
Intensity	Muscle should be stretched beyond its normal length and held for 6–10 sec
Time	3 times

Adapted from Armstrong, N. and Welsman, J. (1993). Training young athletes. In M. Lee (Ed.), *Coaching Children in Sport*. London, Spon, pp. 191–203.

Temperature regulation

The thermoregulatory capacity of the exercising child has been comprehensively documented elsewhere[137, 138, 142] but a brief outline of the key issues regarding child–adult differences in temperature regulation deserves mention as these characteristics leave young, competitive athletes vulnerable to developing heat illness, particularly when exercising in warm, humid environments.

The main physiological and geometric characteristics which predispose children to thermoregulatory stress are summarized in Table 14.2. The key geometric difference between children and adults is the young individual's larger surface area to body mass ratio. Heat transfer between the body and the environment depends upon the surface area exposed to the environment, whereas the production of metabolic heat is proportional to body mass. Therefore, the child absorbs heat from the environment in hot conditions and loses heat to the environment in cold conditions more rapidly than the adult.

A further complication to thermoregulation derives from children's higher production of heat per unit of body mass during both submaximal and maximal exercise. For example, the oxygen cost of running at 10 km·h^{-1} of a 6-year-old girl is some 20% higher than for a 16-year-old.[138] Thus, metabolic heat production is relatively greater in the child than the adolescent or adult placing increased stress upon the heat dissipatory mechanisms. The

Table 14.2. Characteristics of children which influence thermoregulation

- Larger surface area per unit body mass than adults

- Increased metabolic heat production per unit mass during walking and running compared with adults

- Lower sweating rate than adults

situation is aggravated by children's relatively lower cardiac output at any given level of exercise, which may also impede skin perfusion, thus limiting heat loss through convection and radiation.

During exercise in a warm environment, heat dissipation through evaporation of sweat is the main mechanism of thermoregulation in adults. Children have frequently been shown to have much lower sweating rates during exercise than adults[142] amounting to some 60–70% of adult production. It would appear that this is due to a lower sweat production per gland rather than a deficiency in the number of sweat glands in relation to body surface area. Therefore, children are disadvantaged in their ability to dissipate metabolic heat through this mechanism.

Studies have demonstrated that children's thermoregulatory abilities are not challenged by exercise in a thermoneutral environment[399, 662] and the majority of young people thermoregulate adequately during exercise in warm environments.[449, 1169] Problems arise in very hot environments where the child's thermoregulation is seriously compromised.[459, 1587]

Children's problems are compounded by the finding that they take longer to acclimatize to exercise in the heat than adults[1587] and the extent of adjustment is somewhat lower. However, young children appear to acclimatize to exercise in the heat by sitting in a hot environment[750] and this phenomenon does not appear to occur in adults who must experience exercise in the heat to produce the physiological effects of acclimatization (i.e. reduced exercising heart rate, increased sweating rate, and lower core temperature).

These characteristics of children suggest an increased vulnerability to heat illness (heat stroke, heat exhaustion) although the extent of the risk compared with adults is unknown. Adherence to the guidelines for young people exercising and training in the heat presented in Table 14.3 is recommended to prevent the development of heat illness.

In cool environments, children are as able as adults to maintain core temperature and during exercise the metabolic heat generated is usually sufficient to compensate for heat loss to the environment. Appropriate clothing to insulate the body is essential to avoid excessive heat loss and hypothermia during exercise is unlikely to arise. Children do, however, face problems during exercise in water where their higher body surface area to mass ratio predisposes them to rapid heat loss given the 25 times greater heat conductance of water in relation to air.

Menstrual dysfunction

Many female athletes who train intensively for endurance activities, such as distance running, or activities which emphasize leanness, such as ballet, experience menstrual dysfunction. The prevalence and aetiology of aberrant

Table 14.3. Guidelines for young people exercising or training in the heat

---

• Ensure acclimatization

• Ensure full hydration before exercise (e.g. 300–400 mL fluid 20–30 min prior to activity for a 12-year-old)

• Drink periodically throughout prolonged activities
  (e.g. 100 mL every 15 min)

• Fluids should be chilled, flavoured, and not too concentrated
  (e.g. 0.3 g·L^{-1} NaCl and 25 g·L^{-1} glucose)

• Discourage 'making weight' by dehydration

• Make sure activities suit the prevailing climate: take account of children's special problems

• Make sure clothing is appropriate

• Children need to be educated about maintenance of body fluid balance and should learn to drink beyond their subjective needs

---

reproductive endocrinology in adult athletes have been extensively researched and reviewed but studies with adolescents have focused almost exclusively upon the late menarche which is characteristic of athleticism in this population (see Chapter 1), and documentation of other forms of exercise-associated menstrual dysfunction is rare.

Although menarche is a significant event in the maturation of females, its occurrence does not denote the attainment of a fully mature adult reproductive capability. The adolescent menstrual cycle differs in several ways from the adult pattern. For several years after the first menses, the interval between menses varies widely within individual adolescents and this interval progressively reduces over this same period.[1542] Menses which occur in the absence of a released ovum (anovulatory cycles) are also prevalent in adolescence at around 50% of cycles compared with only 5% in the average adult population.[928] The interval between ovulation and menses (the luteal phase) is shorter in adolescents and may take 12 years to decline from a 50% prevalence to 10% in adults.[928] These characteristics of the normal adolescent menstrual cycle are similar to aspects of dysfunction common in adult athletes and thus seriously confound the investigation and interpretation of reproductive function in young athletes.

The exact mechanisms which contribute to the hormonal changes which disrupt the normal adult menstrual cycle remain to be unequivocally established. These have been extensively reviewed elsewhere[719, 929, 1183, 1279] but in brief, gynaecological and chronological age,[583, 1231] intensive exercise participation,[275, 460, 905] inappropriate dietary intake,[427, 1093] and low total body mass and fat levels[36, 112, 719] have been implicated. Recent work has emphasized the concept of energy availability as a causative factor,[774, 928] (i.e. an imbalance between energy intake and expenditure) although the development of menstrual disorders is likely to have a multifactorial aetiology.[719]

The two reproductive disorders which primarily typify the athletic female adult and thus deserve consideration in the adolescent female are luteal suppression (luteal insufficiency) and secondary amenorrhoea. Luteal phase deficiency or luteal suppression describes the occurrence of menstrual cycles in the absence of sufficient progesterone secretion and premature atrophy of the corpus luteum.[927, 928] Thus, in athletic women with menstrual cycles of the same duration as sedentary control subjects, a shortened luteal phase may be present with resultant adverse effects upon fertility.[496, 927] The absence of an abbreviated luteal phase in sedentary control subjects implicates exercise as a causative factor in this dysfunction. The clinical significance of luteal suppression in athletes is not well documented. It may simply represent an appropriate adaptation to strenuous training or may reflect genetic susceptibility to menstrual disturbance. Intensive training in those most susceptible to dysfunction produces amenorrhoea, whereas less susceptible individuals experience luteal suppression.[928] Luteal suppression has been reported in 13–15-year-old adolescent swimmers[217] but this interpretation is confounded by the 7 day shorter duration of the menstrual cycle reported for the swimmers compared with the control subjects.[928]

Amenorrhoea describes the cessation of menses in a post-menarcheal female, although a distinction may be drawn between primary amenorrhoea and secondary amenorrhoea. Primary amenorrhoea may be defined as the occurrence of menarche more than two standard deviations above the average age of menarche in the population.[927] At present this corresponds to approximately 16 years of age.[927, 1617] Secondary amenorrhoea, the focus of the discussion in this chapter, refers to the cessation of menses subsequent to a normal menarche.[927] Published estimates of the prevalence of secondary amenorrhoea in adult athletes range widely, from less than 5% to more than 50% in certain populations.[1595, 1617] This compares with a prevalence less than 5% in the normal population.[1165, 1404] The discrepancies in reported prevalence between studies may be attributed, in part, to the different athletic disciplines represented[927] but will also have been influenced by the particular definition of amenorrhoea. An absence of menses for three consecutive months[26] or fewer than two cycles in the previous 12 months[622] or a complete absence in the past 12 months[932] exemplify the range of definitions used. Such discrepancies are also likely to have contributed to the contention regarding the aetiology of menstrual dysfunction in the female athlete.

Amenorrhoeic athletes display specific hormonal alterations which suppress follicular development and inhibit ovulation. Chronically low levels of oestrogen and progesterone often result.[36] The stress hormone, cortisol, is typically elevated[424, 905] as is melatonin.[774, 887] Conversely, thyroid function is suppressed, particularly triiodothyronine and free thyroxine levels.[973, 1081] Such changes may represent a physiological mechanism for energy conservation in response to insufficient energy status.[1558, 1594]

Whether or not exercise, *per se*, induces these hormonal disruptions has been the subject of debate. Certainly, adolescent ballet dancers have been shown to develop amenorrhoea on resumption of strenuous training following a lay-off.[1593] However, when normally menstruating females undergo a progressive training programme without dietary restriction, amenorrhoea does not normally result.[216, 274, 1231] The addition of a concomitant forced reduction in dietary intake is almost invariably associated with the development of menstrual dysfunction.[275] These data strongly implicate a combination of strenuous exercise and compromised energy intake in the aetiology of athletic amenorrhoea.[928]

Although limited, data from young adolescent females appear to support this hypothesis. Adolescent amenorrhoeic athletes possess many of the same characteristics as observed in amenorrhoeic adults including depressed thyroid function, low oestrogen levels, and a lower energy intake than age-matched groups of either regularly menstruating runners or their sedentary counterparts.[112]

A prolonged absence of regular menstruation in adolescence is of particular concern in view of the unequivocal evidence linking hypo-oestrogenic states to bone mineral depletion with its consequent risk of osteoporotic disease (see Chapter 12). There is widespread documentation of bone mineral densities in amenorrhoeic athletes which are reduced to levels more typical of post-menopausal women.[460, 905, 1082] The period of adolescence and early adulthood is critical for maximizing bone mineral density. Thus, secondary amenorrhoea, particularly when subsequent to a late menarche, may prevent the attainment of peak bone mass[348] and promote the development of stress fractures and scoliosis.[348] As rates of bone loss are faster in the period immediately following the onset of amenorrhoea, approximating 3–5% per year,[190, 301, 461] the early recognition and treatment of hypo-oestrogenic adolescents is crucial for future health.

In recognition of the potentially serious consequences of adolescent menstrual dysfunction, the American Academy of Pediatrics[20] has issued a position statement recommending immediate proactive treatment including hormonal supplementation when appropriate to arrest bone loss. Obviously, hormone replacement therapy is not the ideal management of the condition and adolescent athletes require counselling and education in appropriate nutrition, weight gain if necessary, and a temporary modification of the training programme. These measures may suffice to redress the balance of energy intake and expenditure resulting in a resumption of normal menses[275, 1182, 1183, 1450] but the possibility of any pathological causes for the amenorrhoea must always be evaluated and excluded.[674] Despite the simplicity of this approach acceptance of nutritional or exercise modifications is often resisted by the athlete.[929] Many amenorrhoeic athletes display the characteristics associated with disordered eating, such as fear of fatness, a distorted body image, and a carefully regulated dietary intake.[593, 1492] Such characteristics have been recorded in amenorrhoeic adolescent athletes[112] with these runners scoring significantly higher on questions indicative of latent eating disorders including dissatisfaction with body shape and fear of fatness. The presence of these characteristics confounds rehabilitative attempts and is discussed more fully in the following section.

Eating disorders

Concern with appearance, body mass, and dieting has become increasingly prevalent in Western societies in response to cultural pressures which emphasize and value a slim physique.[566, 899] Substantial evidence confirms these anxieties to be equally true for the normal adolescent population.[314] In a sample of 854 adolescent females, 67% have reported dissatisfaction with their weight.[1062] Another study[1596] reported data from 348 boys and girls aged 12–17 years. Only 5% of the boys and 10% of the girls were currently dieting but of more concern were the 16% of girls who, at less than 95% of recommended body mass, believed themselves to be fat. Data from the United States suggest that dieting is particularly prevalent there with as many as 73% of 14-year-old girls having tried to lose weight at some point.[899] The prevalence of the expressed desire to lose weight is consistently higher in females[315, 713, 1112] and the number of adolescents attempting to diet increases with age.[1112] Even in very early adolescence many boys and girls demonstrate high levels of dietary restraint.[565, 566] In the light of these data, it is not surprising that increasing numbers of adolescents are diagnosed with clinically defined eating disorders.[898]

Eating disorders, particularly anorexia nervosa and bulimia nervosa are predominantly the domain of adolescent and young adult females.[314] Anorexics are characteristically well-educated, high-achieving, compliant individuals from predominantly middle class backgrounds.[600, 677, 890] Although infrequent, anorexia nervosa may develop in children as young as 7 years of age but the incidence increases markedly around puberty[314] peaking in mid to late adolescence.[890, 898] The prevalence of anorexia nervosa in the female population is estimated at between 0.2% and 1.1%[898] and carries a fatality rate of 5–18%.[1664] Adolescent males are much less frequently

Table 14.4. Diagnostic criteria for anorexia nervosa

- Refusal to maintain body mass over a minimal normal mass for age and stature, for example, weight loss leading to maintenance of body weight 15% below that expected; or failure to make expected weight gain during period of growth, leading to body weight 15% below that expected

- Intense fear of gaining weight or becoming fat, even though underweight

- Disturbance in the way in which one's body weight, size, or shape is perceived, undue influence of body mass or shape on self-evaluation, or denial of the seriousness of the current low body mass

- In post-menarcheal females, the absence of at least three consecutive menstrual cycles when otherwise expected to occur (amenorrhoea). A woman is considered to have amenorrhoea if her periods occur only following oestrogen administration

Types of anorexia nervosa

Restricting type   During the current episode of anorexia nervosa, the person has not regularly engaged in binge-eating or purging behaviour (i.e. self-induced vomiting or the misuse of laxatives, diuretics or enemas)

Purging type   During the current episode of anorexia nervosa, the person has regularly engaged in binge-eating or purging behaviour

---

Adapted from American Psychiatric Association. *Diagnostic and Statistical Manual of Mental Disorders, 4th edition (DSM-IV)*. Washington, DC, 1994.

affected representing only 5–10% of reported cases.[561, 695, 755] Anorexics steadfastly refuse to maintain body mass above the minimal level recommended for their age and stature, have a distorted body image, and an extreme fear of gaining weight. Although purging behaviour may be present, weight loss is most frequently achieved through caloric restriction. Despite inadequate nutrition and progressive emaciation, the anorexic will often exercise compulsively and to excess. The clinical criteria for the diagnosis of anorexia nervosa are shown in Table 14.4.

Bulimia nervosa is a more recently recognized condition which typically develops in the late adolescent or young adult and may, in some individuals, supplant prior anorexia nervosa.[374] In bulimia, excessive amounts of food are consumed within a short time period (bingeing) followed by self-induced purging behaviours, such as vomiting and/or the use of laxatives and diuretics, periods of severe dietary restriction or excessive exercise to prevent weight gain. A persistent preoccupation with body shape and fatness, often focused upon specific body areas is typical. Again female

Table 14.5. Diagnostic criteria for bulimia nervosa

- Recurrent episodes of binge-eating. An episode of binge-eating is characterized by both of the following:

    - Eating in a discrete period of time (e.g. within any 2 h period), an amount of food that is definitely larger than most people would eat during a similar period of time and under similar circumstances

    - A feeling of lack of control over eating behaviour during the binge episode (e.g. a feeling that one cannot stop eating or control what or how much one is eating)

- The person regularly engages in either self-induced vomiting, use of laxatives or diuretics, strict dieting or fasting, or vigorous exercise in order to prevent weight gain

- A minimum average of two binge-eating episodes a week for at least three months

- Persistent overconcern with body shape and weight

Types of bulimia nervosa

Purging type During the current episode of bulimia nervosa, the person has regularly engaged in self-induced vomiting or the misuse of laxatives, diuretics, or enemas

Non-purging type During the current episode of bulimia nervosa, the person has used other inappropriate compensatory behaviours, such as fasting or excessive exercise, but has not regularly engaged in self-induced vomiting or the misuse of laxatives, diuretics, or enemas

Adapted from American Psychiatric Association. *Diagnostic and Statistical Manual of Mental Disorders, 4th edition (DSM-IV)*. Washington, DC, 1994.

incidence predominates; accounting for some 90% of cases.[1044] Previous diagnostic criteria have been criticized as insufficiently rigorous[898] thus elevating prevalence rates, but estimates based upon stringent criteria have reported rates which vary between 0.4% and 3.2% in the female population.[1189, 1497] Diagnostic criteria for bulimia nervosa are summarized in Table 14.5.

In parallel with increased concern with diet, body image, and weight control in the normal population has been a growing awareness that eating disorders also pervade the athletic population. Athletes in aesthetic activities such as ballet, where a predetermined 'contract weight' is set,[342, 1580]

Table 14.6. Diagnostic criteria for anorexia athletica

Common features

- Weight loss

- Delayed puberty

- Menstrual dysfunction

- Gastrointestinal complaints

- Absence of medical illness or affective disorder explaining the weight reduction

- Distorted body image

- Excessive fear of becoming obese

- Restriction of food (<1200 kcal·day^{-1})

- Use of purging methods

- Binge-eating

- Compulsive exercise

Adapted from Sundgot-Borgen, J. (1993). Prevalence of eating disorders in female élite athletes. *International Journal of Sport Nutrition*, **3**, 29–40.

gymnastics and synchronized swimming, where appearance is judged, and in endurance sports such as distance running where leanness and low body fat are advantageous for efficient and successful performance,[1490, 1491, 1692] are particularly implicated. Eating disorders of males tend to be associated with sports which require participants to be graded and compete within a weight-class such as wrestling, boxing, and weight-lifting.[1457, 1665]

In recognition of the widespread prevalence of eating behaviours among athletes which share features of, but fail to fulfil, the stringent criteria for clinical diagnosis as anorexia nervosa or bulimia nervosa[337, 1486] a third disorder, 'anorexia athletica', has been described.[1185, 1487] As the diagnostic criteria displayed in Table 14.6 suggest, this condition may be regarded as a subclinical form of the other conditions.[1185, 1488] The essential features of anorexia athletica are an intense fear of gaining weight or becoming fat despite a body mass which is at least 5% lower than expected for age and stature. Weight loss is produced through dietary restriction combined with excessive and compulsive exercise. Binge-eating and purging activities are typically present, but are performed less frequently than in classical bulimia nervosa.

The extent to which disordered eating occurs in the athletic population has not been widely examined although there is evidence to suggest that athletes are more prone to its development than non-athletes.[277, 1490] Summaries of the prevalence of eating disorders in athletes are available elsewhere[1483, 1665] but the following illustrative examples are provided. In female ballet dancers, diagnosable eating disorders have been reported in 6.5%[604]–25.7%[605] of subjects. Prevalences of 33.3% and 27.2% have been observed in élite cross-country skiers and runners, respectively[1483] with amenorrhoeic athletes appearing particularly vulnerable.[254, 593, 1669]

The variation in these estimates may be attributed to the different methods used to obtain data, the size and composition of the subject population and the criteria used to confirm the presence of an eating disorder.[1486] These values may actually underestimate the true extent of these disorders as the identification of an eating disorder within an individual is confounded by the denial which is an adjunct of these conditions.[314, 1392] There are examples where groups of athletes whose responses to established questionnaires have failed to identify them as eating-disordered, have subsequently received medical treatment for anorexia nervosa or bulimia nervosa.[1665] Despite the methodological limitations of documenting the problem, disordered eating is evidently an integral part of athletic life for many individuals.[263]

Given that eating disorders most frequently develop during adolescence and that athletes appear particularly susceptible, young athletes, particularly young female athletes, are likely to represent a particularly vulnerable population. Several other characteristics associated with involvement in intensive training during the adolescent period may be considered to enhance this risk. Young girls and adolescents share close, often intense, relationships with their coaches which are sometimes characterized by domination on the part of the coach and dependence and a sense of lack of control on the part of the athlete.[453] Within such relationships, overt pressure to lose weight or more covert references from the coach regarding 'ideal' body shape or fatness may, in vulnerable individuals, trigger over-concern with body fatness which is ultimately expressed in disordered eating and unhealthy weight-loss practices. Similarly, the ending of these relationships, for whatever reason, may be sufficiently traumatic to precipitate aberrant eating behaviour in the athlete.

A trigger factor for anorexia nervosa is anxiety about puberty, rejection of sexual development, and a perceived inability to cope with sexuality and sexual relationships.[314, 890] Through dieting and extreme weight loss, the anorexic is able to perpetuate a prepubertal body shape. Maturity also creates a paradox for female athletes participating in aesthetic or endurance activities as normal female development represents a deviation from the physique equated with success. Thus, in vulnerable individuals the demands of their chosen sport reinforce the drive to retain a prepubertal body type. Thus, parallels may be drawn between the factors which contribute to the development of classical eating disorders in the normal population and the characteristics, traits, and body images required by many athletic disciplines.

Although data are not extensive, eating disorders have been documented in adolescent athletes. Brooks-Gun *et al.*[254] examined eating attitudes and dietary restraint in female dancers, skaters, swimmers, and non-athletes aged 14–18 years. The dancers and skaters scored higher on measures of dietary restraint, negative attitudes towards food consumption, and bingeing and purging behaviours, although only 5% of the dancers had scores commensurate with clinical populations. A prospective study[605] followed 35 11–14-year-old female ballet students for a period of 2–4 years. At the follow-up, anorexia nervosa was present in 16% of the subjects with 14% suffering from bulimia nervosa or a 'partial syndrome'.

Several authors have demonstrated a high prevalence of preoccupation with weight body dissatisfaction in adolescent female athletes[112, 168] with swimmers also scoring significantly higher on measures reflective of disordered eating than gymnasts or controls.[168] Purging behaviours and claimed anorexia in adolescent athletes are reported to be more common in athletic compared with normal subjects, although the prevalence is less common than in eating-disordered subjects.[971] Although scarce, data from studies of adolescent male wrestlers confirm that aberrant dietary practices including fasting, frequent vomiting, dieting, and bingeing are also prevalent at high rates in this population.[1457, 1641, 1681]

The immediate metabolic complications and longer-term health consequences of eating disorders are well recognized.[1392] Associated conditions range in severity from diarrhoea or constipation to seizures, syncope, severe electrolyte disturbances, muscle weakness, and ketosis.[551, 711] The link with menstrual dysfunction, particularly amenorrhoea, and resultant bone demineralization have been discussed previously and this triad of disorders[1665] represents a serious long-term and not completely reversible condition whose prognosis includes increased risk of fracture or vertebral collapse. The deep-rooted psychological problems experienced by eating-disordered individuals make the conditions particularly resistant to improvement and may continue without complete resolution for many years.[374, 453]

It is imperative that eating disorders are recognized and treated promptly. Table 14.7 summarizes the warning signs which may be indicative of incipient eating disorders in young athletes. Measures to avert the onset of such conditions include dealing sensitively with female adolescents, abolishing contract weights, and not punishing individuals for failing to 'make weight', or being overtly critical of those whose physiques deviate

Table 14.7.   Signs of incipient or developed eating disorder

Anorexia nervosa

• Significant weight loss within a short time period

• Continuation of diet although thin

• Weight-loss goals when reached are immediately set lower for further weight loss

• Dissatisfaction with appearance and individual 'feels fat'

• Cessation of menstrual periods

• Eating is ritualized and very little food is consumed

• Solitary eating is preferred

• Obsessive about exercise

• Appears unhappy

Bulimia nervosa

• Binges regularly

• Purges regularly

• Exercises often but retains or regains weight

• Disappears to the bathroom for long periods

• Suffers from depression

from an unreasonable, unattainable 'ideal'. Where necessary, appropriate nutritional guidance should be given to athletes who wish to lose weight and a slow rate of weight loss promoted to pre-empt rapid weight loss via inappropriate behaviours. By avoiding premature sport specialization and leaving selection for specialized sporting activities until late adolescence, young athletes may be more securely channelled towards those activities that are appropriate to their physique and physiological capabilities.[1489]

Exercise and ergogenic aids

Exogenous performance-enhancing agents

The use of exogenous agents (drugs) to enhance performance has a long history in athletic endeavour and competition. Despite the illegality of the practice adult athletes continue to abuse a variety of substances which they believe will improve their performance despite the risk of serious long-term damage or fatality. Although documentation remains scarce and difficult to interpret due to the necessary reliance upon self-reported data, recent studies indicate a worrying pervasion of performance-enhancing drugs into youth sport.

Pleasure-enhancing drugs are increasingly part of adolescent culture. Over the past two decades their use has been said to have reached epidemic proportions in the United States.[484] Recent data from the United Kingdom support this assertion. By the age of 15–16 years, over 70% of adolescents report personal knowledge of a drug-user, around 30% have used cannabis at least once[125] and many young people report having access to such substances.[125, 1543] Given this 'cultural attunement' to drug use, it may be expected that many young athletes will be amenable to experimentation with illicit chemicals they believe will enhance their athletic performance.[484]

Performance-enhancing agents fall broadly into three categories: (1) anabolic agents; (2) stimulants; and (3) relaxants. Of the anabolic agents, or anabolic-androgenic steroid hormones, synthetic testosterone analogues for injection or oral consumption are most frequently used. More recently, use of growth hormone (GH), which promotes protein anabolism, enhances tissue repair, and increases fat metabolism, and amino acids which may stimulate the release of endogenous GH has become more widespread.[923] Reported benefits of anabolic agents include increased muscle mass, strength, and stamina. Stimulants include drugs such as caffeine, cocaine, and amphetamines. Their ergogenic effect arises from stimulation of the central nervous system which masks fatigue and promotes endurance. Caffeine is also taken for its additional metabolic effects which include increased fat metabolism and utilization, glycogen sparing, and increased muscle contractility. The final group, relaxants, include drugs such as beta blockers, whose relaxant effects facilitate performance in sports, such as archery and shooting, where fine skills are required.

Although stimulant and GH use in young athletes has been reported,[484, 1543] the prevalence of steroid abuse in this population has been researched more extensively.[e.g. 21, 1518, 1670] Even so, studies are scarce and their conclusions limited by the problems inherent with the use of survey techniques to obtain data. These include, difficulties with ensuring random distribution of questionnaires among students and the problems of verifying the honesty of reported answers.[453, 1670]

Estimates of the prevalence of steroid abuse in American, non-athletic teenagers range from less than 1[367]–6.6%.[271] More recent studies have reported prevalences which suggest that steroid abuse is an increasing problem.[1007, 1099, 1518, 1615, 1670] Estimates of the prevalence of steroid abuse in adolescent athletes have varied widely within a range of 1.4[859]–12.5%,[765] but have generally exceeded those in the general adolescent population.[271, 1007, 1670] In view of the problems of obtaining valid and honest responses to questionnaires these values may well underestimate the true prevalence. Several studies have incorporated questions regarding the respondent's knowledge of others who take steroids in an attempt to assess compliance with survey instructions.[1670] Results have invariably indicated others' use to be much higher than the self-reported use[1543, 1670] indicative of a degree of under-reporting.

Given the physiological effects of anabolic steroids, it is not surprising that abuse of these drugs is particularly prevalent in youth sports which require strength and a muscular physique such as American football, weight lifting, and body building.[271, 1670] Resistance training when employed specifically to improve sport performance rather than as a recreation or to promote fitness, may encourage steroid abuse.[200] Studies have consistently reported steroid abuse to be predominantly a male problem, particularly with those in higher socioeconomic groups.[1670] This has led some authors to draw parallels between eating disorders in females and drug abuse in male athletes[453] as both practices involve similar concerns with body appearance and a drive for perfection and success.

Despite contention surrounding the precise mechanisms of the action of exogenous anabolic hormones,[924] the adverse short-term side effects of steroid abuse are well documented. In males, testosterone and subsequently sperm production are suppressed. Steroid users often display increased aggressiveness and irritability, gynaecomastia may appear, or the transient gynaecomastia of male adolescence be aggravated, as is acne. In those with a family susceptibility an irreversible acceleration towards baldness may occur.[1474] The long-term effects of steroid abuse include, in adults, decreased high-density lipoprotein (HDL) levels and consequently worsened coronary heart disease risk and, although rare, hepatic carcinoma.[1474] The main adverse effect specific to young athletes is the risk of an accelerated maturity. Although this may enhance muscularity faster than would otherwise have occurred, premature closure of the epiphyses of the long bones may significantly reduce the ultimate stature obtained.[923, 1474] Furthermore, obtaining steroid drugs from non-physician sources leaves the athlete open to the effects of an uncontrolled steroid dosage and added impurities.

In addition to the apparently increased prevalence of steroid abuse, these studies have identified several other features which give serious cause for concern. Many young people report knowing where to obtain drugs,[1007] and their availability to young athletes appears to be on the increase.[1543] The belief that steroids are beneficial to performance is prevalent among athletic adolescents[1615] and many, not currently taking steroids, would consider using them to further their athletic career in the future.[453, 1615] Indeed, some feel their chances of success are compromised by not taking drugs.[453] Of particular concern are the reports of pressure placed upon young athletes to take steroids by significant others such as coaches and parents;[453] as many as 20% of requests for steroids for adolescents are reported to be made by parents.[1319]

In conclusion, it would appear that drugs are a familiar feature of adolescent culture. The growing infiltration of youth culture by soft and hard drugs and young people's growing awareness of them suggest that abuse of performance-enhancing agents is likely to increase in the adolescent athletic population. Steroid abuse is a particular concern in young athletes given their potential for adverse effects upon normal growth.

Summary

Regular physical activity confers many positive health outcomes but intensive exercise participation may have adverse physiological and health consequences. The immature musculoskeletal system is particularly vulnerable to overuse injury arising from unresolved, repeated microtrauma. Repetitive damage to the epiphyseal plates can arrest growth of the involved limbs, inappropriate training techniques or equipment can induce stress fractures, and apophyseal damage, such as Osgood–Schlatter's disease, is increasingly evident. Appropriate training, including flexibility training can minimize the risk of overuse injury.

Children are at particular risk of developing heat illness during exercise due to their higher body surface area to mass ratio, higher metabolic heat production, and lower sweating rate. Similarly in cold environments, particularly water, these same characteristics cause children to lose heat rapidly. During exercise in environmental extremes appropriate acclimatization, clothing, and fluid replacement are essential.

Many young female athletes in intensive training experience disruption to the normal menstrual cycle with luteal suppression and secondary amenorrhoea being the disorders most frequently experienced. Identification of the precise causative factors remains elusive but training volume, low body fat, dietary restriction, and hormonal alterations have been implicated. It is essential that amenorrhoea is investigated and treated given the negative effect of prolonged low levels of oestrogen upon bone mass.

The prevalence of eating disorders, notably anorexia nervosa and bulimia nervosa, in the young female athletic population is increasing. Young women participating in sports which emphasize leanness are particularly affected. The condition 'anorexia athletica' has been defined to categorize the aberrant eating behaviours strongly associated with athletic participation but which do not fulfil the stringent diagnostic criteria for anorexia or bulimia. Adolescent athletes may be particularly vulnerable to developing eating disorders, given their association with anxieties about puberty and sexuality, and the conflict many girls experience as their normal female development produces a physique incompatible with success in their chosen sport. Eating disorders are associated with serious immediate and longer-term negative health outcomes and are often present in amenorrhoeic athletes. Leaving sport specialization until puberty would enable more appropriate matching of physical and physiological characteristics to a given sport.

Throughout history, athletes have taken exogenous substances which they believe enhance performance. Pleasure-enhancing drugs are increasingly part of adolescent culture therefore the permeation into youth sport of drug use to increase performance is not surprising. Anabolic agents, including synthetic testosterone analogues, stimulants, and relaxants are the three categories of drug most widely employed. Steroid abuse occurs most frequently in young athletes, particularly in those sports requiring strength and muscularity. The adverse health consequences of steroid abuse are well documented, with the risk of accelerated puberty and premature epiphyseal closure of particular concern in young athletes.

Part IV

Physical activity: benefits,
correlates, and promotion

In Part III we reviewed the potential health benefits of physical activity during childhood and adolescence and came to the following conclusions.

Children's and adolescents' habitual physical activity has little or no relationship with their aerobic fitness, probably because young people rarely experience the volume of physical activity required to promote aerobic fitness. Exercise training programmes of the appropriate frequency, intensity, and duration will enhance the aerobic fitness of both boys and girls, although the magnitude of the increase may be less than that expected with adult subjects. As with all exercise training programmes once training ceases the dependent variable, in this case aerobic fitness, will gradually return to pre-training level.

Muscular strength increases with growth and maturation but a well-designed resistance training programme will induce further increases in the muscular strength of both children and adolescents. Prepubescent children and adolescent girls can improve their muscular strength with an appropriate resistance training programme but they are less likely to demonstrate significant muscle hypertrophy than adolescent boys.

There is evidence to indicate that exercise training, aerobic fitness, and high levels of habitual physical activity are associated with favourable blood lipid and lipoprotein profiles. However, the few prospective studies carried out to date have not provided any significant support for a positive relationship between physical activity and blood lipids or lipoproteins during childhood and adolescence. Similarly, with normotensive young people the evidence that physical activity will induce significant changes in blood pressure is not convincing. Aerobic exercise training does appear to be effective in reducing both diastolic blood pressure (DBP) and systolic blood pressure (SBP) of hypertensive children and adolescents. Attempts to establish a cause and effect relationship between young people's physical activity and a low incidence of cigarette smoking have been unsuccessful. The argument that physical activity has a significant role to play in reducing the prevalence of young smokers is intuitively appealing but unproven.

Increased physical activity may promote significant reductions in children's and adolescents' body fat particularly when combined with dietary modification. In contrast to obesity management programmes based upon dietary restriction alone, the inclusion of physical activity promotes the maintenance of muscle mass. Physical activity also appears to improve adverse blood lipid levels and elevated blood pressure if they are present in obese young people.

In conjunction with dietary modification and insulin administration, the beneficial effects of physical activity upon diabetes mellitus have long been recognized. Although not directly ameliorating diabetic control as reflected by levels of glycolysated haemoglobin, regular physical activity may enhance insulin sensitivity thus reducing exogenous insulin requirement and improve an adverse lipid profile in diabetic children and adolescents.

Risk of osteoporosis in adult life can be reduced by enhancing peak bone mineral density (BMD) developed during growth and maturation. Bone responds positively to appropriate skeletal loading and both general body mass-supporting activities and resistance training may increase BMD. Immobilization and inactivity have adverse effects on BMD and should be avoided whenever possible.

The causal mechanism or mechanisms of any relationship between physical activity and young people's psychological well-being are not well understood but physical activity has been associated with improvements in self-esteem, and reductions in anxiety, stress, and depression. Appropriate physical activity may also promote academic achievement. There is no evidence to suggest that physical activity may induce psychological harm in children and adolescents.

It appears, however, that many young people seldom experience the volume of physical activity associated with health-related outcomes. Despite the methodological problems associated with the estimation of young people's physical activity the data are remarkably consistent. Boys are more physically active than girls during childhood and girls' activity levels decline more rapidly than those of boys as they progress through adolescence. No prospective study of physical activity patterns has followed children through adolescence into adult middle age and beyond. However, data from retrospective surveys and relatively short-term prospective studies support the premise that inactive young people are unlikely to become physically active adults. The challenge with children and adolescents is therefore to promote and foster active lifestyles which are likely to be sustained into adult life.

Young people's physical activity patterns are influenced by a variety of interacting psychological, social, and environmental factors, the relative importance of which will vary with age, gender, growth, and maturation. In Part IV, we will analyse factors which are correlated with physical activity and comment on ways of promoting, fostering, and sustaining active lifestyles.

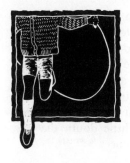

15
Promoting physical activity

There may be a genetic predisposition towards being more or less physically active[1339, 1648, 1649] but if so, it is mediated by a wide range of other factors.[1063, 1158, 1159] The myriad of interacting factors which may influence young people's physical activity is not fully understood but the consensus view is that no single correlate explains physical activity behaviour.[447, 1303, 1313] To identify and categorize the principal factors involved we will develop the framework described by Sallis[1302] and examine the promotion of children's and adolescents' physical activity in terms of biological, psychological, social, and environmental issues. This approach is simplistic but it provides a means of isolating key correlates which may be important in the promotion of young people's physical activity.

Biological factors

The biological factors which may influence physical activity were reviewed in earlier chapters and will only be briefly revisited here. Readers are referred to the appropriate chapter for applicable references.

In Chapter 6, the plethora of methods used to estimate physical activity were analysed and the difficulties involved in accurately determining the amount of physical activity experienced by young people were outlined. Regardless of methodology, however, the data remain remarkably consistent. Age is negatively correlated with physical activity and gender differences are readily apparent. Both boys and girls reduce their level of physical activity as they progress through childhood and adolescence into adult life. Boys are generally more active than girls from an early age but between the ages of 6 and 17 years the gender differences become more pronounced as the rate of decline in physical activity is about 2.5 times greater in girls than in boys. The goals of programmes designed to promote physical activity should therefore be tailored to specific age groups and particular attention should be paid to the needs of girls.

Gender differences in physical activity may be related to boys' higher aerobic fitness (see Chapter 4) but any relationship between aerobic fitness and habitual physical activity is tentative (see Chapter 7). The structural and functional changes with growth and maturation which leave males with greater stature, more body mass, larger muscle to mass ratio, longer limbs, and wider shoulders than females were described in Chapter 1. These characteristics provide boys with a marked advantage in many organized activities and also contribute to gender differences in aspects of motor performance (see ref. 241 for a review). The structural and functional differences between boys and girls may be a significant factor in explaining gender differences in physical activity but there is little doubt that the effects are magnified by social and environmental influences.[76, 487, 1524]

Psychological factors

Data on psychological factors which may influence physical activity are accumulating but they are often difficult to interpret. Definitions of factors vary from study to study and the self-report techniques utilized lack precision, especially with young children[1303] (and see Chapter 6).

Attitudes about physical activity[284, 1429] and personality characteristics[282, 409] appear to be weakly or not at all associated with young people's physical activity behaviour. However, research into goal orientations[1103] has indicated that task-orientation (where success is self-referenced and the experiences of learning and personal improvement occasion feelings of success) is more likely than ego-orientation (where perceptions of competence are most often founded on normative or peer comparison) to promote young people's physical activity and/or sustained sports participation.[413, 464, 564]

Several behavioural models of physical activity have been proposed but a detailed analysis of the extant literature is beyond the scope of this text and readers are referred elsewhere for extensive reviews.[445, 446, 1434] No single model has emerged as capable of explaining or predicting children's and adolescents' physical activity patterns[1302, 1303] but the most extensively researched models/theories are the health belief model,[159] the theory of reasoned action,[10] and social cognitive theory.[130]

The health belief model proposes that the likelihood of engaging in health-related behaviour is dependent upon perceived benefits of behaviour, perceived barriers to that behaviour, and perceived threat posed by not engaging in the behaviour. Knowledge of the effect of physical activity on health apparently has little influence on children's and adolescents' physical activity[547, 1113] but knowledge about how to exercise may be beneficial.[423, 642] Perceived barriers to engaging in physical activity have been identified in adolescents as time constraints, lack of equipment or facilities, job responsibilities, unsuitable weather, school and schoolwork, and lack of interest.[1507] Wanting to do other things with their time was the most relevant barrier among girls whereas the most important barriers among boys included having a girlfriend, and the use of alcohol and other drugs.[1507]

The theory of reasoned action states that behaviour is influenced by the intention to act and that the intention is determined by the individual's attitudes toward the action and his/her perception of social norms toward the action. Several studies have demonstrated that intention to exercise is correlated with physical activity[547, 654, 1202] but studies with adolescents show either weak or non-significant correlations between attitude measures and either intended or actual physical activity.[628, 629, 654] The interpretation of studies investigating what children or adolescents perceive others want them to do is complex[1302] and data are sparse.[628]

Social cognitive theory suggests that self-efficacy (confidence in one's ability to perform a task) is the primary psychological determinant of behaviour but also acknowledges the influence of social factors and role models. Data supporting self-efficacy as a predictor of children's and adolescents' physical activity are scarce although a recent prospective study which estimated adolescents' physical activity at baseline, 4 months, and 16 months later provides some support for the concept. Higher levels of self-efficacy were related to higher levels of physical activity in both boys and girls, and self-efficacy measured at baseline was a significant predictor of boys' physical activity 4 months later and girls' physical activity 16 months later.[1202] Social influences, which are central to social cognitive theory, are addressed in the following section.

Although models and theories are useful for organizing concepts and some psychological variables are clearly correlated with physical activity, psychological factors have been unable to clarify fully variations in young people's physical activity patterns. The evidence indicates the importance of children gradually building a repertoire of motor skills and participating in activities appropriate to their development. This approach will increase the chances of children experiencing success in physical activities and promote enjoyment. Activities which encourage children to initially compete with themselves and reward participation rather than beating opponents, are more likely to engender positive physical activity behaviour in the majority of children.

Promoting young people's physical activity solely through interventions aimed at changing knowledge, attitudes, and beliefs about physical activity is unlikely to be successful and consideration of variables outside the person is required.[1303]

Social factors

Physical activity behaviour is influenced by a variety of social variables and role models the relative significance of which change as young people progress through childhood and adolescence. Family influences on physical activity during childhood and adolescence are well documented but vary with age, gender, maturity, and race.[272, 642, 651, 654, 1286] Adults such as teachers,[628, 930, 1637] physicians,[18, 22, 1480] and other health-care providers[49, 469] may be influential in promoting young people's physical activity but data are relatively sparse and further research is required before their roles can be fully evaluated. As children get older adult influence declines and same-sex peers, and then opposite-sex peers impact upon behaviour.[272] The combined support of both family and peers has been found to be a significant predictor of adolescents' physical activity in at least one study.[1202]

Family

Early influences of parental behaviour on children's physical activity patterns are well documented. Two studies from the same research group have demonstrated how parental encouragement and discouragement have an almost immediate effect on 20–46-month-old children's physical activity levels.[828, 832] The mere presence of mother has been reported to stimulate physical activity in a group of 5-year-olds but interestingly not in 3- or 4-year-old children.[1250] Primary schoolchildren's physical activity has been significantly correlated with their parents' activity levels in most[575, 1138, 1309, 1311, 1649] but not all[413] studies. Parents' inactivity may exert more influential modelling behaviour than physical activity.[575]

Fewer studies have been carried out with young adolescents and the data are equivocal with some studies supporting a correlation between parental and offspring activity[31, 1063, 1385] and others unable to detect a significant relationship.[630, 1043] Parental physical activity behaviour may have a stronger influence on physical activity among girls than boys.[642, 1482] Whether mother[654, 1311] or father[629, 641] or either parent[1159] provides the most significant role model is unclear and probably varies with age, maturity, and gender. Both parents should therefore provide positive role models for their children's physical activity. Parents should encourage their offspring to be physically active but be cautious about pressuring their children to exercise vigorously as this may have the effect of spoiling children's pleasure in being physically active.[1001]

Boys appear to receive more parental support and encouragement to be physically active than girls[31, 266] although when they do receive support, girls may be more responsive than boys.[31] Lewko and Greendorfer[900] have catalogued evidence which clearly demonstrates that from infancy boys and girls receive differential treatment in this context. Boys are allowed more freedom to display aggressive behaviour and to engage in more vigorous activities whereas girls are encouraged to be more dependent and less exploratory in their behaviour. Both parents elicit gross motor behaviour more from their sons than daughters. However, if girls do adopt active lifestyles and/or engage in sporting activities they tend to receive the support they need.[31] Parental influence is probably a contributory factor to girls being less physically active than boys and parents need to offer their children equitable physical activity opportunities.

Peers

Peer influence on physical activity is less well researched than family influence but the available evidence is unequivocal and indicates that peers play a pivotal role in determining adolescents' level of physical activity.[31, 641, 654] In one study the support of peers was found to be more important for 11-year-old boys than girls of the same age.[1482] The promotion of co-operative, group physical activities (e.g. cycling, walking) as well as organized activities and sports may positively influence peer pressure on physical activity.

Environmental factors

A variety of environmental factors influence children's and adolescents' physical activity behaviour and in this section we will focus on independent mobility, television watching, the community, and the school.

Independent mobility

Time spent outdoors is strongly correlated with physical activity in young children[829] but Hillman's research has clearly demonstrated that children's freedom to participate in many outdoor activities, or, as he terms it their 'independent mobility', has declined with time.[723, 724] In 1971, Hillman surveyed children (7–11-year-olds) and adolescents (11–15-year-olds) from five areas in England chosen to provide geographical and social diversity. He repeated the survey in the same areas in 1990 and a comparison of findings revealed a marked decline in young people's independent mobility (Fig. 15.1). In 1971, two-thirds of cycle owners were allowed to use them on the roads, by 1990 the proportion had fallen to one-quarter. Four times as many children were chauffeured to school in 1990 as in 1971, thus losing an excellent opportunity for both individual and family physical activity.[50] Hillman's findings clearly demonstrate the importance of traffic-calming schemes, the provision of safe walkways, and the development of an extensive array of cycle paths. To increase the number of young people cycling to school secure storage facilities for bicycles need to be provided by the school.

Hillman's data[723, 724] also revealed significant gender differences in independent mobility. Boys enjoyed far more independence than girls in each of the situations studied. For example, in 1990 one-third of cycle owning

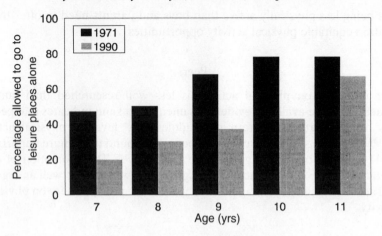

Fig. 15.1. Percentage of English junior schoolchildren allowed to go to leisure places alone according to age (1971 and 1990). Figure redrawn from Hillman, M. (Ed.) (1993). *Children, Transport and the Quality of Life*. London, Policy Studies Institute. Reprinted with permission.

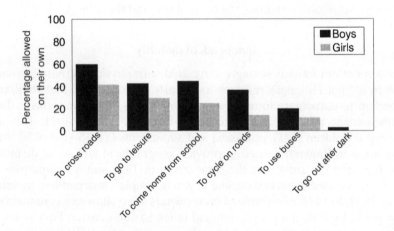

Fig. 15.2. Independent mobility of English junior girls and boys. Figure redrawn from Hillman, M., Adams, J. and Whitelegg, J. (1990). *One False Move*. London, Policy Studies Institute. Reprinted with permission.

boys were allowed to cycle on the roads, whereas only one in nine of cycle owning girls were allowed to do so. Selected gender differences in independent mobility are summarized in Fig. 15.2 and the differential impact on children's physical activity behaviour is readily apparent.

Television

Watching television is a popular pastime among children, at least in Europe and North America. The number of hours of television viewed by young people appears to average about two to three per day[124, 1220, 1240] but it varies with age and gender, and from country to country.[703, 820] For example, 2 hours viewing per day has been reported by 87% of 11-year-old boys and 13-year-old girls and boys in Hungary, compared with only 38% of 11-year-old Norwegian girls.[820]

Data relating television viewing to physical activity are conflicting. Two studies of the impact of the introduction of television into small communities in Scotland[255] and Canada[1662] reported a negative correlation between physical activity and television viewing. A significant negative relationship between television viewing and physical fitness among 379 male adolescents has been reported[1545] although physical activity was not assessed in this study. In a national survey parents' (but not teachers') ratings of the level of physical activity of primary schoolchildren were negatively associated with television viewing time.[1241] Conversely, a well-controlled study of 671 adolescent girls cross-sectionally and subsequently 279 of them longitudinally for 2 years reported television viewing time to have only a weak association with physical activity.[1220] Similar findings have been reported with young children aged 3–8 years.[467, 1508] Nevertheless, time spent watching television is time during which physical activity is likely to be low and, of course, what young people watch may be more related to their physical activity behaviour than the length of time they watch television. Broadcasters have a responsibility to balance the many negative messages they transmit with encouragement, perhaps through role model characters in popular programmes, for youngsters to adopt active lifestyles.

Community

Economic differences both between[201] and within countries[438, 806, 1377] affect young people's physical activity patterns. Impoverished children's and adolescents' habitual physical activity may be adversely affected through less access to resources, such as bicycles, skates, and balls, than more affluent young people. They may not have the money for entry to leisure facilities or for membership of youth or sports clubs. They may have restricted leisure time through the need to work after school and during holidays to supplement family income. Teachers, youth leaders, and senior members of sports clubs and similar community organizations should be sensitive to the difficulties of young people from deprived backgrounds and make every effort to facilitate their physical activity needs.

Seasonal differences in physical activity have been observed in a large North American survey.[1237] Activity time peaked in the summer, fell off rapidly in the autumn and winter and then rose towards the summer level during the spring. The physical activity patterns of girls and younger students were disproportionately affected by changes in the weather. A smaller European study in a less variable climate reported no differences in the level of physical activity of 10- and 11-year-old children in the summer and autumn school terms.[63] Nevertheless, planners and managers need to be aware of any seasonal differences in young people's physical activity and to ensure that facilities operate in a way which promotes and sustains youth participation during inclement weather.

Few secure data are available on youngsters' physical activity patterns during the summer vacation when they are unrestricted by school attendance. Whether children and adolescents are more active at weekends than during weekdays which include school attendance is unclear and may vary with age.[57, 64, 1386] Lack of attractive, safe play areas near to home may limit children's physical activity opportunities. The availability of appropriate equipment and the accessibility and cost of using leisure facilities such as swimming pools, sports halls, and playing fields may impose restrictions on adolescents' physical activity behaviour.[284, 1482] Young people should be given some priority to use leisure facilities at times when they can easily attend, such as early evenings, weekends and school holidays, at a cost they can afford.

Youth clubs, sports clubs, and a variety of community organizations provide an important focus for organized physical activity and sport in a community setting.[1236, 1443] There is evidence to suggest that girls have fewer opportunities to participate in community-organized physical activity and sport,[1442, 1445] fewer girls than boys are members of sports clubs and, unlike boys, girls' membership of sports clubs declines in late adolescence.[1444] The gender difference in club membership may be related to the nature of many girls' interests. In out of school time boys tend to opt for competitive and/or team-oriented activities which are generally well supported in the community, whereas girls often choose to participate in individual and less competitive activities which may carry lower prestige.[75, 1237, 1444]

There are a range of ways in which youth leaders and senior members of sports clubs could enhance young people's participation in their organizations. Young people should be consulted and involved in drawing up appropriate plans for the club. Plans should address issues of equity, give equal prestige to all agreed activities, and facilitate membership of all socioeconomic groups in the community. Effective working relationships should be developed with schools and other organizations that provide for young people. Senior personnel should identify with youth sections of a club, be aware of what is offered in local schools, and promote school-to-community links. To encourage young people to sustain club membership mechanisms to facilitate progress through youth sections into adult sections should be established.[1442]

School

All children attend school from an early age and the school setting provides perhaps the most promise for influencing young people's physical activity behaviour. A number of school-based intervention programmes have been mounted with the objective of increasing children's physical activity but they have met with only limited success, sometimes because they were geared towards an outcome of enhancing physical fitness rather than promoting physical activity (reviewed in refs 820, 1298, 1415). In schools, physical activity should not be divorced from other aspects of a healthy lifestyle and special provision should be made for a 'whole-school' cross-curricular approach to promoting healthy lifestyles. Science, home economics, physical education, health education, school meals, and school nursing staff should all be involved in a multidisciplinary, integrated approach. As the role of the school nurse moves towards health promotion he/she could occupy a pivotal role in developing and co-ordinating a school policy for the promotion of physical activity.

The school should explore ways of using resources such as playgrounds and of making equipment (e.g. jump ropes) available at break times in order to promote equitable physical activity which is not dominated by boys' games. Partnerships with families, physicians, and community organizations should be developed, facilities shared where appropriate, and school policy should be sensitive not only to current but also to post-school physical activity needs of its pupils.

Physical education

The value of promoting enjoyable early life experiences of physical activity has been supported by several studies[547, 629, 1399] and primary school physical education is therefore a potentially important vehicle for fostering an appreciation of physical activity. The primary school should provide an ideal environment for promoting an active lifestyle but concerns have been expressed in both Europe and North America over facilities for physical education and access to fully qualified physical education teachers.[321, 1242] Initial teacher training and in-service courses devote an inadequate amount of time to physical education and the time allocated tends to be dominated by team games.[310, 321] This often creates a feeling of inadequacy among primary school staff.[812, 1650] In primary schools, it is unlikely that specialist physical education teachers will always be available but at the very least each school should identify a physical education curriculum leader with responsibility for the subject. The curriculum leader's continuing professional development in the subject should be supported through in-service courses and visiting specialists.

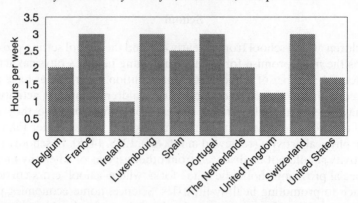

Fig. 15.3. Hours per week of physical education in primary schools (5–11 years). Figure drawn from data extracted from an unpublished survey by the European Physical Education Associations and Ross, J.G., Pate, R.R., Corbin, C.B., Delpy, L.A. and Gold, R.S. (1987). What is going on in the elementary physical education programme? *Journal of Physical Education, Recreation and Dance*, **58**, 78–84.

The weekly quota of school curriculum time for primary school physical education varies between countries (see Fig. 15.3) but the United Kingdom and Ireland allocate less time than other comparable countries. Curriculum content is, however, more important than time and the primary school physical education curriculum is generally very popular with children.[1240] It tends to focus upon individual motor skills and co-operative rather than competitive activities,[1240, 1445] although the recently introduced and prescribed National Curriculum in the United Kingdom promotes an increased emphasis upon competition and generates concern over the possible loss of the fun element of the programme.[415, 767, 1652]

Concerns have been expressed over the activity content of physical education lessons[1073, 1416, 1417] and although there appear to be no significant gender differences in physical activity during structured lesson content girls have been observed to be less active than boys during free play within lessons.[1006] However, although the provision of a high-activity content should be an important component of physical education lessons it is much more important to build a foundation of motor skills and to make children's early activity experiences enjoyable in order to foster future participation. Recommendations for, 'a daily session of vigorous physical activity in each primary school'[1345, p. 27] need to be viewed with caution because children's resistance to participation in regimented, compulsory exercise is well documented.[267, 268, 361]

The transition from primary school to secondary school has been associated with a precipitous drop in children's physical activity.[1092, 1522] This

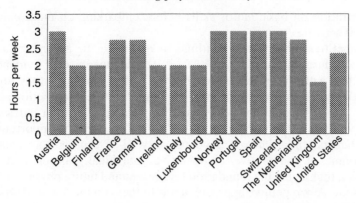

Fig. 15.4. Hours per week of physical education in secondary schools (11–16 years). Figure drawn from data extracted from an unpublished survey by the European Physical Education Associations and Ross, J.G., Dotson, C.O., Gilbert, G.G. and Katz, S.J. (1985). What are kids doing in school physical education? *Journal of Physical Education, Recreation and Dance,* **56**, 73–6.

may be prevented by good primary–secondary school liaison and a more gradual change of emphasis. In most countries more time appears to be devoted to physical education in secondary schools than in primary schools and all countries on which we have data average at least 2 h per week, except in the United Kingdom (see Fig. 15.4). In the United Kingdom only a minority of young people receive 2 h per week of curriculum physical education[1354, 1444] and, despite recommendations for more time to be allocated to physical education from the Government,[421, 488] professional associations,[1167, 1354] and royal colleges of medicine,[320] there has been a marked reduction in recent years.[1355] This is compounded by a growing concern over diminishing resources and the apparent necessity for schools to sell playing fields in order to remain financially viable.[1167, 1355]

The 'moderate to vigorous physical activity' content of lessons has been questioned in both Europe[824, 1471, 1472] and North America[901, 1401, 1469] but it appears that curriculum content and enjoyment and not high-activity content are the most influential factors in developing positive or negative attitudes towards physical education.[930] These factors appear to be particularly important to females less inclined to physical activity and point to the need to create programmes that capture students' interest. In one study of 488 adolescents, both boys and girls indicated that being successful and competent in required activities gave them a positive attitude towards physical education and that a lack of competence and success gave them a negative attitude.[930] These findings emphasize the importance of early concentration on basic motor skills before embarking on more complex physical activities.

Competitive team games continue to dominate the secondary school physical education curriculum[415, 1167, 1238] despite unequivocal evidence to show that, with the possible exception of football for boys, they are not transferring to out-of-school participation.[1307, 1444, 1513] Competitive team games are a valuable component of the physical education curriculum. Many youngsters enjoy team sport and should be given the opportunity to fulfil their potential but young people need to be exposed to a balanced programme of competitive, co-operative, individual, partner, and team activities, thus laying the foundation for present and future physical activity behaviour. A competitive approach tends to focus on the few students with high ability and may alienate the majority of young people. Early maturing boys tend to excel[42, 154, 245] but there is little evidence to suggest that early specialization is necessary for the nurturing of sporting talent.[504, 552] In fact, early specialization may turn young people off lifetime physical activity,[114, 516] especially if through extrinsic teacher/coach domination they have not internalized the motivation to be active and achieved 'activity independence'.[45]

A competitive ethos appears to be more acceptable to boys, but, notably, not acceptable to low-exercising boys.[612] Many girls reject competition, even the high exercisers.[612] Individual sports and activities are far more popular with girls than competitive team games.[242, 1237, 1444] The dislike of many girls for team games should not be confused with inability or disinterest in physical activity but team game dominance of the curriculum may well contribute to girls' low levels of physical activity.[51, 1014] Physical educators need to take a more pensive view of the balance, organization, and presentation of their programmes in order to challenge the gender ideologies reflected in many physical education curricula.[75]

Despite a change in emphasis from physical fitness to physical activity in physical education programmes in both the United Kingdom[47, 248] and the United States,[576, 1268] and regular challenges, over the last decade in the United Kingdom[40, 1168] and more recently in the United States,[576, 1266] most secondary schools in both countries include compulsory fitness testing within their physical education curriculum.[686, 1238] Yet, tests that are suitable for use in the school environment and that provide valid and objective measures of fitness are not available.[41, 43] Fitness tests simply determine the obvious, at best only distinguishing the mature and/or motivated youngster from the immature and/or unmotivated child or adolescent.[55, 62] The use of norm tables promotes ego orientation[413] and confounds the issue of relative fitness because tables constructed on the basis of chronological age cannot be used to classify legitimately young people at different levels of maturity (see Chapter 1). Furthermore, having different norms for boys and girls results in different expectations. Norms are based on performances rather than capabilities and if teachers accept lower norms for girls as reflecting acceptable performances, girls will tend to meet these lower expectations.[1524, 1526] Students view fitness testing unfavourably and as a major contribution to negative attitudes towards physical education.[930] Teachers must ask themselves why they are testing young people's fitness, and if the answer is for classification purposes, then we suggest that they would be better employed seriously addressing the problem of young people's sedentary lifestyles.

Other factors relating to the physical education curriculum which may provide barriers to adopting active lifestyles include the availability of private showering facilities and the compulsory wearing of perceived unattractive 'gym kit'. Clothing has been identified as a determinant of negative attitudes for both males and females but it is a major problem for some girls since notions of femininity and body image are more intensely bound together for them. 'Looking good' remains a significant motivator for girls' participation in physical activity.[930, 1385, 1445] A dialogue between staff and students should be able to solve this perceived problem.

In the United Kingdom there has been a marked decline in school-related extra-curricular physical activities and sport over recent years.[1355] Competitive team games continue to dominate remaining extra-curricular time and a wider choice of activities are on offer to boys than to girls.[1445] Girls' games, such as hockey and netball, appear to carry less prestige in the social life of the school than boys' games, such as football and rugby, and this may reinforce the relative unimportance of physical activity in the lives of adolescent girls. More balanced extra-curricular programmes which appeal to, and are open to, the whole spectrum of young people need to be developed.

Summary

Correlates of physical activity

Young people's physical activity is influenced by a myriad of interacting biological, psychological, social, and environmental factors. Boys are generally more active than girls during childhood and the level of physical activity of both sexes declines as they progress through adolescence. The rate of decline is 2.5 times greater in girls than in boys. Some of the gender difference in physical activity may be explained by biological and psychological factors but the contention that the difference is augmented by social and environmental influences cannot easily be dismissed.

Parental activity habits are likely to influence those of their offspring and parental behaviour in offering, from an early age, more encouragement to be active to sons than to daughters is probably a contributory factor to girls being less active than boys. Peer pressure on young people's physical activity patterns appears to be important but few data are available. Data on the effects of television viewing on physical activity are equivocal and although adverse effects of television watching on physical activity are intuitively plausible the case remains to be proven.

Children's and adolescents' independent mobility has markedly declined over the last two decades but boys continue to enjoy far more freedom of movement than girls. Girls have fewer opportunities to participate in community organized physical activity and sport, and both school physical education curricular and extra-curricular activities appear to be more attractive to boys than girls.

Promoting physical activity

To promote young people's physical activity parents should adopt active lifestyles themselves and support and encourage equally their sons and daughters to be more active. Parents should campaign on behalf of their children for traffic-calming schemes, safe walkways, extensive cycle paths, attractive play areas, and subsidised and easily accessible leisure facilities. Local authorities and community leaders should explore the provision and attraction to young people of youth clubs, sports clubs, and other similar community organizations, always addressing issues of equity.

School governing bodies should appraise the resource they devote to physical education and evaluate their success in building school–community links which are likely to promote post-school physical activities among their pupils. Physical education teachers should examine their curriculum and extra-curricular provision and confirm that, within the constraints within which they are working, they are offering a balanced programme that provides opportunities for all children and facilitates the adoption of active lifestyles which are likely to be sustained into adult life.

References

1. Aaron, D.J., Kriska, A.M., Dearwater, S.R., Andersen, R.F.L., Olsen, T.L. and Cauley, J.A. (1993). The epidemiology of leisure physical activity in an adolescent population. *Medicine and Science in Sports and Exercise*, **25**, 847–53.
2. Abraham, S., Collins, G. and Nordsieck, M. (1971). Relationship of childhood weight status to morbidity in adults. *Public Health Reports*, **86**, 273–84.
3. Abraham, G.E., Stevenson, G.W. and Chiamori, N.Y. (1982). Clinical indications for serum DHEA-S measurements. *Clinical Laboratory Products*, **11**, 8.
4. Acheson, R.M. (1954). A method of assessing maturity from radiographs. A report from the Oxford child health survey. *Journal of Anatomy*, **88**, 488–508.
5. Acheson, R.M. (1966). Maturation of the skeleton. In F. Falkner (Ed.), *Human Development*. Philadelphia, Saunders, pp. 465–502.
6. Activity and Health Research (1992). *Allied Dunbar National Fitness Survey*. London, Sports Council and Health Education Authority.
7. Adams, J.E. (1965). Injury to the throwing arm: a study of traumatic changes in the elbow joint of boy baseball players. *California Medicine*, **102**, 127–32.
8. Adeniran, S.A. and Toriola, A.L. (1988). Effects of continuous and interval running programmes on aerobic and anaerobic capacities in schoolgirls aged 13 to 17 years. *Journal of Sports Medicine and Physical Fitness*, **28**, 260–6.
9. Aherne, W., Ayyar, D.R., Clarke, P.A. and Walton, J.N. (1971). Muscle fiber size in normal infants, children and adolescents: an autopsy study. *Journal of the Neurological Sciences*, **14**, 171–82.
10. Ajzen, I. and Fishbein, M. (1980). *Understanding Attitudes and Predicting Social Behaviour*. Englewood Cliffs, NJ, Prentice-Hall.
11. Akerblom, H., Viikari, J., Uhari, M., Rasanen, L., Dahl, M., Lahde, P-L. *et al.* (1984). Multicenter study of atherosclerosis precursors in Finnish children: report of two pilot studies. In J. Ilmarinen and I. Valimaki (Eds.), *Children and Sport*. Berlin, Springer, pp. 219–30.
12. Albanese, S.A., Palmer, A.K., Kerr, D.R., Carpenter, C.W., Lisi, D. and Levinsohn, E.M. (1989). Wrist pain and distal growth plate closure of the radius in gymnasts. *Journal of Pediatric Orthopedics*, **9**, 23–8.
13. Alexander, R.M., Jayes, A.S., Maloiy, G.M.O. and Wathuta, E.M. (1981). Allometry of the leg muscles of mammals. *Journal of Zoology*, London, **194**, 539–52.
14. Al-Hazzaa, H.M. and Sulaimen, M.A. (1993). Maximal oxygen uptake and daily physical activity in 7- to-12-year-old boys. *Pediatric Exercise Science*, **5**, 357–66.

15. Al-Hazzaa, H.M., Sulaimen, M.A., Al-Matar, A.J. and Al-Mobaireek, K.F. (1994). Cardiorespiratory fitness, physical activity patterns and coronary risk factors in preadolescent boys. *International Journal of Sports Medicine*, **15**, 267–72.

16. Alpert, B.S. and Wilmore, J.H. (1994). Physical activity and blood pressure in adolescents. *Pediatric Exercise Science*, **6**, 361–80.

17. Alter, M.J. (1988). *Science of Stretching*. Champaign, IL, Human Kinetics.

18. American Academy of Pediatrics (1976). Fitness in the pre-school child. *Pediatrics*, **58**, 88–9.

19. American Academy of Pediatrics (1990). Strength training, weight and power lifting, and body building by children and adolescents. *Pediatrics*, **86**, 801–3.

20. American Academy of Pediatrics, Committee on Sports Medicine (1989). Amenorrhea in adolescent athletes. *Pediatrics*, **84**, 394–5.

21. American Academy of Pediatrics, Committee on Sports Medicine (1989). Anabolic steroids and the adolescent athlete. *Pediatrics*, **83**, 127–8.

22. American College of Sports Medicine (1988). Opinion statement on physical fitness in children and youth. *Medicine and Science in Sports and Exercise*, **20**, 422–3.

23. American College of Sports Medicine (1990). Position stand on the recommended quantity and quality of exercise for developing and maintaining cardiorespiratory and muscular fitness in healthy adults. *Medicine and Science in Sports and Exercise*, **22**, 265–74.

24. American College of Sports Medicine (1991). *Guidelines for Exercise Testing and Prescription*. Philadelphia, Lea and Febiger.

25. American Health Foundation (1983). Conference on blood lipids in children: optimal levels for early prevention of coronary artery disease. *Preventive Medicine*, **12**, 741–97.

26. American Psychiatric Association (1994). *Diagnostic and Statistical Manual of Mental Disorders, Fourth edition (DSM-IV)*. Washington, DC.

27. Andersen, K.L., Ilmarinen, J., Rutenfranz, J., Ottman, W., Berndt, I., Kylian, H. *et al.* (1984). Leisure time sport activities and maximal aerobic power during late adolescence. *European Journal of Applied Physiology*, **52**, 431–6.

28. Andersen, K.L., Masironi, R., Rutenfranz, J. and Seliger, V. (1978). *Habitual Physical Activity and Health*. (World Health Organization Regional Publications, European Series, No. 6). Copenhagen, World Health Organization.

29. Andersen, K.L., Seliger, V., Rutenfranz, J. and Skrobak-Kaczynske, J. (1976). Physical performance capacity of children in Norway. Part IV – The rate of growth in maximal aerobic power and the influence of improved physical education of children in a rural community. *European Journal of Applied Physiology*, **35**, 49–58.

30. Anderson, J.J.B. (1991). Nutritional biochemistry of calcium and phosphorus. *Journal of Nutritional Biochemistry*, **2**, 300–7.

31. Anderssen, N. and Wold, B. (1992). Parental and peer influences on leisure-time physical activity in young adolescents. *Research Quarterly for Exercise and Sport*, **63**, 341–8.

32. Andrews, J.R. (1985). Bony injuries about the elbow in the throwing athlete. *American Academy of Orthopedic Surgery Instructional Course Lectures*, **34**, 323.

33. Antonutto, G. and di Prampero, P.E. (1995). The concept of lactate threshold. A short review. *Journal of Sports Medicine and Physical Fitness*, **35**, 6–12.

34. Apple, D.F. (1985). Adolescent runners. *Clinics in Sports Medicine*, **4**, 641–55.

35. Arce, J.C. and de Souza, M.J. (1993). Exercise and male infertility. *Sports Medicine*, **15**, 146–69.

36. Arena, B., Maffulli, N., Maffulli, F. and Morleo, M.A. (1995). Reproductive hormones and menstrual changes with exercise in female athletes.. *Sports Medicine*, **19**, 278–87.

37. Arensman, F.W., Christiansen, J.L. and Strong, W.B. (1989). Juvenile hypertension and exercise. In O. Bar-Or (Ed.), *Advances in Pediatric Sport Sciences, Vol. 3*. Champaign, IL, Human Kinetics, pp. 203–20.

38. Arkin, A.M. and Katz, J.F. (1956). The effects of pressure on epiphyseal growth. *Journal of Bone and Joint Surgery*, **38A**, 1056–76.

39. Armamento-Villereal, R., Villereal, D.T., Avioli, L. and Civitelli, R. (1992). Estrogen status and heredity are major determinants of premenopausal bone mass. *Journal of Clinical Investigations*, **90**, 2464–71.

40. Armstrong, N. (1986). A comment on physical fitness testing. *British Journal of Physical Education*, **17**, 34.

41. Armstrong, N. (1987). A critique of fitness testing. In S. Biddle (Ed.), *Foundations of Health-Related Fitness in Physical Education*. London, Ling Publishing House, pp. 136–8.

42. Armstrong, N. (1987). Health and fitness programmes in schools: a physiological rationale. In S. Biddle (Ed.), *Foundations of Health-Related Fitness in Physical Education*. London, Ling Publishing House, pp. 19–27.

43. Armstrong, N. (1989). Is fitness testing either valid or useful? *British Journal of Physical Education*, **20**, 66–7.

44. Armstrong, N. (1989). Children are fit but not active. *Education and Health*, **7**, 28–32.

45. Armstrong, N. (1990). Children's physical activity patterns – the implications for physical education. In N. Armstrong (Ed.), *New Directions in Physical Education, Vol. 1*. Champaign, IL, Human Kinetics, pp. 1–16.

46. Armstrong, N. (1991). Health-related physical activity. In N. Armstrong and A. Sparkes (Eds.), *Issues in Physical Education*. London, Cassells, pp. 139–54.

47. Armstrong, N. (1992). Are British children and youth fit? *Research Quarterly for Exercise and Sport*, **63**, 449–50.

48. Armstrong, N. (1992). The development of training programmes for children. *Athletics Coach*, **26**, 5–9.

49. Armstrong, N. (1993). Promoting physical activity in schools. *Health Visitor*, **66**, 362–4.

50. Armstrong, N. (1993). Independent mobility and children's physical development. In M. Hillman (Ed.), *Children, Transport and Quality of Life*. London, Policy Studies Institute, pp. 35–43.

51. Armstrong, N. (1995). The challenge of promoting physical activity. *Journal of the Royal Society of Health*, **115**, 187–92.

52. Armstrong, N. (1995). Children, physical activity and health. In. F.J. Ring (Ed.), *Children in Sport*. Bath, Centre for Continuing Education, pp. 5–16.

53. Armstrong, N. (1995). Children's cardipulmonary fitness and physical activity patterns – the European scene. In O. Bar-Or and C.M.J. Blimkie (Eds.), *New Horizons in Pediatric Exercise Science*. Champaign, IL, Human Kinetics, pp. 177–89.

54. Armstrong, N. (1995). Physical education at the crossroads. In M. Darmody and G. O'Donovan (Eds.), *Physical Education at the Crossroads*. Limerick, PEAI, pp. 36–43.

55. Armstrong, N. (1995). The assessment of health-related fitness in schools. In M. Darmody and G. O'Donovan (Eds.), *Physical Education at the Crossroads*. Limerick, PEAI, pp. 44–8.

56. Armstrong, N., Balding, J., Bray, S., Gentle, P. and Kirby, B. (1990). The physical activity patterns of 10 and 13 year old children. In G. Beunen, J. Ghesquiere, R. Reybrouck and A.L. Claessens (Eds.), *Children and Exercise XIV*. Stuttgart, Enke, pp. 152–7.

57. Armstrong, N., Balding, J., Gentle, P. and Kirby, B. (1990). Patterns of physical activity among 11 to 16 year old British children. *British Medical Journal*, **301**, 203–5.

58. Armstrong, N., Balding J., Gentle, P. and Kirby, B. (1990). Estimation of coronary risk factors in British schoolchildren: a preliminary report. *British Journal of Sports Medicine*, **24**, 61–6.

59. Armstrong, N., Balding, J., Gentle, P. and Kirby, B. (1992). Serum lipids and blood pressure in relation to age and sexual maturity. *Annals of Human Biology*, **19**, 477–87.

60. Armstrong, N., Balding, J., Gentle, P., Williams, J. and Kirby, B. (1990). Peak oxygen uptake and habitual physical activity in 11 to 16 year olds. *Pediatric Exercise Science*, **2**, 349–58.

61. Armstrong, N., Bellew, B., Biddle, S., Bray, S., Gardonyi, P. and Winter, E. (1990). Health-related physical activity in the national curriculum. *British Journal of Physical Education*, **21**, 225.

62. Armstrong, N. and Biddle, S. (1992). Health-related physical activity in the national curriculum. In N. Armstrong (Ed.), *New Directions in Physical Education, Vol. 2, Towards a National Curriculum*. Champaign, IL, Human Kinetics, pp. 71–110.

63. Armstrong, N. and Bray, S. (1990). Primary schoolchildren's physical activity patterns during Autumn and Summer. *Bulletin of Physical Education*, **26**, 23–6.

64. Armstrong, N. and Bray, S. (1991). Physical activity patterns defined by heart rate monitoring. *Archives of Disease in Childhood*, **66**, 245–7.

65. Armstrong, N., Chedzoy, S., Welsman, J. and Withers, S. (unpublished). Aerobic training in 10-year-old and adult females.

66. Armstrong, N. and Davies, B. (1980). The prevalence of coronary risk factors in children. *Acta Paediatrica Belgica*, **33**, 209–17.

67. Armstrong, N. and Davies, B. (1981). An ergometric analysis of age group swimmers. *British Journal of Sports Medicine*, **15**, 20–6.

68. Armstrong, N. and Davies, B. (1982). High density lipoprotein cholesterol and physical activity patterns in children. *Australian Journal of Sports Medicine*, **14**, 53–9.

69. Armstrong, N. and Davies, B. (1984). The metabolic and physiological responses of children to exercise and training. *Physical Education Review*, **7**, 90–105.

70. Armstrong, N., Davies, B. and Heal, M. (1983). The specificity of energy utilization by trained and untrained adolescent boys. *British Journal of Sports Medicine*, **17**, 193–9.

71. Armstrong, N. and Ellard, R. (1984). The measurement of alactic anaerobic power in trained and untrained adolescent boys. *Physical Education Review*, **7**, 73–9.

72. Armstrong, N., Kirby, B., McManus, A. and Welsman, J. (1995). Aerobic fitness of pre-pubescent children. *Annals of Human Biology*, **22**, 427–41.

73. Armstrong, N., Kirby, B., McManus, A. and Welsman, J. (1996). Physical activity patterns and aerobic fitness among pre-pubescents. *European Physical Education Review*, **2**, 19–29.

74. Armstrong, N., Kirby, B.J. and Welsman, J.R. (manuscript under review). *Young people, aerobic fitness, physical activity, and fatness.*

75. Armstrong, N. and McManus, A. (1994). Children's fitness and physical activity – a challenge for physical education. *British Journal of Physical Education*, **25**, 20–6.

76. Armstrong, N. and McManus, A. (1996). Growth, maturation and physical education. In N. Armstrong (Ed.), *New Directions in Physical Education, Vol. 3, Change and Innovation*. London, Cassells, pp. 19–32.

77. Armstrong, N., McManus, A. and Welsman, J. (1994). The assessment of aerobic fitness in children. *British Journal of Physical Education*, **25**, 9–11.

78. Armstrong, N. and Simons-Morton, B. (1994). Physical activity and blood lipids in adolescents. *Pediatric Exercise Science*, **6**, 381–405.

79. Armstrong, N. and Welsman, J. (1993). Training young athletes. In M.J. Lee (Ed.), *Coaching Children in Sport*. London, Spon, pp. 191–203.

80. Armstrong, N. and Welsman, J. (1993). Children's physiological responses to exercise. In M. Lee (Ed.), *Coaching Children in Sport*. London, Spon, pp. 64–77.

81. Armstrong, N. and Welsman, J. (1994). Assessment and interpretation of aerobic function in children and adolescents. *Exercise and Sport Sciences Reviews*, **22**, 435–76.

82. Armstrong, N. and Welsman, J. (1994). Laboratory testing in young athletes. In N. Maffuli (Ed.), *A Colour Atlas of Sports Medicine in Childhood and Adolescence*. London, Mosby-Wolfe, pp. 109–22.

83. Armstrong, N. and Welsman, J. (1994). Today's children: fitness, fatness, and physical activity. *Education and Health*, **12**, 66–9.

84. Armstrong, N., Welsman, J. and Winsley, R. (1996). Is peak $\dot{V}O_2$ a maximal index of children's aerobic fitness? *International Journal of Sports Medicine*, **17**, 356–9.

85. Armstrong, N., Wiliams, J., Balding, J., Gentle, P. and Kirby, B. (1991). The peak oxygen uptake of British children with reference to age, sex and sexual maturity. *European Journal of Applied Physiology*, **62**, 369–75.

86. Armstrong, N., Williams, J., Balding, J., Gentle, P. and Kirby, B. (1991). Cardiopulmonary fitness, physical activity patterns, and selected coronary risk factor variables in 11 to 16 year olds. *Pediatric Exercise Science*, **3**, 219–28.

87. Aro, A., Suimakallio, S., Voutailainen, E., Enholm, C. and Wiljasalo, M. (1986). Lipoprotein lipid levels as indicators of the severity of angiographically assessed coronary artery disease. *Atherosclerosis*, **62**, 219–75.

88. Arroll, B. and Beaglehole, R. (1992). Does physical activity lower blood pressure: a critical review of the clinical trials. *Journal of Clinical Epidemiology*, **45**, 439–47.

89. Asano, H. and Hirakoba, S. (1984). Respiratory and circulatory adaptation during prolonged exercise in 10–12 year old children and adults. In J. Ilmarinen and I. Valimaki (Eds.), *Children and Sport*. Berlin, Springer, pp. 119–28.

90. Ashton, N.G. (1983). Relationship of chronic physical activity levels to physiologic and anthropometric variables in 9–10 year old girls. *Medicine and Science in Sports and Exercise*, **15**, 143.

91. Ashwell, M., Cole, T.J. and Dixon, A.K. (1985). Obesity: a new insight into the anthropometric classification of fat distribution shown by computed tomography. *British Medical Journal*, **290**, 1692–4.

92. Asmussen, E. (1962). Muscular performance. In K. Rodahl and S.M. Horvath (Eds.), *Muscle as a Tissue*. New York, McGraw-Hill, pp. 161–75.

93. Asmussen, E. (1973). Growth in muscular strength and power. In G. Rarick (Ed.), *Physical Activity, Human Growth and Development*. London: Academic Press, pp. 60–80.

94. Asmussen, E. and Christensen, E.H. (1967). Kompendium i legemsövelsernes specielle teori, Köbenhavns Universitets Fond til Tilvejebringelse af Läremidler, Köbenhavn, 1967. Cited in P.O. Astrand and K. Rodahl (1986). *Textbook of Work Physiology (3rd edition)*. New York, McGraw-Hill, p. 398.

95. Asmussen, E. and Heeboll-Nielsen, K. (1955). A dimensional analysis of physical performance and growth in boys. *Journal of Applied Physiology*, **7**, 593–603.

96. Asmussen, E., Secher, N.H. and Andersen, E.S. (1981). Heart rate and ventilatory frequency as dimension-dependent variables. *European Journal of Applied Physiology*, **46**, 379–86.

97. Assmann, G. and Funke, H. (1993). HDL metabolism and atherosclerosis. *Journal of Cardiovascular Pharmacology*, **16** (Suppl. 9), S15–S20.

98. Astrand, P.O. (1952). *Experimental Studies of Physical Working Capacity in Relation to Sex and Age*. Copenhagen, Munksgaard.

99. Astrand, P.O. (1971). Personal communication. Cited by R.J. Shephard (Ed.), *Frontiers of Fitness*. Springfield, IL, Charles C. Thomas, p. 336.

100. Astrand, P.O. (1976). The child in sport and physical activity – physiology. In J.G. Albinson and G.M. Andrew (Eds.), *Child in Sport and Physical Activity*. Baltimore, University Park Press, pp. 19–33.

101. Astrand, P.O., Engstrom, L., Eriksson, B.O., Karlberg, P., Nylander, I., Saltin, B. *et al.* (1963). Girl swimmers. *Acta Paediatrica*, **147** (Suppl.), 3–75.
102. Astrand, P.O. and Rodahl, K. (1986). *Textbook of Work Physiology*. New York, McGraw-Hill.
103. Atha, J. (1982). Strengthening muscle. *Exercise and Sport Sciences Reviews*, **9**, 1–73.
104. Atomi, Y., Fukunaga, T., Hatta, H. and Yamamoto, Y. (1987). Relationship between lactate threshold during running and relative gastrocnemius area. *Journal of Applied Physiology*, **63**, 2343–7.
105. Atomi, Y., Fukunaga, T., Yamamoto, Y. and Hatta, H. (1986). Lactate threshold and $\dot{V}O_2$ max of trained and untrained boys relative to muscle mass and composition. In J. Rutenfranz, R. Mocellin and F. Klimt (Eds.), *Children and Exercise XII*. Champaign, IL, Human Kinetics, pp. 53–8.
106. Atomi, Y., Iwaoka, K., Hatta, H., Miyashita, M. and Yamamoto, Y. (1986). Daily physical activity levels in preadolescent boys related to $\dot{V}O_2$ max and lactate threshold. *European Journal of Applied Physiology*, **55**, 156–61.
107. Atomi, Y., Kuroda, Y., Asami, T. and Kawahara, T. (1986). HDL_2-cholesterol of children (10 to 12 years of age), related to $\dot{V}O_2$ max body fat and sex. In J. Rutenfranz, R. Mocellin and F. Klimt (Eds.), *Children and Exercise XII*. Champaign, IL, Human Kinetics, pp. 167–72.
108. August, F., Grumback, M. and Kaplan, S. (1972). Hormonal changes in puberty: III. Correlation of plasma testosterone, LH, FSH, and testicular size, and bone age with pubertal development. *Journal of Clinical Endocrinology and Metabolism*, **34**, 319–26.
109. Austin, A., Warty, V., Janosky, J. and Arslanian, S. (1993). The relationship of physical fitness to lipid and lipoprotein (a) levels in adolescents with IDDM. *Diabetes Care*, **16**, 421–5.
110. Ayalon, A., Inbar, O. and Bar-Or, O. (1974). Relationships among measurements of explosive strength and anaerobic power. In E. Nelson and C.A. Morehouse (Eds.), *International Series on Sports Sciences, Vol. I, Biomechanics IV*. Baltimore, MD, University Park Press, pp. 527–32.
111. Bachrach, L.K., Katzman, D.K. and Litt, I.F. (1991). Recovery from osteopenia in adolescent girls with anorexia nervosa. *Journal of Clinical Endocrinology and Metabolism*, **72**, 602–6.
112. Baer, J.T. (1993). Endocrine parameters in amenorrheic and eumenorrheic adolescent female runners. *International Journal of Sports Medicine*, **14**, 191–5.
113. Bahrke, M.S. and Smith, R.G. (1985). Alterations in anxiety of children after exercise and rest. *American Corrective Therapy Journal*, **39**, 90–4.
114. Bailey, D.A. (1982). Sport and the child: physiological considerations. In R.A. Magill, M.J. Ash and F.L. Smoll (Eds.), *Children in Sport*. Champaign, IL, Human Kinetics, pp. 97–105.
115. Bailey, D.A. (1995). The role of mechanical loading in the regulation of skeletal development during growth. In C.J.R. Blimkie and O. Bar-Or (Eds.), *New Horizons in Pediatric Exercise Science*. Champaign, IL, Human Kinetics, pp. 97–108.

116. Bailey, D., Daniels, K., Dzus, A., Yong-Hing, K., Drinkwater, D., Wilkinson, A. *et al.* (1992). Bone mineral density in the proximal femur of children with Legg Calve Perthes Disease. *Journal of Bone Mineral Research,* **7** (Suppl.), S287.

117. Bailey, D., Drinkwater, D., Faulkner, R. and McKay, H. (1993). Proximal femur bone mineral changes in growing children: dimensional considerations. *Pediatric Exercise Science,* **5**, 388.

118. Bailey, D.A. and Martin, A.D. (1994). Physical activity and skeletal health in adolescents. *Pediatric Exercise Science,* **6**, 330–47.

119. Bailey, D.A. and Mirwald, R.L. (1984). The effect of training on the growth and development of the child. In R.M. Malina (Ed.), *Young Athletes.* Champaign, IL, Human Kinetics, pp. 33–47.

120. Bailey, D.A., Ross, W.D., Mirwald, R.L. and Weese, C. (1978). Size dissociation of maximal aerobic power during growth in boys. *Medicine Sport,* **11**, 140–51.

121. Bailey, D.A., Wedge, J.H., McCulloch, R.G. and Martin, A.D. (1988). The relationship of fractures of the distal radius to growth velocity in children. *Canadian Journal of Sports Sciences,* **3**, 40P–41P.

122. Bailey, R.C., Olson, J., Pepper, S.L., Porszasz, J., Barstow, T.T. and Cooper, D.M. (1995). The level and tempo of children's physical activities: an observational study. *Medicine and Science in Sports and Exercise,* **27**, 1033–41.

123. Balding, J. (1995). Weighing the worry, measuring the mind. *Education and Health,* **12**, 73–6.

124. Balding, J. (1995). *Young People in 1994.* Exeter, University Press.

125. Balding, J. (1995). Drugs: all our children are close to sources. *Education and Health,* **13**, 21–7.

126. Bale, P. (1981). Pre- and post-adolescents' physiological response to exercise. *British Journal of Sports Medicine,* **15**, 246–9.

127. Bale, P. (1992). The functional performance of children in relation to growth, maturation and exercise. *Sports Medicine,* **13**, 151–9.

128. Ball, T.E., Going, S.B. and Lohman, T. (1987). The relationship of muscle cross-sectional area to height in six to eighteen year old children. *Canadian Journal of Sports Sciences,* **12**, 3P.

129. Ballor, D.L., Burke, L.M., Knudson, D.V., Olson, J.R. and Montoye, H.J. (1989). Comparison of three methods of estimating energy expenditure: caltrac, heart rate, and video analysis. *Research Quarterly for Exercise and Sport,* **60**, 362–8.

130. Bandura, A. (1986). *Social Foundations of Thought and Action.* Englewood Cliffs, NJ, Prentice-Hall.

131. Baranowksi, T., Bouchard, C., Bar-Or, O., Bricker, T., Heath, G., Kimm, S.Y.S. *et al.* (1992). Assessment, prevalence, and cardiovascular benefits of physical activity and fitness in youth. *Medicine and Science in Sports and Exercise,* **24**, S237–S247.

132. Baranowski, T., Dworkin, R.J., Cieslik, C., Hooks, P., Clearman, D.R., Ray, L. *et al.* (1984). Reliability and validity of self report of aerobic activity: Family Health Report. *Research Quarterly for Exercise and Sport,* **55**, 309–17.

133. Baranowski, T. and Simons-Morton, B.G. (1991). Dietary and physical activity assessment in school-aged children: measurement issues. *Journal of School Health*, **61**, 195–7.

134. Baranowski, T., Thompson, W.O., DuRant, R.H., Baranowski, J. and Puhl, J. (1993). Observations on physical activity in physical locations: age, gender, ethnicity and month effects. *Research Quarterly for Exercise and Sport*, **64**, 127–33.

135. Baranowski, T., Tsong, Y., Hooks, P., Cieslik, C. and Nader, P.R. (1987). Aerobic physical activity among third to sixth grade children. *Journal of Developmental and Behavioural Pediatrics*, **8**, 203–6.

136. Barnard, R.J. and Wen, S.J. (1994). Exercise and diet in the prevention and control of the metabolic syndrome. *Sports Medicine*, **18**, 218–28.

137. Bar-Or, O. (1980). Climate and the exercising child – a review. *International Journal of Sports Medicine*, **1**, 53–60.

138. Bar-Or, O. (1983). *Pediatric Sports Medicine for the Practioner*. New York, Springer.

139. Bar-Or, O. (1984). The growth and development of children's physiologic and perceptional responses to exercise. In J. Ilmarinen and I. Valimaki (Eds.), *Children and Sport*. Berlin, Springer, pp. 3–17.

140. Bar-Or, O. (1985). Physical conditioning in children with cardiorespiratory disease. *Exercise and Sport Sciences Reviews*, **13**, 305–34.

141. Bar-Or, O. (1987). The Wingate anaerobic test an update on methodology, reliability and validity. *Sports Medicine*, **4**, 381–91.

142. Bar-Or, O. (1989). Temperature regulation during exercise in children and adolescents. In C.V. Gisolfi and D.R. Lamb (Eds.), *Perspectives in Exercise Science and Sports Medicine, Vol. 2, Youth, Exercise, and Sport*. Indianapolis, IN, Benchmark Press, pp. 335–67.

143. Bar-Or, O. (1989). Trainability of the prepubescent child. *The Physician and Sports Medicine*, **17**, 65–82.

144. Bar-Or, O. (1993). Noncardiopulmonary pediatric exercise tests. In T.W. Rowland (Ed.), *Pediatric Laboratory Exercise Testing*. Champaign, IL, Human Kinetics, pp. 165–86.

145. Bar-Or, O. (1995). Obesity. In B. Goldberg (Ed.), *Sports and Exercise for Children with Chronic Health Conditions*. Champaign, IL, Human Kinetics, pp. 335–54.

146. Bar-Or, O. and Baranowski, T. (1994). Physical activity, adiposity and obesity among adolescents. *Pediatric Exercise Science*, **6**, 348–60.

147. Bar-Or, O., Dotan, R. and Inbar, O. (1977). A 30-second all-out ergometric test – its reliability and validity for anaerobic capacity. *Israel Journal of Medical Sciences*, **13**, 326.

148. Bar-Or, O., Dotan, R., Inbar, O., Rotschtein, A., Karlsson, J. and Tesch, P. (1980). Anaerobic capacity and muscle fiber type distribution in man. *International Journal of Sports Medicine*, **1**, 89–92.

149. Bar-Or, O. and Inbar, O. (1978). Relationships among anaerobic capacity, sprint and middle distance running of school children. In R.J. Shephard and H. Lavallée (Eds.), *Physical Fitness Assessment*. Springfield, IL, Charles C. Thomas, pp. 142–7.

150. Bar-Or, O. and Malina, R.M. (1995). Activity, fitness, and health of children and adolescents. In L.W.Y. Cheung and J.B. Richmond (Eds.), *Child Health, Nutrition and Physical Activity*. Champaign, IL, Human Kinetics, pp. 79–123.

151. Bar-Or, O. and Zwiren, L.D. (1973). Physiological effects of increased frequency of physical education classes and of endurance conditioning on 9 to 10 year old girls and boys. In O. Bar-Or (Ed.), *Pediatric Work Physiology*. Natanya, Israel, Wingate Institute, pp. 183–98.

152. Barr, S.I. (1995). Nutritional factors in bone growth and development. In C.J.R. Blimkie and O. Bar-Or (Eds.), *New Horizons in Pediatric Exercise Science*. Champaign, IL, Human Kinetics, pp. 109–20.

153. Barta, L., Czinner, A., Tichy, M. and Bedo, M. (1986). Risk factors in childhood diabetes mellitus. *Acta Paediatrica Hungarica*, **27**, 9–13.

154. Baxter-Jones, A.D.G. (1995). Growth and development of young athletes. *Sports Medicine*, **20**, 59–64.

155. Baxter-Jones, A., Goldstein, H. and Helms, P. (1993). The development of aerobic power in young athletes. *Journal of Applied Physiology*, **75**, 1160–7.

156. Bazzano, C., Cunningham, L.N., Varrassi, G. and Falcanio, T. (1992). Health-related fitness and blood pressure in boys and girls ages 10 to 17 years. *Pediatric Exercise Science*, **4**, 128–35.

157. Beaglehole, R., Trost, D.C., Tamir, I., Kwiterovich, P.P., Glueck, C.J., Insull, W. *et al.* (1980). Plasma high density lipoprotein cholesterol in children and young adults. The lipid research clinics prevalence study. *Circulation*, **62** (Suppl.), 83–92.

158. Becker, D.M. and Vaccaro, P. (1983). Anaerobic threshold alterations caused by endurance training in young children. *Journal of Sports Medicine and Physical Fitness*, **23**, 445–9.

159. Becker, M.H. and Maiman, L.A. (1975). Sociobehavioural determinants of compliance with medical care recommendations. *Medical Care*, **13**, 10–24.

160. Becque, M.D., Katch, V.L., Rocchini, A.P., Marks, C.R. and Moorehead, C. (1988). Coronary risk incidence of obese adolescents: reduction by exercise plus diet intervention. *Pediatrics*, **81**, 605–12.

161. Bedale, E.M. (1923). Energy expenditure and food requirements of children at school. *Proceedings of the Royal Society (London)*, **94**, 368–404.

162. Behnke, A.R. and Wilmore, J.H. (1974). *Evaluation and Regulation of Body Build and Composition*. Englewood Cliffs, NJ, Prentice Hall.

163. Belanger, A.Y. and McComas, A.J. (1981). Extent of motor unit activation during effort. *Journal of Applied Physiology*, **57**, 1131–5.

164. Bell, R.D., Macek, M., Rutenfranz, J. and Saris, W.H.M. (1986). Health indicators and risk factors of cardiovascular diseases during childhood and adolescence. In J. Rutenfranz, R. Mocellin and F. Klimt (Eds.), *Children and Exercise XII*. Champaign, IL, Human Kinetics, pp. 19–27.

165. Bell, R.D., MacDougall, J.D., Billeter, R. and Howald, H. (1980). Muscle fibre types and morphometric analysis of skeletal muscles in six year old children. *Medicine and Science in Sports and Exercise*, **12**, 28–31.

166. Benedict, G., Vaccaro, P. and Hatfield, B.D. (1985). Physiological effects of an eight week precision jump rope program in children. *American Corrective Therapy Journal*, **5**, 108–11.

167. Ben-Ezra, V. and Gallagher, K. (1989). Blood lipid profiles of 8–10 year old children: the effect of diet and exercise. *Medicine and Science in Sports and Exercise*, **21**, 584.

168. Benson, J.E., Allemann,Y., Theintz, G.E. and Howald, H. (1990). Eating problems and calorie intake levels in Swiss adolescent athletes. *International Journal of Sports Medicine*, **11**, 249–52.

169. Benton, J.W. (1983). Epiphyseal fractures in sports. *The Physician and Sports Medicine*, **10**, 63–71.

170. Berenson, G.S. (1980). *Cardiovascular Risk Factors in Children*. New York, Oxford University Press.

171. Berenson, G.S. (1986). *Causation of Cardiovascular Risk Factors in Childhood*. New York, Raven Press.

172. Berg, A., Kim, S.S. and Keul, J. (1986). Skeletal muscle enzyme activities in healthy young subjects. *International Journal of Sports Medicine*, **7**, 236–9.

173. Berg, A., Ringwald, G. and Keul, J. (1980). Lipoprotein-cholesterol in well trained athletes. *International Journal of Sports Medicine*, **1**, 137–8.

174. Berg, M.S., Rogers, R.K.L., Ryschon, T.W. and Vaccaro, P. (1995). Standard criteria for $\dot{V}O_2$ max determination can be used in healthy very active children. *Pediatric Exercise Science*, **7**, 109.

175. Bergen, G. and Christensen, E.H. (1950). Heart rate and body temperature as indices of metabolic rate during work. *Arbeitsphysiologie*, **14**, 255–60.

176. Berger, B.G., Friedman, E. and Eaton, M. (1988). Comparison of jogging, the relaxation response, and group interaction for stress reduction. *Journal of Sport and Exercise Psychology*, **10**, 431–47.

177. Berger, M., Cuppers, H.-J., Hegner, H., Jorgens, V. and Berchtold, P. (1982). Absorption kinetics and biological effects of subcutaneously injected insulin preparations. *Diabetes Care*, **5**, 77–91.

178. Berger, M., Halban, J.P., Assal, R.E., Offord, M., Vranic, M. and Renold, A.E. (1979). Pharmacokinetics of subcutaneously injected tritiated insulin: effects of exercise. In M. Vranic, J. Wahren and S. Horvath (Eds.), Proceedings of a Conference on Diabetes and Exercise. *Diabetes*, **28** (Suppl. 1), 53–7.

179. Bergh, U., Sjodin, B., Forsberg, A. and Svedenhag, J. (1991). The relationship between body mass and oxygen uptake during running in humans. *Medicine and Science in Sports and Exercise*, **23**, 205–11.

180. Berk, M.A., Clutter, W.E., Skor, D.A., Shah, S.D., Gingerich, R.P. and Cryer, P.E. (1985). Enhanced glycemic responsiveness to epinephrine in insulin dependent diabetes mellitus is the result of the inability to secrete insulin. *Journal of Clinical Investigation*, **75**, 1842–51.

181. Berlin, J.A. and Colditz, G.A. (1990). A meta-analysis of physical activity in the prevention of coronary heart disease. *American Journal of Epidemiology*, **132**, 612–28.

182. Beunen, G. (1989). Biological age in pediatric exercise research. In O. Bar-Or (Ed.), *Advances in Pediatric Sport Sciences, Vol. 3*. Champaign, IL, Human Kinetics, pp. 1–40.

183. Beunen, G. and Malina, R.M. (1988). Growth and physical performance relative to the timing of the adolescent spurt. *Exercise and Sport Sciences Reviews*, **16**, 503–40.

184. Beunen, G.P., Malina, R.M., Renson, R., Simons, J., Ostyn, M. and Lefevre, J. (1992). Physical activity and growth, maturation and performance: a longitudinal study. *Medicine and Science in Sports and Exercise*, **24**, 576–85.

185. Beunen, G.P., Malina, R.M., Van't Hof, M.A., Simons, J., Ostyn, M., Renson, R. *et al.* (1988). *Adolescent Growth and Motor Performance*. Champaign, IL, Human Kinetics.

186. Beyer, H.G. (1896). The influence of exercise on growth. *Journal of Experimental Medicine*, **1**, 546–58.

187. Biddle, S. and Armstrong, N. (1992). Children's physical activity: an exploratory study of psychological correlates. *Social Science and Medicine*, **34**, 325–31.

188. Biddle, S., Mitchell, J. and Armstrong, N. (1991). The assessment of physical activity in children: a comparison of continuous heart rate monitoring, self-report and interview techniques. *British Journal of Physical Education Research Supplement*, **10**, 4–8.

189. Billat, V., Gratas-Delamarche, A., Monnier, M. and Delamarche, P. (1995). A test to approach maximal lactate steady state in 12-year-old boys and girls. *Archives of Physiology and Biochemistry*, **102**, 1–8.

190. Biller, B.M.K., Coughlin, J.F., Saxe, V., Schoenfeld, D., Spratt, D.I. and Klibanski, A. (1991). Osteopenia in women with hypothalamic amenorrhea: a prospective study. *Obstetrics and Gynecology*, **78**, 996–1001.

191. Billewicz, W.Z., Fellowes, H.M. and Hytten, C.A. (1976). Comments on the critical metabolic mass and the age of menarche. *Annals of Human Biology*, **3**, 51–9.

192. Billewicz, W.Z., Fellowes, H.M. and Thomson, A.M. (1981). Pubertal changes in boys and girls in Newcastle-upon-Tyne. *Annals of Human Biology*, **8**, 211–19.

193. Binkhorst, R.A., Saris, W.H.M., Noordeloos, A.M., Van't Hof, M.A. and de Haan, A.F.J. (1986). Maximal oxygen consumption of children (6 to 18 years) predicted from maximal and submaximal values in treadmill and bicycle tests. In J. Rutenfranz, R. Mocellin and I. Klimt (Eds.), *Children and Exercise XII*. Champaign, IL, Human Kinetics, pp. 227–32.

194. Birk, T., Quan, A., Schroeder, R., Wight, D. and Fahey, T. (1981). Effects of different exercise intensities and durations on selected lipoproteins, lipids and body composition. *Medicine and Science in Sport and Exercise*, **13**, 97.

195. Bjorntorp, P. (1991). Abdominal adiposity as a generator of risk factors for cardiovascular disease and diabetes. *Briefs in Metabolic Investigation*, **11**, 1–2.

196. Bland, J.M. and Altman, D.G. (1986). Statistical methods for assessing agreement between two methods of clinical measurement. *Lancet*, **i**, 307–10.

197. Blanksby, B. and Gregor, J. (1981). Anthropometric, strength and physiological changes in male and female swimmers with progressive resistance training. *Australian Journal of Sports Sciences*, **1**, 3–6.

198. Blimkie, C.J.R. (1989). Age and sex-associated variation in strength during childhood: anthropometric, morphological, neurologic, biomechanical,

endocrinologic, genetic and physical activity correlates. In C.V. Gisolfi and D.R. Lamb (Eds.), *Perspectives in Exercise Science and Sports Medicine, Vol. 2, Youth, Exercise, and Sport.* Indianapolis, IN, Benchmark Press, pp. 99–161.

199. Blimkie, C.J.R. (1993). Resistance training during preadolescence. *Sports Medicine*, **15**, 389–407.

200. Blimkie, C.J.R. (1993). Benefits and risks of resistance training in children. In B.R. Cahill and A.J. Pearl (Eds.), *Intensive Participation in Children's Sports.* Champaign, IL, Human Kinetics, pp. 133–65.

201. Blimkie, C.J.R. and Bar-Or, O. (Eds.) (1995). *New Horizons in Pediatric Exercise Science.* Champaign, IL, Human Kinetics.

202. Blimkie, C.J., Cunningham, D.A. and Leung, F.Y. (1977). Urinary catecholamine excretion and lactate concentrations in competitive hockey players aged 11 to 23 years. In H. Lavallée and R.J. Shephard (Eds.), *Frontiers of Activity and Child Health.* Quebec, Editions du Pelican, pp. 313–22.

203. Blimkie, C.J.R., Martin,J., Ramsay, J., Sale, D. and MacDougall, D. (1989). The effects of detraining and maintenance weight training on strength development in prepubertal boys. *Canadian Journal of Sports Sciences*, **14**, 102P.

204. Blimkie, C.J.R., Ramsay, J., Sale, D., MacDougall, D., Smith, K. and Garner, S. (1989). Effects of 10 weeks of resistance training on strength development in prepubertal boys. In S. Oseid and K.-H. Carlsen (Eds.), *Children and Exercise XIII.* Champaign, IL, Human Kinetics, pp. 183–97.

205. Blimkie, C.J.R., Rice, S., Webber, C., Martin, J., Levy, D. and Gordon, C. (1993). Effects of resistance training on bone mass and density in adolescent females. *Medicine and Science in Sports and Exercise*, **25** (Suppl.), S48.

206. Blimkie, C.J.R., Rice, S., Webber, C., Martin, J., Levy, D. and Parker, D. (1992). Bone density, physical activity, fitness, anthropometry, gynecologic, endocrine and nutrition status in adolescent girls. In J. Coudert and E. Van Praagh (Eds.), *Pediatric Work Physiology.* Paris, Masson, pp. 201–4.

207. Blimkie, C.J.R., Roche, P. and Bar-Or, O. (1986). The anaerobic-to-aerobic power ratio in adolescent boys and girls. In J. Rutenfranz, R. Mocellin and F. Klimt (Eds.), *Children and Exercise XII.* Champaign, IL, Human Kinetics, pp. 31–8.

208. Block, G. (1982). A review of validations of dietary assessment methods. *American Journal of Epidemiology*, **115**, 492–505.

209. Blomqvist, C.G. and Saltin, B. (1983). Cardiovascular adaptations to physical training. *Annual Reviews in Physiology*, **45**, 169–89.

210. Blount, W.P. and Clark, G.R. (1949). Control of bone growth by epiphyseal stapling. *Journal of Bone and Joint Surgery*, **31A**, 464–78.

211. Boden, G., Master, R.W. and Gordon, S.S. (1980). Monitoring metabolic control in diabetic outpatients with glycosylated haemoglobin. *Annals of Internal Medicine*, **92**, 357–60.

212. Bogardus, C., Thuillez, P., Ravissin, E., Vasquez, B., Narimiga, M. and Azhar, S. (1983). Effect on muscle glycogen depletion on in vivo insulin action in man. *Journal of Clinical Investigation*, **72**, 1605–10.

213. Boileau, R.A., Bonen, A., Heyward, V.H. and Massey, B.H. (1977). Maximal aerobic capacity on the treadmill and bicylcle ergometer of boys 11–14 years of age. *Journal of Sports Medicine and Physical Fitness*, **17**, 153–62.

214. Boileau, R.A., Lohman, T.G., Slaughter, M.H., Horswill, G.A. and Stillman, R.J. (1986). Problems associated with determining body composition in maturing youngsters. In E.W. Brown and C.F. Branta (Eds.), *Competitive Sports for Children and Youth*. Champaign, IL, Human Kinetics, pp. 3–16.

215. Bonanno, J.A. and Lies, J.E. (1974). Effects of physical training on coronary risk factors. *American Journal of Cardiology*, **33**, 760–4.

216. Bonen, A. (1992). Recreational exercise does not impair menstrual cycles: a prospective study. *International Journal of Sports Medicine*, **13**, 110–20.

217. Bonen, A., Belcastro, A.N., Ling, W.Y. and Simpson, A.A. (1981). Profiles of selected hormones during menstrual cycles of teenage athletes. *Journal of Applied Physiology*, **50**, 545–51.

218. Bonjour, J.-P., Theintz, G., Buchs, B., Slosman, D. and Rizzoli, R. (1991). Critical years and stages of puberty for spinal and femoral bone mass accumulation during adolescence. *Journal of Clinical Endocrinology and Metabolism*, **73**, 555–63.

219. Bookwalter, K.W., Bruce, B., Cameron, C., Fox, G.I., Hoffman, V.L., Newquist, P. *et al.* (1950). Grip strength norms for males. *Research Quarterly*, **21**, 249–73.

220. Boreham, C.A.G., Primrose, E.D., Savage, J.M., Cran, G.W. and Strain, J.J. (1992). Selected atherosclerotic risk indicators in schoolchildren from Northern Ireland. In J. Coudert and E. Van Praagh (Eds.), *Pediatric Work Physiology*. Paris, Masson, pp. 93–6.

221. Borer, K.T. (1994). Neurohumoral mediation of exercise-induced growth. *Medicine and Science in Sports and Exercise*, **26**, 741–54.

222. Borms, J. (1986). The child and exercise: an overview. *Journal of Sports Science*, **4**, 3–20.

223. Bouchard, C. (1986). Genetics, growth and physical activity. In F. Landry and W.A.R. Orban (Eds.), *Physical Activity and Human Well-Being*. Miami, FL, Symposium Specialists, pp. 29–45.

224. Bouchard, C., Boulay, M.R., Dionne, F.T., Pérusse, L., Thibault, M.-C. and Simoneau, J.-A. (1990). Genotype, aerobic performance to training. In G. Beunen, J. Ghesquiere, T. Reybrouck and A.L. Claessens (Eds.), *Children and Exercise*. Stuttgart, Enke, pp. 124–35.

225. Bouchard, C., Lesage, R., Lortie, G., Simoneau, J.-A., Hamel, P., Boulay, M.R. *et al.* (1986). Aerobic performance in brothers, dizygotic and monozygotic twins. *Medicine and Science in Sports and Exercise*, **18**, 639–46.

226. Bouchard, C. and Lortie, G. (1984). Heredity and endurance performance. *Sports Medicine*, **1**, 38–64.

227. Bouchard, C. and Malina, R.M. (1983). Genetics of physiological fitness and motor performance. *Exercise and Sport Sciences Reviews*, **11**, 306–37.

228. Bouchard, C., Shephard, R.J., Stephens, T., Sutton, J.R. and McPherson, B.D. (1990). Exercise, fitness and health: the consensus statement. In C. Bouchard,

R.J. Shephard, T. Stephens, J.R. Sutton and B.D. McPherson (Eds.), *Exercise, Fitness and Health*. Champaign, IL, Human Kinetics, pp. 3–28.

229. Bouchard, C., Shephard, R.J., Stephens, T., Sutton, J.R. and McPherson, B.D. (Eds.) (1990). *Exercise, Fitness and Health: a Consensus of Current Knowledge*. Champaign, IL, Human Kinetics.

230. Bouchard, C., Simoneau, J.-A., Lortie, G., Boulay, M.R., Marcotte, M. and Thibault, M.C. (1986). Genetic effects in human skeletal muscle fibre type distribution and enzyme activities. *Canadian Journal of Physiology and Pharmacology*, **64**, 1245–51.

231. Bouchard, C., Taylor, C., Simoneau, J.-A. and Dulac, S. (1991). Testing anaerobic power and capacity. In J.D. MacDougall, H.A. Wenger and H.J. Green (Eds.), *Physiological Testing of the High-Performance Athlete*. Champaign, IL, Human Kinetics, pp. 175–222.

232. Bouchard, C., Tremblay, A., Leblanc, C., Lortie, G., Savard, R. and Theriault, G. (1983). Method to assess energy expenditure in children and adults. *American Journal of Clinical Nutrition*, **37**, 461–7.

233. Boulton, J. (1981). Nutrition in childhood and its relationships to early somatic growth, body fat, blood pressure, and physical fitness. *Acta Paediatrica Scandinavica*, **284**, 30–46.

234. Bourey, R.E. and Santoro, S.A. (1988). Interactions of exercise, coagulation, platelets and fibronolysis – a brief review. *Medicine and Science in Sports and Exercise*, **20**, 439–46.

235. Braden, D.S. and Strong, W.B. (1989). Cardiovascular responses and adaptations to exercise in childhood. In C.V. Gisolfi and D.R. Lamb (Eds.), *Perspectives in Exercise Science and Sports Medicine, Vol. 2, Youth, Exercise, and Sport*. Indianapolis, IN, Benchmark Press, pp. 293–334.

236. Bradfield, R.B., Chan, H., Bradfield, N.E. and Payne, R.R. (1971). Energy expenditures and heart rates of Cambridge boys at school. *American Journal of Clinical Nutrition*, **24**, 1461–6.

237. Bradfield, R.B., Paulos, J. and Grossman, L. (1971). Energy expenditure and heart rate of obese high school girls. *American Journal of Clinical Nutrition*, **24**, 1482–4.

238. Brady, T.A., Cahill, B. and Bodnar, L. (1982). Weight training related injuries. *American Journal of Sports Medicine*, **10**, 1–5.

239. Brahms, M.A., Fumich, R.M. and Ippolito, V.D. (1980). Atypical stress fracture of the tibia in a professional athlete. *American Journal of Sports Science*, **8**, 131–2.

240. Brambilla, P., Manzoni, P., Sironi, P., Del Maschio, A., Di Natale, B. and Chiumello, G. (1994). Peripheral and abdominal adiposity in childhood obesity. *International Journal of Obesity*, **18**, 795–800.

241. Branta, C., Haubenstricker, J. and Seefeldt, V. (1984). Age changes in motor skills during childhood and adolescence. *Exercise and Sport Sciences Reviews*, **12**, 467–520.

242. Branta, C.F., Painter, M. and Kiger, J.E. (1987). Gender differences in play patterns and sport participation of North American youth. In D. Gould and M.R. Weiss (Eds.), *Advances in Pediatric Sport Sciences, Vol. 2*. Champaign, IL, Human Kinetics, pp. 25–42.

243. Bray, G.A. (1990). Exercise and obesity. In C. Bouchard, R.J. Shephard, T. Stephens, J.R. Sutton and B.D. McPherson (Eds.), *Exercise, Fitness and Health*. Champaign, IL, Human Kinetics, pp. 497–510.

244. Bray, M.S., Morrow, J.R., Pivarnik, J.M. and Bricker, J.T. (1992). Caltrac validity for estimating caloric expenditure with children. *Pediatric Exercise Science*, **4**, 166–79.

245. Brewer, J., Balsom, P. and Davis, J. (1995). Seasonal birth distribution amongst European soccer players. *Sports Exercise and Injury*, **1**, 154–7.

246. Brier, C., Drexel, H., Lisch, H.J., Mulhberger, V. and Herold, M. (1985). Essential role of post-heparin lipoprotein lipase activity and of plasma testosterone in coronary artery disease. *Lancet*, **i**, 1242–4.

247. Brisson, G.R., Dulac, S., Peronnet, F. and Ledoux, M. (1982). The onset of menarche: a late event in pubertal progression to be affected by physical training. *Canadian Journal of Applied Sport Sciences*, **7**, 61–7.

248. British Association of Sports Sciences, Health Education Authority and Physical Education Association (1990). Health-related physical activity in the National Curriculum. *British Journal of Physical Education*, **21**, 225.

249. Brodie, D.A. (1988). Techniques of measurement of body composition. Part I. *Sports Medicine*, **5**, 11–40.

250. Brodie, D.A. (1988). Techniques of measurement of body composition. Part II. *Sports Medicine*, **5**, 74–98.

251. Brodie, D.A. and Eston, R.G. (1992). Body fat estimations by electrical impedance and infra-red interactance. *International Journal of Sports Medicine*, **13**, 319–25.

252. Brody, S., Proctor, R.C. and Ashworth, U.S. (1934). Basal metabolism, endogenous nitrogen, creatine and neutral sulphur excretions as functions of body weight. *University of Missouri Agriculture Experiment Station Research Bulletin*, **220**, 1–40.

253. Brooks, G.A. (1985). Anaerobic threshold: review of the concept and directions for future research. *Medicine and Science in Sports and Exercise*, **17**, 22–31.

254. Brooks-Gunn, J., Burrow, C. and Warren, M.P. (1988). Attitudes toward eating and body weight in different groups of female adolescent athletes. *International Journal of Eating Disorders*, **7**, 749–57.

255. Brown, J.R., Cramond, J.K. and Wilde, R.J. (1974). Displacement effects of television and the child's functional orientation to media. In J.G. Blumler and E. Katz (Eds.), *The Uses of Mass Communications: Current Perspectives on Gratifications Research*. Beverley Hills, CA, Sage, pp. 93–112.

256. Brown, C.H., Harrower, J.R. and Deeter, M.F. (1972). The effects of cross-country running on pre-adolescent girls. *Medicine and Science in Sports*, **4**, 1–5.

257. Brown, D.R. (1990). Exercise, fitness, and mental health. In C. Bouchard, R.J. Shephard, T. Stephens, J.R. Sutton and B.D. McPherson (Eds.), *Exercise, Fitness and Health*. Champaign, IL, Human Kinetics, pp. 607–26.

258. Brown, E.W. and Kimball, R.G. (1983). Medical history associated with adolescent powerlifting. *Pediatrics*, **72**, 636–44.

259. Brown, J.D. and Lawton, M. (1986). Stress and well-being in adolescence: the moderating role of physical exercise. *Journal of Human Stress*, **12**, 125–31.

260. Brown, J.D. and Seigel, J.M. (1988). Exercise as a buffer of life stress: a prospective study of adolescent health. *Health Psychology*, **7**, 341–53.

261. Brown, R.S. (1982). Exercise and mental health in the pediatric population. *Clinics in Sports Medicine*, **1**, 515–27.

262. Brown, S.W., Welch, M.C., Labbe, E.E., Vitulli, W.F. and Kulkarni, P. (1992). Aerobic exercise in the psychological treatment of adolescents. *Perceptual and Motor Skills*, **74**, 755–60.

263. Brownell, KD., Rodin, J. and Wilmore, J.H. (1988). Eat, drink and be worried? *Runner's World*, 28 August.

264. Brozek, J., Grande, F., Anderson, J.T. and Keys, A. (1963). Densitometric analysis of body composition: revision of some quantitative assumptions. *Annals of the New York Academy of Science*, **110**, 113–40.

265. Brunner, B.C. (1969). Personality and motivating factors influencing adult participation in vigorous physical activity. *Research Quarterly*, **40**, 464–9.

266. Brustad, R.J. (1993). Who will go out and play? Parental and psychological influences on children's attraction to physical activity. *Pediatric Exercise Science*, **5**, 210–23.

267. Bryant, J.G., Garett, H.L. and Dean, M.S. (1984). Coronary heart disease: the beneficial effects of exercise to children. *Louisiana State Medical Journal*, **136**, 15–17.

268. Bryant, J.G., Garett, H.L. and Dean, M.S. (1984). The effects of an exercise programme on selected risk factors to coronary heart disease in children. *Social Science and Medicine*, **19**, 765–6.

269. Buchanan, J., Meyers, C., Lloyd, T., Leuenberger, P. and Derners, L. (1988). Determinants of peak trabecular bone density in women: the role of androgens, estrogen, and exercise. *Journal of Bone Mineral Research*, **3**, 673–80.

270. Bucher, C.A. (1974). National adult physical fitness survey: some implications. *Journal of Health Physical Education and Recreation*, **45**, 25–8.

271. Buckley, W.E., Yesalis, C.E., Friedl, K.E., Anderson, W.A., Streit, A.L. and Wright, J.E. (1988). Estimated prevalence of anabolic steroid use among male high school seniors. *Journal of the American Medical Association*, **260**, 3441–5.

272. Buhrmester, D. and Furman, W. (1987). The development of companionship and intimacy. *Child Development*, **58**, 1101–13.

273. Bullen, B.A., Reed, R.B. and Mayer, J. (1964). Physical activity of obese and non-obese adolescent girls appraised by motion picture sampling. *American Journal of Clinical Nutrition*, **14**, 211–23.

274. Bullen, B.A., Skrinar, G.S., Beitins, I.Z., Carr, D.B., Reppert, S.M., Dotson, C.O. *et al.* (1984). Endurance training effects on plasma hormonal responsiveness and sex hormone excretion. *Journal of Applied Physiology*, **56**, 1453–63.

275. Bullen, B.A., Skrinar, G.S., Beitins, I.Z., von Mering, G., Turnbull, B.A. and McArthur, J.W. (1985). Induction of menstrual disorders by strenuous exercise in untrained women. *New England Journal of Medicine*, **312**, 1349–53.

276. Buono, M.J., Roby, J.J., Micale, F.G. and Sallis, J.F. (1989). Predicting maximal oxygen uptake in children: modification of the Astrand-Rhyming test. *Pediatric Exercise Science*, 1, 278–83.

277. Burckes-Miller, M.E. and Black, D.R. (1988). Black, male and female college athletes. Prevalence of anorexia nervosa and bulimia nervosa. *Athletic Training*, 23, 137–40.

278. Burke, V., Beilin, L.J., Milligan, R. and Thompson, C. (1995). Assessment of nutrition and physical activity education programmes in children. *Clinical and Experimental Pharmacology and Physiology*, 22, 212–16.

279. Burnie, J. and Brodie, D.A. (1986). Isokinetic measurement in preadolescent males. *International Journal of Sports Medicine*, 7, 205–9.

280. Burstein, R., Polychronakos, C., Toews, C.J., MacDougall, J.D., Guyda, H.J. and Posner, B.I. (1985). Acute reversal of the enhanced insulin action in trained athletes: association with insulin receptor changes. *Diabetes*, 34, 756–60.

281. Buskirk, E.R. (1961). Underwater weighing and body density: a review of procedures. In J. Brozek and A. Henschel (Eds.), *Techniques for Measuring Body Composition*. Washington, DC, National Academy of Science.

282. Buss, D.M., Block, J.H. and Block, J. (1980). Preschool activity level: personality correlates and developmental implications. *Child Development*, 51, 401–8.

283. Busse, M.W., Muller, M. and Boning, D. (1983). A method of continuous treadmill testing. International Congress on Sports and Health Maastricht, The Netherlands, 22–24 September. *International Journal of Sports Medicine*, (abstract suppl.), 2.

284. Butcher, J. (1983). Socialization of adolescent girls into physical activity. *Adolescence*, 18, 753–66.

285. Butler, G.E., Walker, R.F., Walker, R.V., Teague, P., Riad-Fahmy, D. and Ratcliffe, S.G. (1989). Salivary testosterone levels and the progress of puberty in the normal boy. *Clinical Endocrinology*, 30, 587–96.

286. Cahill, B.R. and Griffith, E.H. (1978). Effect of pre-season conditioning on the incidence and severity of high school football knee injuries. *American Journal of Sports Medicine*, 6, 180–4.

287. Cahill, B.R. and Pearl, A.J. (Eds.) (1993). *Intensive Participation in Children's Sports*. Champaign, IL, Human Kinetics.

288. Caine, D.J. (1990). Growth plate injury and bone growth: an update. *Pediatric Exercise Science*, 2, 209–29.

289. Caizzo, V.J. and Kyle, C.R. (1980). The effects of external loading upon power output in stair climbing. *European Journal of Applied Physiology*, 44, 217–22.

290. Calder, W.A. III. (1987). Scaling energetics of homeothermic vertebrates: an operational allometry. *Annual Reviews in Physiology*, 49, 107–20.

291. Calderone, G., Leglise, M., Giampietro, M. and Berlutti, G. (1986). Anthropometric measurements, body composition, biological maturation and growth predictions in young female gymnasts of high agonistic level. *Journal of Sports Medicine*, 26, 263–73.

292. Cale, L. and Almond, L. (1992). Physical activity levels of young children: a review of the evidence. *Health Education Journal*, 51, 94–9.

293. Calfas, K.J. and Taylor, W.C. (1994). Effects of physical activity on psychological variables in adolescents. *Pediatric Exercise Science*, **6**, 406–23.

294. Calvo, M., Kumar, R. and Heath, H. (1990). Persistently elevated parathyroid hormone secretion and action in young women after four weeks of ingesting high-phosphorus, low-calcium diets. *Journal of Clinical and Endocrinological Metabolism*, **70**, 1334–40.

295. Cameron, N. (1976). Weight and skinfold variation at menarche and the critical body weight hypothesis. *Annals of Human Biology*, **3**, 279–82.

296. Campaigne, B.N., Gilliam, T.B., Spencer, M.L. and Gold, E.R. (1984). Heart rate holter monitoring of 6- and 7-year-old children with insulin dependent diabetes mellitus cardiovascular and short-term metabolic response to exercise: a pilot study. *Research Quarterly for Exercise and Sport*, **55**, 69–73.

297. Campaigne, B.N., Gilliam, T.B., Spencer, M.L., Lampman, R.M. and Schork, M.A. (1984). Effects of a physical activity program on metabolic control and cardiovascular fitness in children with insulin-dependent diabetes mellitus. *Diabetes Care*, **7**, 57–62.

298. Campaigne, B.N., Landt, K.W., Mellies, M.J., James, F.W., Glueck, C.J. and Sperling, M.A. (1985). The effects of physical training on blood lipid profiles in adolescents with insulin-dependent diabetes mellitus. *The Physician and Sports Medicine*, **13**, 83–9.

299. Canada Fitness Survey (1983). *Canadian Youth and Physical Activity*. Ottawa, Canada, Fitness Canada.

300. Canada Fitness Survey (1985). *Physical Fitness of Canadian Youth*. Ottawa, Canada, Fitness Canada.

301. Cann, C.E., Martin, M.C. and Jaffe, R.B. (1985). Duration of amenorrhea affects rate of bone loss in women runners: implications for therapy. *Medicine and Science in Sports and Exercise*, **17**, 214.

302. Capozzo, A. (1983). Force actions in the human trunk during running. *Journal of Sports Medicine and Physical Fitness*, **23**, 14–22.

303. Carew, T.E., Koschinsky, T., Hayes, S.B. and Steinberg, D. (1976). A mechanism by which high density lipoproteins may slow the atherogenic process. *Lancet*, **i**, 1315–17.

304. Carli, G., Martelli, G., Viti, A., Baldi, L., Bonifazi, M. and Lupo di Prisco, C. (1983). The effect of swim training on hormonal levels in girls. *Journal of Sports Medicine and Physical Fitness*, **23**, 45–51.

305. Carli, G., Martelli, G., Viti, A., Baldi, L., Bonifazi, M. and Lupo di Prisco, C. (1983). Modulation of hormone levels in male swimmers during training. In A.P. Hollander, P.A. Huijing and C. de Groot (Eds.), *Biomechanics and Medicine in Swimming*. Champaign, IL, Human Kinetics, pp. 33–40.

306. Carlson, J.S. and Naughton, G.A. (1992). Determination of the maximal accumulated oxygen deficit in male children. In J. Coudert and E. Van Praagh (Eds.), *Pediatric Work Physiology*. Paris, Masson, pp. 23–5.

307. Carlson, J.S. and Naughton, G.A. (1993). An examination of the anaerobic capacity of children using maximal accumulated oxygen deficit. *Pediatric Exercise Science*, **5**, 60–71.

308. Carlson, J.S. and Naughton, G.A. (1994). Performance characteristics of children using various braking resistances on the Wingate anaerobic test. *Journal of Sports Medicine and Physical Fitness*, **34**, 362–9.

309. Carlson, L. and Bottiger, A. (1972). Ischemic heart disease in relation to fasting values of plasma triglycerides and cholesterol. Stockholm Prospective Study. *Lancet*, **i**, 865–8.

310. Carney, C. and Armstrong, N. (1996). The provision of physical education in primary initial teacher training courses in England and Wales. *European Physical Education Review*, **2**, 64–74.

311. Carron, A.V. and Bailey, D.A. (1974). Strength development in boys from 10 through 16 years. *Monographs of the Society for Research in Child Development*, **39**, 1–37.

312. Carter, S.R., Aldridge, M.J., Fitzgerald, R. and Davis, A.M. (1988). Stress changes of the wrist in adolescent gymnasts. *British Journal of Radiology*, **61**, 109–12.

313. Caspari, A.F. and Ewing, L.D. (1985). Severe hypoglycemia in diabetic patients: frequency, causes, prevention. *Diabetes Care*, **8**, 141–5.

314. Casper, R.C. (1995). Fear of fatness and anorexia nervosa in children. In L.W.Y. Cheung and J.B. Richmond (Eds.), *Child Health, Nutrition, and Physical Activity*. Champaign, IL, Human Kinetics, pp. 211–34.

315. Casper, R.C. and Offer, D. (1990). Weight and dieting concerns in adolescents, fashion or symptom? *Pediatrics*, **86**, 385–90.

316. Casperson, C.J. (1989). Physical activity epidemiology: concepts, methods and applications to exercise science. *Exercise and Sport Sciences Reviews*, **17**, 423–74.

317. Casperson, C.J., Powell, K. and Christenson, G. (1985). Physical activity, exercise and physical fitness: definitions and distinctions of health-related research. *Public Health Reports*, **100**, 126–31.

318. Cassady, S.L., Neilsen, D.H., Janz, K.F., Wu, Y.T., Cook, J.S. and Hansen, J.R. (1993). Validity of near infrared body composition analysis in children and adolescents. *Medicine and Science in Sports and Exercise*, **25**, 1185–91.

319. Cassell, C., Benedict, M., Uetrect, G., Ranz, J., Ho, M. and Specker, B. (1993). Bone mineral density in young gymnasts and swimmers. *Medicine and Science in Sports and Exercise*, **25** (Suppl.), S49.

320. Central Council for Physical Recreation (1994). *A Charter for School Sport*. London, Central Council for Physical Recreation.

321. Central Council for Physical Recreation and National Association of Headteachers (1992). *National Survey of Physical Education in Primary Schools*. London, Central Council for Physical Recreation.

322. Cerretelli, P., Pendergast, D., Paganelli, W.C. and Rennie, D.W. (1979). Effects of specific muscle training on $\dot{V}O_2$ on response and early blood lactate. *Journal of Applied Physiology*, **47**, 761–9.

323. Chan, G.M. (1991). Dietary calcium and bone mineral status of children and adolescents. *American Journal of Diseases of Children*, **146**, 631–4.

324. Chan, O.L., Duncan, M.T., Sundsten, J.W., Thinakaran, T., Noh, M.N.B.C. and Klissouras, V. (1976). The maximum aerobic power of the Temiars. *Medicine and Science in Sports*, **8**, 235–8.

325. Chandler, T.J., Kibler, W.B., Uhl, T.L., Wooten, B., Kiser, A.M. and Stone, E. (1990). Shoulder strength, power, and endurance in college tennis players. *American Journal of Sports Medicine*, **20**, 455–8.

326. Charney, E., Chamblee Goodman, H., McBride, M., Lyon, B. and Pratt, R. (1976). Childhood antecedents of adult obesity. Do chubby infants become obese adults? *New England Journal of Medicine*, **295**, 6–9.

327. Chatterjee, S., Banerjee, P.K., Chatterjee, P. and Maitra, S.R. (1979). Aerobic capacity of young girls. *Indian Journal of Medical Research*, **69**, 327–33.

328. Chausow, S.A., Riner, W.F. and Boileau, R.A. (1984). Metabolic and cardiovascular responses of children during prolonged physical activity. *Research Quarterly for Exercise and Sport*, **55**, 1–7.

329. Chestnut, C. (1991). Theoretical overview: bone development, peak bone mass, bone loss, and fracture risk. *American Journal of Medicine*, **91** (Suppl. 5B), 2S–4S.

330. Cheung, L.W.Y. and Richmond, J.B. (1995). *Child Health, Nutrition and Physical Activity*. Champaign, IL, Human Kinetics.

331. Chilibeck, P.D., Sale, D.G. and Webber, C.E.(1995). Exercise and bone mineral density. *Sports Medicine*, **19**, 103–22.

332. Choay, P. and Morla, S. (1981). The "Know Your Body" program in France. *Preventive Medicine*, **10**, 149–58.

333. Chow, K., Harrison, J.E. and Notarius, C. (1987). Effect of two randomized exercise programmes on bone mass of healthy postmenopausal women. *British Medical Journal*, **295**, 1441–4.

334. Christakis, G., Sajeckie, S., Hillman, R.W., Miller, E., Blumenthal, S. and Archer, M. (1966). Effect of a combined nutrition education – physical fitness program on weight status of obese high school boys. *Federation Proceedings*, **25**, 15–19.

335. Claessens, A.L., Malina, R.M., Lefevre, J., Beunen, G., Stijnen, V., Maes, H. et al. (1992). Growth and menarcheal status of elite female gymnasts. *Medicine and Science in Sports and Exercise*, **24**, 755–63.

336. Clain, M.R. and Hershman, E.B. (1989). Overuse injuries in children and adolescents. *The Physician and Sports Medicine*, **17**, 111–22.

337. Clark, N., Nelson, M. and Evans, W. (1988). Nutrition education for elite female runners. *The Physician and Sports Medicine*, **16**, 124–36.

338. Clarke, H.H. (1974). National adult physical fitness survey. *Physical Fitness Research Digest*, **4**, 2.

339. Clarke, W.R., Schrott, H.G., Leaverton, P.E., Connor, W.E. and Lauer, R.M. (1978). Tracking of blood lipids and blood pressures in school-age children: the Muscatine Study. *Circulation*, **58**, 626–34.

340. Clausen, J.P. (1977). Effect of physical training on cardiovascular adjustments to exercise in man. *Physiological Reviews*, **57**, 779–815.

341. Coates, T.J. and Thoresen, C.E. (1978). Treating obesity in children and adolescents: a review. *American Journal of Public Health*, **68**, 143–51.

342. Cohen, J.L., Potosnak, L., Frank, O. and Baker, H. (1985). A nutritional and hematologic assessment of elite ballet dancers. *The Physician and Sports Medicine*, **13**, 43–54.

343. Cohen, M.V. (1983). Coronary and collateral blood flows during exercise and myocardial vascular adaptations to training. *Exercise and Sport Sciences Reviews*, **11**, 55–98.

344. Colling-Saltin, A.-S. (1980). Skeletal muscle development in the human fetus and during childhood. In K. Berg and B.O. Eriksson (Eds.), *Children and Exercise IX*. Baltimore, MD, University Park Press, pp. 193–207.

345. Conroy, B.P., Kraemer, W.J., Maresh, C.M., Fleck, S.J., Stone, M.H., Frey, A.C. et al. (1993). Bone mineral density in elite junior Olympic weightlifters. *Medicine and Science in Sports and Exercise*, **25**, 1103–9.

346. Consensus Development Conference (1991). Diagnosis, prophylaxis and treatment of osteoporosis. *American Journal of Medicine*, **90**, 170–210.

347. Consolazio, C.F., Johnson, R.E. and Pecora, L.J. (Eds.). (1963). *Physiological Measurements of Metabolic Functions in Man*. New York, McGraw-Hill.

348. Constantini, N.W. (1994). Clinical consequences of athletic amenorrhoea. *Sports Medicine*, **17**, 213–23.

349. Conway, J.M. and Norris, K.H. (1984). A new approach for the estimation of body composition: Infrared interactance. *American Journal of Clinical Nutrition*, **40**, 1123–30.

350. Cook, D.L. (1962). The Hawthorne Effect in educational research. *Phi Delta Kappa*, **44**, 116–22.

351. Cook, J., Altman, D.G., Moore, D.M.C., Topp, S.G. and Holland, W.W. (1973). A survey of the nutritional status of schoolchildren. *British Journal of Preventive and Social Medicine*, **27**, 91–9.

352. Cook, T.C., LaPorte, R.E., Washburn, R.A., Traven, N.D., Slemenda, C.W. and Metz, K.F. (1986). Chronic low-level physical activity as a determinant of high-density lipoprotein cholesterol and subfractions. *Medicine and Science in Sports and Exercise*, **18**, 653–7.

353. Cooper, C., Cawley, M., Bhalla, A., Egger, P., Ring, F., Morton, L. et al. (1995). Childhood growth, physical activity and peak bone mass in women. *Journal of Bone and Mineral Research*, **10**, 940–7.

354. Cooper, D.M. (1989). Development of the oxygen transport system in normal children. In O. Bar-Or (Ed.), *Advances in Pediatric Sports Sciences, Vol. 3*. Champaign, IL, Human Kinetics, pp. 67–100.

355. Cooper, D.M. and Berman, N. (1995). Ratios and regressions in body size and function: a commentary. *Journal of Applied Physiology*, **77**, 2015–17.

356. Cooper, D.M., Berry, C., Lamarra, N. and Wasserman, K. (1985). Kinetics of oxygen uptake and heart rate at onset of exercise in children. *Journal of Applied Physiology*, **59**, 211–17.

357. Cooper, D.M., Kaplan, M.R., Baumgarten, L., Weiler-Ravell, D., Whipp, B.J. and Wasserman, K. (1987). Coupling of ventilation and CO_2 production during exercise in children. *Pediatric Research*, **21**, 568–72.

358. Cooper, D.M., Poage, J., Barstow, T.J. and Springer, C. (1990). Are obese children truly unfit? Minimizing the confounding effect of body size on the exercise response. *Journal of Pediatrics*, **116**, 223–30.

359. Cooper, D.M., Weiler-Ravell, D., Whipp, B.J. and Wasserman, K. (1984). Aerobic parameters of exercise as a function of body size during growth. *Journal of Applied Physiology*, **56**, 628–34.

360. Cooper, K.H., Pollock, M.L., Martin, R.P., White, S.R., Linnerud, A.C. and Jackson, A. (1976). Physical fitness levels vs selected coronary risk factors. *Journal of the American Medical Association*, **236**, 166–9.

361. Cooper, K.H., Purdy, J.G., Friedman, A., Bohannon, R.L., Harris, R.A. and Arrends, J.A. (1975). An aerobics conditioning programme for the Fort Worth TX school district. *Research Quarterly*, **46**, 345–50.

362. Corbin, C.B. and Lindsay, R. (1984). *The Ultimate Fitness Book*. New York, Leisure Press.

363. Corbin, C.B. and Lindsey, R. (1985). *Concepts of Physical Fitness*. Dubuque, IA, Brown.

364. Corbin, C.B. and Lindsey, R. (1990). *Fitness for Life*. Glenview, IL, Scott, Foresman and Co.

365. Corbin, C.B. and Pletcher, P. (1968). Diet, physical activity patterns of obese and non-obese elementary schoolchildren. *Research Quarterly*, **39**, 922–8.

366. Cordain, L., Whicker, R.E. and Johnson, J.E. (1988). Body composition determination in children using bioelectrical impedance. *Growth, Development and Ageing*, **52**, 37–40.

367. Corder, B.W., Dezelsky, T.L., Toohey, J.V. *et al.* (1975). An analysis of trends in drug use behavior at ten central Arizona high schools. *Arizona Journal of Health, Physical Education, Recreation and Dance*, **18**, 10–11.

368. Coronary Prevention Group (1989). *Should the Prevention of Coronary Heart Disease Begin in Childhood?* London, Coronary Prevention Group.

369. Costello, J. and Laubach, S.A. (1978). Student behaviour. In W.C. Anderson and G.T. Barrette (Eds.), What's going on in gym: descriptive studies of physical education classes. *Motor Skills Theory into Practice Monograph*, **1**, 11–24.

370. Coward, W.A. (1988). The doubly-labelled-water ($^2H_2{}^{18}O$) method: principles and practice. *Proceedings of the Nutrition Society*, **47**, 209–18.

371. Crasslet, W. (1988). Somatic development in children aged 7–18 years. In A. Dirix, H.G. Knuttgen and K. Tittel (Eds.), *The Olympic Book of Sports Medicine, Vol. 1*. Oxford, Blackwell, pp. 286–99.

372. Crawford, J.D. and Ostler, D.C. (1975). Body composition at menarche: the Frisch-Revelle hypothesis revisited. *Pediatrics*, **56**, 449–58.

373. Crielaard, J.M., Piront, B., Franchimont, P., Pirnay, F. and Petit, J.M. (1986). Evolution de la capacité anaérobie lactique au cours de la croissance. *Médicine du Sport*, **60**, 8–14.

374. Crisp, A.H., Kalucy, R.S., Lacey, J.H. and Harding, B. (1977). The long-term prognosis in anorexia nervosa: some factors predictive of outcome. In R. Vigersky (Ed.), *Anorexia Nervosa*. New York, Raven Press, pp. 55–65.

375. Cumming, G.R. (1967). Current levels of fitness. *Canadian Medical Association Journal*, **88**, 351–5.

376. Cumming, G.R. (1971). Personal communication. Cited by R.J. Shephard (Ed.), *Frontiers of Fitness*. Springfield, IL, Charles C. Thomas, p. 336.

377. Cumming, G.R. (1974). Correlation of athletic performance and anaerobic power in 12–17 year old children with bone age, calf muscle and total body potassium, heart volume and two indices of anaerobic power. In O. Bar-Or (Ed.), *Pediatric Work Physiology*. Israel, Wingate Institute, pp. 109–34.

378. Cumming, G.R., Hastman, L., McCort, J. and McCullough, S. (1980). High serum lactates do occur in children after maximal work. *International Journal of Sports Medicine*, **1**, 66–9.

379. Cumming, G.R. and Langford, S. (1985). Comparison of nine exercise tests used in pediatric cardiology. In R.A. Binkhorst, H.C.G. Kemper and W.H.M. Saris (Eds.), *Children and Exercise XI*. Champaign, IL, Human Kinetics, pp. 58–68.

380. Cunningham, D.A. (1980). Physical working capacity of children and adolescents. In G.A. Stull (Ed.), *Encyclopedia of PE, Fitness and Sports*. Utah, Brighton Publishing Co., pp. 481–94.

381. Cunningham, D.A. and Enyon, R.B. (1973). The working capacity of young competitive swimmers, 10–16 years of age. *Medicine and Science in Sports*, **5**, 227–31.

382. Cunningham, D.A. and Faulkner, J.A. (1969). The effect of training on aerobic and anaerobic metabolism during a short exhaustive run. *Medicine and Science in Sports*, **1**, 65–9.

383. Cunningham, D.A., MacFarlane, B., Waterschoot, V., Paterson, D.H., Lefcoe, M. and Sangal, S.P. (1977). Reliability and reproducibility of maximal oxygen uptake measurement in children. *Medicine and Science in Sports*, **9**, 104–8.

384. Cunningham, D.A., Paterson, D.H. and Blimkie, C.J.R. (1984). The development of the cardiorespiratory system with growth and physical activity. In R.A. Boileau (Ed.), *Advances in Pediatric Sport Sciences, Vol. 1*. Champaign, IL, Human Kinetics, pp. 85–116.

385. Cunningham, D.A., Paterson, D.H., Blimkie, C.J.R. and Donner, A.P. (1984). Development of cardiorespiratory function in circumpubertal boys: a longitudinal study. *Journal of Applied Physiology*, **56**, 302–7.

386. Cunningham, D.A., Stapleton, J.J., MacDonald, I.C. and Paterson, D.H. (1981). Daily energy expenditure of young boys as related to maximal aerobic power. *Canadian Journal of Appied Sports Science*, **6**, 207–11.

387. Cunningham, D.A., Telford, P. and Swart, G.T. (1976). The cardiopulmonary capacities of young hockey players: age 10. *Medicine and Science in Sports*, **8**, 23–5.

388. Cureton, K.J. (1987). Commentary on children and fitness: a public health perspective. *Research Quarterly for Exercise and Sport*, **58**, 315–20.

389. Currey, J.D. and Butler, G. (1975). The mechanical properties of bone tissue in children. *Journal of Bone and Joint Surgery*, **57**, 810–17.

390. Dahl, M., Uhari, M., Viikari, J., Akerblom, H.K., Lahde, P.L., Pesonen, E. *et al.* (1985). Athersclerosis precursors in Finnish children and adolescents. III. Blood pressure. *Acta Paediatrica Scandinavia*, **318**, 89–102.

391. Dahl-Jørgensen, K., Meen, H.D., Hanssen, Kr.F. and Aagenaes, O. (1980). The effect of exercise on diabetic control and hemoglobin A_1 (HbA$_1$) in children. *Acta Paediatrica Scandinavica*, **283** (Suppl.), 53–6.

392. Dalsky, G., Stocke, K.S. and Ehsani, A.A. (1988). Weight-bearing exercise training and lumbar bone mineral content in postmenopausal women. *Annals of Internal Medicine*, **108**, 824–8.

393. Danforth, J.S., Allen, K.D., Fitterling, J.M., Danforth, J.A., Farrar, D., Brown, M. and Drabman, R.S. (1990). Exercise as a treatment for hypertension in low-socioeconomic-status black children. *Journal of Consulting Clinical Psychology*, **58**, 237–9.

394. Daniels, J.T., Oldridge, N., Nagle, F. and White, B. (1978). Differences and changes in $\dot{V}O_2$ among young runners 10 to 18 years of age. *Medicine and Science in Sports*, **3**, 200–3.

395. Danilevicius, Z. (1974). Editorial. When does coronary heart disease start? *Journal of the American Medical Association*, **230**, 1565–6.

396. Danner, F., Noland, M., McFadden, M., DeWalt, K. and Kotchen, J.M. (1991). Description of the physical activity of young children using movement sensor and observation methods. *Pediatric Exercise Science*, **3**, 11–20.

397. Dauncey, M.J. and James, W.P.T. (1979). Assessment of the heart rate method for determining energy expenditure in man, using a whole body calorimeter. *British Journal of Nutrition*, **42**, 1–13.

398. Davies, C.E., Gordon, D., Larosa, J., Wood, P.D.S. and Halperin, M. (1980). Correlations of plasma high-density lipoprotein cholesterol levels with other plasma lipid and lipoprotein concentrations. *Circulation*, **62**, 24–30.

399. Davies, C.T.M. (1981). Thermal responses to exercise in children. *Ergonomics*, **24**, 55–61.

400. Davies, C.T.M. (1985). Strength and mechanical properties of muscle in children and young adults. *Scandinavian Journal of Sports Science*, **7**, 11–15.

401. Davies, C.T.M., Barnes, C. and Godrey, S. (1972). Body composition and maximal exercise in children. *Human Biology*, **44**, 195–214.

402. Davies, C.T.M., Few, J., Foster, K.G. and Sargeant, A.J. (1974). Plasma catecholamine concentration during dynamic exercise involving different muscle groups. *European Journal of Applied Physiology*, **32**, 195–206.

403. Davies, C.T.M., Godrey, S., Light, M., Sargeant, A.J. and Zeidifard, E. (1975). Cardiopulmonary response to exercise in obese girls and young women. *Journal of Applied Physiology*, **38**, 373–6.

404. Davies, K.M., Recker, R.R., Stegman, M.R., Heaney, R.P., Kimmel, D.B. and Leist, J. (1990). Third decade bone gain in women. In D.V. Cohn, F.H. Glorieux and T.J. Martin (Eds.), *Calcium Regulation and Bone Metabolism*. Amsterdam, Elsevier, pp. 497–550.

405. Davies, P.S.W., Preece, M.A., Hicks, C.J. and Halliday, D. (1988). The prediction of TBW using bioelectrical impedance in children and adolescents. *Annals of Human Biology*, **15**, 237–40.

406. Davis, J.A. (1985). Anaerobic threshold: review of the concept and directions for future research. *Medicine and Science in Sports and Exercise*, **17**, 6–18.

407. DeBusk, R.F., Stenestrand, U., Sheehan, M. and Haskell, W.L. (1990). Training effects of long versus short bouts of exercise in healthy subjects. *American Journal of Cardiology*, **65**, 1010–13.

408. de Hass, J.H. (1978). Risk factors of coronary heart disease in children – a retrospective view of the Westland study. *Postgraduate Medical Journal*, **54**, 187–9.

409. Dekker, H., Ritmeester, J.W. and Snel, J. (1985). Personality traits and school attitude. In H.C.G. Kemper (Ed.), *Growth, Health and Fitness of Teenagers*. New York, Karger, pp. 137–47.

410. Delany, J.P., Harsha, D.W., Kime, J.C., Kumler, J., Melancon, L. and Bray, G.A. (1995). Energy expenditure in lean and obese prepubertal children. *Obesity Research*, **3** (Suppl. 1), 67–72.

411. DeLorme, T.L., Ferris, B.G. and Gallagher, J.R. (1952). Effect of progressive resistance exercise on muscle contraction time. *Archives of Physical Medicine and Rehabilitation*, **33**, 86–92.

412. de Man, S.A., van Stiphout, W.-A., H.J., Grobbee, D.E., Hofman, A. and Valkenburg, H.A. (1989). Is blood pressure in children related to physical fitness? In S. Oseid and K.-H. Carlsen (Eds.), *Children and Exercise XIII*. Champaign, IL, Human Kinetics, pp. 261–8.

413. Dempsey, J.M., Kimiecik, J.C. and Horn, T.S. (1993). Parental influence of children's moderate to vigorous physical activity participation: an expectancy-value approach. *Pediatric Exercise Science*, **5**, 151–67.

414. Dennison, B.A., Straus, J.H., Mellitus, E.D. and Chamey, E. (1988). Childhood physical fitness tests: predictor of adult physical activity levels? *Pediatrics*, **82**, 324–30.

415. Department for Education (1995). *Physical Education in the National Curriculum*. London, Her Majesty's Stationery Office.

416. Department of Health (1989). The Diets of British Schoolchildren. *Report on Health and Social Subjects 36*. London, Her Majesty's Stationery Office.

417. Department of Health (1992). *The Health of the Nation*. London, Her Majesty's Stationery Office.

418. Department of Health (1994). *On the State of the Public Health 1993*. London, Her Majesty's Stationery Office.

419. Department of Health (1995). *Health of the Young Nation Fact Sheet*. London, Department of Health.

420. Department of Health (1995). *Health of the Nation: Obesity, Reversing the increasing problem of obesity in England*. London, Department of Health.

421. Department of National Heritage (1995). *Sport: Raising the Game*. London, Department of National Heritage.

422. de Ridder, C.M., de Boer, R.W., Seidell, J.C., Nieuwenhoff, C.M., Jeneson, J.A.L., Bakker, C.J.G. *et al.* (1992). Body fat distribution in pubertal girls quantified by magnetic resonance imaging. *International Journal of Obesity*, **16**, 443–9.

423. Desmond, S.M., Price, J.H., Lock, R.S., Smith, D. and Stewart, P.W. (1990). Urban black and white adolescents' physical fitness status and perceptions of exercise. *Journal of School Health*, **60**, 220–5.

424. de Souza, M.J. and Metzger, D.A. (1991). Reproductive dysfunction in amenorrheic athletes and anorexic patients: a review. *Medicine and Science in Sports and Exercise*, **23**, 995–1007.

425. Després, J.-P., Bouchard, C. and Malina, R.M. (1990). Physical activity and coronary heart disease risk factors during childhood and adolescence. *Exercise and Sport Sciences Reviews*, **18**, 243–61.

426. Deurenberg, P., Westrate, J.A., Paymeans, I. and van der Kooy, K. (1988). Factors affecting bioelectrical impedance measurements in humans. *European Journal of Clinical Nutrition*, **42**, 1017–22.

427. Deuster, P.A., Kyle, S.B., Moser, P.B., Vigersky, R.A., Singh, A. and Schoomaker, E.B. (1986). Nutritional survey of highly trained women runners. *American Journal of Clinical Nutrition*, **45**, 954–62.

428. Deutsch, M.I., Mueller, W.H. and Malina, R.M. (1985). Androgyny in fat patterning is associated with obesity in adolescents and young adults. *Annals of Human Biology*, **12**, 275–86.

429. Devas, M. (1975). *Stress Fractures*. Edinburgh, Churchill Livingstone.

430. Deveaux, K.F., Bell, R.D. and Laxdal, V.A. (1986). The effects of a season of competitive soccer on the serum lipid and lipoprotein cholesterol profile of adolescent boys. In J. Rutenfranz, R. Mocellin and F. Klimt (Eds.), *Children and Exercise XII*. Champaign, IL, Human Kinetics, pp. 173–83.

431. Devlin, J.T. and Horton, E.S. (1985). Effects of prior high-intensity exercise on glucose metabolism in normal and insulin-resistant men. *Diabetes*, **34**, 973–8.

432. deWeir, J.B. (1949). New methods for calculating metabolic rate with special reference to protein metabolism. *Journal of Physiology*, **109**, 1–9.

433. Dhuper, S., Warren, M.P., Brooks-Gunn, J. and Fox, R. (1990). Effects of hormonal status on bone density in adolescent girls. *Journal of Clinical Endocrinology and Metabolism*, **71**, 1083–8.

434. Dickenson, B. (1986). Report on children's activity patterns and their perceptions of physical education and activity. *British Journal of Physical Education*, **17**, ii.

435. Dickenson, B. (1986). The physical activity patterns of young people – the implications for P.E. *Bulletin of Physical Education*, **22**, 36–9.

436. Dietz, W.H. (1983). Childhood obesity: susceptibility, cause and management. *Journal of Pediatrics*, **103**, 676–85.

437. Dietz, W.H. (1994). Childhood obesity. In L.W.Y. Cheung and J.B. Richmond (Eds.), *Child Health, Nutrition, and Physical Activity*. Champaign, IL, Human Kinetics, pp. 155–70.

438. Dietz, W. and Gortmaker, S. (1984). Factors within the physical environment associated with childhood obesity. *American Journal of Clinical Nutrition*, **39**, 619–24.

439. Dimsdale, J.E., Graham, R.M., Zeigler, M.G., Zusman, R.M. and Berry, C.C. (1987). Age, race, diagnosis and sodium effects on the pressor response to infused hypertension. *Hypertension*, **10**, 564–9.

440. DiNubile, N.A. (1990). Strength training. *Clinics in Sports Medicine*, **10**, 33–62.

441. di Prampero, P.E. and Ceretelli, P. (1969). Maximal muscular power (aerobic and anaerobic) in African natives. *Ergonomics*, **12**, 51–9.

442. Dishman, R.K. (1986). Mental health. In V. Seefeldt (Ed.), *Physical Activity and Well-Being*. Retson, VA, American Alliance for Health, Physical Education, Recreation and Dance, pp. 303–41.

443. Dishman, R.K. (1988). Supervised and free living physical activity: no differences in former athletes and non-athletes. *American Journal of Preventive Medicine*, **4**, 153–60.

444. Dishman, R.K. (1989). Exercise and sport psychology in youth 6 to 18 years of age. In C.V. Gisolfi and D.R. Lamb (Eds.), *Perspectives in Exercise Science and Sports Medicine, Vol. 2, Youth, Exercise, and Sport*. Indianapolis, IN, Benchmark Press, pp. 47–98.

445. Dishman, R.K. (1990). Determinants of participation in physical activity. In C. Bouchard, R.J. Shephard, T. Stephens, J.R. Sutton and B.D. McPherson (Eds.), *Exercise, Fitness and Health*. Champaign, IL, Human Kinetics, pp. 75–101.

446. Dishman, R.K. and Dunn, A.L. (1988). Exercise adherence in children and youth: implications for adulthood. In R.K. Dishman (Ed.), *Exercise Adherence*. Champaign, IL, Human Kinetics, pp. 155–200.

447. Dishman, R.K., Sallis, J.F. and Orenstein, O.R. (1985). The determinants of physical activity and exercise. *Public Health Reports*, **100**, 158–71.

448. Dissamarn, R., Kirtiputra, N. and Leeyavanija, U. (1981). Risk factors for chronic disease in Thai schoolchildren. *Preventive Medicine*, **10**, 226–34.

449. Docherty, D., Eckerson, J.S. and Hayward, J.S. (1986). Physique and thermoregulation in prepubertal males during exercise in a warm, humid environment. *American Journal of Physical Anthropology*, **70**, 19–23.

450. Docherty, D. and Gaul, C.A. (1991). Relationship of body size, physique and composition to physical performance in young boys and girls. *International Journal of Sports Medicine*, **12**, 525–32.

451. Docherty, D., Wenger, H.A. and Collis, M.L. (1987). The effects of resistance training on aerobic and anaerobic power of young boys. *Medicine and Science in Sports and Exercise*, **19**, 389–92.

452. Docherty, D., Wenger, H.A., Collis, M.L. and Quinney, H.A. (1987). The effects of variable speed resistance training on strength development in prepubertal boys. *Journal of Human Movement Studies*, **13**, 377–82.

453. Donnelly, P. (1993). Problems associated with youth involvement in high-performance sport. In B.R. Cahill and A.J. Pearl (Eds.), *Intensive Participation in Children's Sports*. Champaign, IL, Human Kinetics, pp. 95–126.

454. Dorchy, H. and Poortmans, J. (1989). Sport and the diabetic child. *Sports Medicine*, **7**, 248–62.

455. Dotan, R. and Bar-Or, O. (1983). Load optimisation for the Wingate Anaerobic Test. *European Journal of Applied Physiology*, **51**, 409–17.

456. Dotson, C.O. and Ross, J.G. (1985). Relationship between activity patterns and fitness. *Journal of Physical Education, Recreation and Dance*, **56**, 86–90.

457. Drinkwater, B.L. (1990). Physical exercise and bone health. *Journal of the American Medical Women's Association*, **45**, 91–7.

458. Drinkwater, B.L. (1994). Does physical activity play a role in preventing osteoporosis? *Research Quarterly for Exercise and Sport*, **65**, 197–206.

459. Drinkwater, B.L., Kupprat, I.C., Denton, J.E., Crist, J.L. and Horvath, S.M. (1977). Response of prepubertal girls and college women to work in the heat. *Journal of Applied Physiology*, **43**, 1046–53.

460. Drinkwater, B.L., Nilson, K., Chesnut, C.H. III., Bremner, W.J., Shainholtz, S. and Southworth, M.B. (1984). Bone mineral content of amenorrheic and eumenorrheic athletes. *New England Journal of Medicine*, **31**, 277–81.

461. Drinkwater, B.L., Nilson, K., Ott, S. and Chesnut, C.H. (1986). Bone mineral density after resumption of menses in amenorrheic athletes. *Journal of the American Medical Association*, **256**, 380–2.

462. Driscoll, D., Staats, B.A. and Beck, K.C. (1989). Measurement of cardiac output in children during exercise: a review. *Pediatric Exercise Science*, **1**, 102–15.

463. Duché, P., Falgairette, G., Bedu, M., Lac, G., Robert, A. and Coudert, J. (1992). Longitudinal approach of bioenergetic profile in boys before and during puberty. In J. Coudert and E. Van Praagh (Eds.), *Pediatric Work Physiology*. Paris, Masson, pp. 43–6.

464. Duda, J.L., Fox, K.R., Biddle, S.J.H. and Armstrong, N. (1992). Children's achievement goals and beliefs about success in sport. *British Journal of Educational Psychology*, **62**, 313–23.

465. Duda, M. (1986). Prepubescent strength training gains support. *The Physician and Sports Medicine*, **14**, 157–61.

466. Duke, P.M., Litt, I.F. and Gross, R.T. (1980). Adolescents' self assessment of sexual maturation. *Pediatrics*, **66**, 918–20.

467. DuRant, R.H., Baranowski, T., Johnson, M. and Thompson, W.O. (1994). The relationship among television watching, physical activity and body composition of young children. *Pediatrics*, **94**, 449–55.

468. DuRant, R.H., Baranowski, T., Rhodes, T., Gutin, B., Thompson, W.O., Carroll, R. *et al.* (1993). Association among serum lipid and lipoprotein concentrations and physical activity: physical fitness and body composition in young children. *Journal of Pediatrics*, **123**, 185–92.

469. DuRant, R.H. and Hergenroeder, A.C. (1994). Promotion of physical activity among adolescents by primary health care providers. *Pediatric Exercise Science*, **6**, 448–63.

470. DuRant, R.H., Linder, C.W., Harkness, J.W. and Gray, R.G. (1983). The relationship between physical activity and serum lipids and lipoproteins in black children and adolescents. *Journal of Adolescent Health Care*, **4**, 55–60.

471. DuRant, R.H., Linder, C.W. and Mahoney, O.M. (1983). Relationship between habitual activity and serum lipoprotein levels in white male adolescents. *Journal of Adolescent Health Care*, **4**, 235–40.

472. Durnin, J.V.G.A. (1967). Activity patterns in the community. *Canadian Medical Association Journal*, **96**, 882–6.

473. Durnin, J.V.G.A. (1982). Energy consumption and its measurement in physical activity. *Annals of Clinical Research*, **14**, (Suppl. 34), 6–11.

474. Durnin, J.V.G.A. (1990). Assessment of physical activity during leisure and work. In C. Bouchard, R.J. Shephard, T. Stephens, J.R. Sutton and B.D. McPherson (Eds.), *Exercise, Fitness and Health*. Champaign, IL, Human Kinetics, pp. 63–70.

475. Durnin, J.V.G.A. (1992). Physical activity levels past and present. In N. Norgan (Ed.), *Physical Activity and Health*. Cambridge University Press, pp. 20–7.

476. Durnin, J.V.G.A., Lonergan, M.E., Good, J. and Ewan, A. (1974). A cross-sectional nutritional and anthropometrical study, with an interval of 7 years

on 611 young adolescent schoolchildren. *British Journal of Nutrition*, **32**, 169–79.

477. Durnin, J.V.G.A. and Passmore, R. (1967). *Energy, Work and Leisure*. London, Heineman.

478. Durstine, J.L. and Haskell, W.L. (1994). Effects of exercise training on plasma lipids and lipoproteins. *Exercise and Sport Sciences Reviews*, **22**, 477–521.

479. Dux, L., Dux, E. and Guba, F. (1982). Further data on the androgenic dependency of the skeletal musculature. The effect of prepubertal castration of the structural development of the skeletal muscles. *Hormone and Metabolic Research*, **14**, 191–4.

480. Dux, L., Dux, E., Mazareau, H. and Guba, F. (1979). A non-neural regulatory effect on the metabolic differentiation of the skeletal muscle. Effect of castration and testosterone administration on the skeletal muscles of the rat. *Comparative Biochemistry and Physiology*, **64A**, 177–83.

481. Dwyer, T., Coonan, W.E., Leitch, D.R., Hetzel, B.S. and Baghurst, R.A. (1983). An investigation of the effects of daily physical activity on the health of primary school students in South Australia. *International Journal of Epidemiology*, **12**, 308–13.

482. Dwyer, T. and Gibbons, L.E. (1994). Physical fitness related to blood pressure but not lipoproteins. *Circulation*, **89**, 1539–44.

483. Dyer, J.B. and Crouch, J.G. (1987). Effects of running on moods: a time series study. *Perceptual and Motor Skills*, **64**, 783–9.

484. Dyment, P.G. (1989). Stimulant drug abuse by young athletes. In N.J. Smith (Ed.), *Common Problems in Pediatric Sports Medicine*. Chicago, Year Book Medical Publishers, pp. 125–30.

485. Eakin, B.L., Serwer, G.A. and Rosenthal, A. (1995). Sex differences in oxygen consumption and heart rate plateau characteristics at maximal exercise in children. *Medicine and Science in Sports and Exercise*, **27** (Suppl.), S116.

486. Eaton, C.B. (1992). Relation of physical activity and cardiovascular fitness to coronary heart disease, part 1: a meta-analysis of the independent relation of physical activity and coronary heart disease. *Journal of American Board of Family Practitioners*, **5**, 31–42.

487. Eaton, W.O. and Enns, L.R. (1986). Sex differences in human motor activity level. *Psychological Bulletin*, **100**, 19–28.

488. Education, Science and Arts Committee (1991). *Sport in Schools*. London, Her Majesty's Stationery Office.

489. Eidsmoe, R.M. (1951). The facts about the academic performance of high school athletes. *Journal of Health, Physical Education and Recreation*, **32**, 20.

490. Eisenman, P.A. and Golding, G.A. (1975). Comparisons of effects of training on VO_2 max in girls and young women. *Medicine and Science in Sports*, **7**, 136–8.

491. Eisman, J.A., Sambrook, P.N., Kelly, P.J. and Pocock, N.A. (1991). Exercise and its interaction with genetic influences in the determination of bone mineral density. *American Journal of Medicine*, **91** (Suppl. 5B), 5S–9S.

492. Ekblom, B. (1969). Effect of physical training in adolescent boys. *Journal of Applied Physiology*, **27**, 350–5.

493. Elliot, D.L., Goldberg, L., Kuehl, K.S. and Hanna, C. (1989). Metabolic evaluation of obese and nonobese siblings. *Journal of Pediatrics*, **114**, 957–62.

494. Ellison, P.T. (1981). Threshold hypotheses, developmental age, and menstrual function. *American Journal of Physical Anthropology*, **54**, 337–40.

495. Ellison, R.C., Freedson, P.S., Zevallos, J.C., White, M.J., Marmor, J.K., Garrahie, E.J. *et al.* (1992). Feasibility and costs of monitoring physical activity in young children using the Caltrac accelerometer. *Pediatric Exercise Science*, **4**, 136–41.

496. Ellison, P.T. and Lager, C. (1986). Moderate recreational running is associated with lower salivary progesterone profiles in women. *American Journal of Obstetrics and Gynecology*, **154**, 1000–3.

497. Elo, O., Hirvonen, L., Peltonen, T. and Valimaki, I. (1965). Physical working capacity of normal and diabetic children. *Annales Paediatricae Fenniae*, **11**, 25–31.

498. El-Sayed, M.S., George, K.P., Wilkinson, D., Mullan, N., Fenoglio, R. and Flannigan, J. (1992). Fingertip and venous blood lactate concentration in response to graded treadmill exercise. *Journal of Sports Science*, **11**, 139–43.

499. Emans, J.B. (1984). Upper extremity injuries in sports. In L.J. Micheli (Ed.), *Pediatric and Adolescent Sports Medicine*. Boston, Little Brown and Co., pp. 49–79.

500. Emons, H.J.G., Groenenboom, D.C., Westerterp, K.R. and Saris, W.H.M. (1992). Comparison of heart rate monitoring combined with indirect calorimetry and the doubly labelled water ($^2H_2{}^{18}O$) method for the measurement of energy expenditure in children. *European Journal of Applied Physiology*, **65**, 99–103.

501. Engstrom, I., Eriksson, B.O., Karlberg, P., Saltin, B. and Thoren, G. (1971). Preliminary report on the development of lung volumes in young girl swimmers. *Acta Paediatrica Scandinavica*, **217** (Suppl.), 73–6.

502. Engstrom, L.-M. (1980). Physical activity of children and youth. *Acta Pediatrica Scandinavica*, **283** (Suppl.), 101–5.

503. Engstrom, L.-M. (1986). The process of socialisation into keep-fit activities. *Scandinavian Journal of Sports Science*, **8**, 89–97.

504. Engstrom, L.-M. (1990). *Importance and influence of behavioural aspects on the participation and attrition of youth in sport*. Paper presented to the International Congress on Youth, Leisure and Physical Activity, Brussels, Belgium.

505. Engstrom, L.-M. and Fischbein, S. (1977). Physical capacity in twins. *Acta Geneticae Medicae et Gemellologiae*, **26**, 159–65.

506. Enos, W.F., Beyer, J.C. and Holmes, R.H. (1955). Pathogenesis of coronary disease in American soldiers killed in Korea. *Journal of the American Medical Association*, **158**, 912–14.

507. Enos, W.F., Holmes, R.H. and Beyer, J.C. (1953). Coronary disease among United States soldiers killed in action in Korea. Preliminary report. *Journal of the American Medical Association*, **152**, 1090–3.

508. Epstein, L.H., Valoski, A., Wing, R.R. and McCurley, J. (1990). Ten-year follow-up of behavioural, family-based treatment for obese children. *Journal of the American Medical Association*, **264**, 2519–23.

509. Epstein, L.H., Wing, R.R., Koeske, R., Ossip, D.J. and Beck, S. (1982). A comparison of lifestyle change and programmed aerobic exercise on weight and fitness changes in obese children. *Behavior Therapy*, **13**, 651–65.

510. Epstein, L.H., Wing, R.R., Koeske, R. and Valoski, A. (1985). A comparison of lifestyle exercise, aerobic exercise and calisthenics on weight loss in obese children. *Behavior Therapy*, **16**, 345–56.

511. Epstein, L.H., Woodall, K., Goreczny, A.J., Wing, R.R. and Robertson, R.J. (1984). The modification of activity patterns and energy expenditure in obese young girls. *Behavior Therapy*, **15**, 101–8.

512. Eriksson, B.O. (1972). Physical training, oxygen supply and muscle metabolism in 11–13 year old boys. *Acta Physiologica Scandinavica*, **384** (Suppl.), 1–48.

513. Eriksson, B.O. (1978). Physical activity from childhood to maturity: medical and pediatric considerations. In F. Landry and W.A.R. Orban (Eds.), *Physical Activity and Human Well-Being*. Miami, Symposia Specialists, pp. 47–55.

514. Eriksson, B.O. (1980). Muscle metabolism in children – a review. *Acta Paediatrica Scandinavica*, **283** (Suppl.), 20–8.

515. Eriksson, B.O., Berg, K. and Taranger, J. (1978). Physiological analysis of young boys starting intensive training in swimming. In B.O. Eriksson and B. Furberg (Eds.), *Swimming Medicine IV*. Baltimore, MD, University Park Press, pp. 147–59.

516. Eriksson, B.O., Engstrom, I., Karlberg, P., Saltin, B. and Thoren, C. (1971). A physiological analysis of former girl swimmers. *Acta Paediatrica Scandinavica*, **217**, 68–72.

517. Eriksson, B.O., Freychuss, U., Lundin, A. and Thoren, C.A.R. (1980). Effect of physical training in former female top athletes in swimming. In K. Berg and B.O. Eriksson (Eds.), *Children and Exercise IX*. Baltimore, MD, University Park Press, pp. 116–27.

518. Eriksson, B.O., Gollnick, P.D. and Saltin, B. (1973). Muscle metabolism and enzyme activities after training in boys 11–13 years old. *Acta Physiologica Scandinavica*, **87**, 485–97.

519. Eriksson, B.O., Gollnick, P.D. and Saltin, B. (1974). The effect of physical training on muscle enzyme activities and fiber composition in 11 year old boys. *Acta Paediatrica Belgica*, **28** (Suppl.), 245–52.

520. Eriksson, B.O., Grimby, G. and Saltin, B. (1971). Cardiac output and arterial blood gases during exercise in pubertal boys. *Journal of Applied Physiology*, **32**, 348–52.

521. Eriksson, B.O., Karlsson, J. and Saltin, B. (1971). Muscle metabolites during exercise in pubertal boys. *Acta Paediatrica Scandinavica*, **217** (Suppl.), 154–7.

522. Eriksson, B.O. and Koch, G. (1973). Effect of physical training on hemodynamic response during submaximal and maximal exercise in 11–13 year old boys. *Acta Physiologica Scandinavica*, **87**, 27–39.

523. Eriksson, B.O. and Koch, G. (1973). Cardiac output and intra-arterial blood pressure at rest and during submaximal and maximal exercise in 11 to 13 year old boys before and after physical training. In O. Bar-Or (Ed.), *Pediatric Work Physiology*. Natanya, Israel, Wingate Institute, pp. 139–50.

524. Eriksson, B.O., Persson, B. and Thorell, J.I. (1971). The effects of repeated prolonged exercise on plasma growth hormone, insulin, glucose, free-fatty acids, glycerol, lactate and beta-hydroxybutyric acid in 13 year old boys and in adults. *Acta Paediatrica Scandinavica*, **217** (Suppl.), 142–6.

525. Eriksson, B.O. and Saltin, B. (1974). Muscle metabolism during exercise in boys aged 11–16 years compared to adults. *Acta Paediatrica Belgica*, **28** (Suppl.), 257–65.

526. Eriksson, B.O. and Thoren, C. (1978). Training girls for swimming from medical and physiological points of view, with special reference to growth. In B.O. Eriksson and B. Furberg (Eds.), *Swimming Medicine IV*. Baltimore, MD, University Park Press, pp. 3–15.

527. European Atherosclerosis Society (1987). Strategies for the prevention of coronary heart disease: a policy statement of the European Atherosclerosis Society. *European Heart Journal*, **8**, 77–88.

528. Evans, J.A. and Quinney, H.A. (1981). Determination of resistance settings for anerobic power testing. *Canadian Journal of Applied Sport Science*, **6**, 53–6.

529. Fagard, R. (1985). Habitual physical activity, training and blood pressure in normo- and hypertension. *International Journal of Sports Medicine*, **6**, 57–67.

530. Fahey, T.D., Del Valle-Zuris, A., Oehlsen, G., Trieb, M. and Seymour, J. (1979). Pubertal stage differences in hormonal and haematological responses to maximal exercise in males. *Journal of Applied Physiology*, **46**, 823–7.

531. Faigenbaum, A.D., Zaichkowsky, L.D., Westcott, W.L., Micheli, L.J. and Fehlandt, A.F. (1993). The effects of a twice-a-week strength training program on children. *Pediatric Exercise Science*, **5**, 339–46.

532. Falgairette, G., Bedu, M., Fellmann, N., Van-Praagh, E. and Coudert, J. (1991). Bioenergetic profile in 144 boys age from 6 to 15 years with special reference to sexual maturation. *European Journal of Applied Physiology*, **62**, 151–6.

533. Falgairette, G., Bedu, M., Fellmann, N., Van Praagh, E., Jarrige, J.F. and Coudert, J. (1990). Modifications of aerobic and anaerobic metabolisms in active boys during puberty. In G. Beunen, J. Ghesquiere, T. Reybrouck and A.L. Claessens (Eds.), *Children and Exercise*. Stuttgart, Enke, pp. 42–9.

534. Falgairette, G., Duché, P., Bedu, M., Fellmann, N. and Coudert, J. (1993). Bioenergetic characteristics in prepubertal swimmers. *International Journal of Sports Medicine*, **14**, 444–8.

535. Falk, B. and Bar-Or, O. (1993). Longitudinal changes in peak aerobic and anaerobic mechanical power of circumpubertal boys. *Pediatric Exercise Science*, **5**, 318–31.

536. Fardy, P.S., Maresh, C.M., Abbot, R. and Kristiansen, T. (1978). A comparison of habitual lifestyle, aerobic power, and systolic time intervals in former athletes and non-athletes. *Journal of Sports Medicine and Physical Fitness*, **18**, 287–99.

537. Fassler, A.L.C. and Bonjour, J.P. (1995). Osteoporosis as a pediatric problem. *Pediatric Clinics of North America*, **42**, 811–24.

538. Faulkner, B. (1987). Is there a black hypertension? *Hypertension*, **10**, 551–4.

539. Faulkner, R.A., Houston, C.S., Bailey, D.A., Drinkwater, D.T., McKay, H.A. and Wilkinson, A.A. (1993). Comparison of bone mineral content and bone mineral density between dominant and nondominant limbs in children 8–16 years of age. *American Journal of Human Biology*, **5**, 491–9.

540. Faust, M.S. (1977). Somatic development of adolescent girls. *Monographs of the Society for Research in Child Development*, **42**, 1–90.

541. Fehily, A., Coles, R., Evans, W. and Elwood, P. (1992). Factors affecting bone density in young adults. *American Journal of Clinical Nutrition*, **56**, 579–86.

542. Fein, F.S. and Sonnenblick, E.H. (1985). Diabetic cardiomyopathy. *Progress in Cardiovascular Disease*, **27**, 255–70.

543. Feldman, H.A. and McMahon, T.A. (1983). The 3/4 mass exponent for energy metabolism is not a statistical artifact. *Respiration Physiology*, **52**, 149–63.

544. Fellman, N., Bedu, M., Spielvogel, H., Falgairette, G., Van Praagh, E., Jarrige, J. *et al.* (1988). Anaerobic metabolism during pubertal development at high altitude. *Journal of Applied Physiology*, **64**, 1382–6.

545. Fenster, J., Freedson, P., Washburn, R.A. and Ellison, R.C. (1989). The relationship between physical activity and peak $\dot{V}O_2$ in 6 to 8-year-old children. *Pediatric Exercise Science*, **1**, 81–2.

546. Fentem, P.H., Bassey, E.J. and Turnbull, N.B. (1988). *The New Case for Exercise*. London, Sports Council and Health Education Authority.

547. Ferguson, K.J., Yesalis, C.E., Pomrehn, P.R. and Kirkpatrick, M.B. (1989). Attitudes, knowledge, and belief as predictors of exercise intent and behaviour in schoolchildren. *Journal of School Health*, **59**, 112–15.

548. Fernqvist, E., Linde, B., Ostman, J. and Gunnarsson, R. (1986). Effects of physical exercise on insulin absorption in insulin-dependent diabetics. A comparison between human and porcine insulin. *Clinical Physiology*, **6**, 489–98.

549. Finkelstein, J.S., Neer, R.M., Biller, B.M., Crawford, J.D. and Klibanski, A. (1992). Osteopenia in men with a history of delayed puberty. *New England Journal of Medicine*, **326**, 600–4.

550. Fisher, A.G. and Brown, M. (1982). The effects of diet and exercise on selected coronary risk factors in children. *Medicine and Science in Sports and Exercise*, **14**, 2.

551. Fisher, M. (1992). Medical complications of anorexia and bulimia nervosa. *Adolescent Medicine State of the Art Reviews*, **3**, 486–502.

552. Fisher, R. (1996). Gifted children and young people in physical education and sport. In N. Armstrong (Ed.), *New Directions in Physical Education, Vol. 3, Change and Innovation*. London, Cassell, pp. 131–43.

553. Fixler, D.E. (1978). Epidemiology of childhood hypertension. In W.B. Strong (Ed.), *Atherosclerosis: Its Pediatric Aspects*. New York, Grune & Stratton, pp. 177–92.

554. Fleck, S.J. and Kraemer, W.J. (1988). Resistance training: physiological responses and adaptations. *The Physician and Sports Medicine*, **16**, 63–6, 69, 72–4.

555. Florini, J.R. (1985). Hormonal control of muscle cell growth (review). *Journal of Animal Sciences*, **61**, 21–38.

556. Florini, J.R. (1987). Hormonal control of muscle growth. *Muscle and Nerve*, **10**, 577–98.

557. Folkins, C.H., Lynch, S. and Gardner, M.M. (1972). Psychological fitness as a function of physical fitness. *Archives of Physical and Medical Rehabilitation*, **53**, 503–8.

558. Folkins, C.H. and Sime, W.E. (1981). Physical fitness training and mental health. *American Psychologist*, **9**, 380–9.

559. Forbes, G.B. (1986). Body composition in adolescence. In F. Falkner and J.M. Tanner (Eds.), *Human Growth, A Comprehensive Treatise, 2nd edition*. New York, Plenum Press, pp. 119–45.

560. Forbes, G.B. (1987). *Human Body Composition*. New York, Springer.

561. Fosson, A., Knibbs, J., Bryant-Waugh, R. and Lake, B. (1987). Early onset anorexia nervosa. *Archives of Disease in Childhood*, **62**, 114–18.

562. Fournier, M., Ricci, J., Taylor, A.W., Ferguson, R.J., Montpetit, R.R. and Chaitman, B.R. (1982). Skeletal muscle adaptation in adolescent boys: sprint and endurance training and detraining. *Medicine and Science in Sports and Exercise*, **14**, 453–6.

563. Fox, E.L. and Mathews, D.K. (1981). *The Physiological Basis of Physical Education and Athletics, 3rd edition*. Philadelphia, PA, Saunders College Publishing.

564. Fox, K., Goudas, M., Biddle, S., Duda, J. and Armstrong, N. (1994). Children's task and ego goal profiles in sport. *British Journal of Educational Psychology*, **64**, 253–61.

565. Fox, K., Page, A., Armstrong, N. and Kirby, B. (1994). Dietary restraint and self-perceptions in early adolescence. *Personality and Individual Differences*, **17**, 87–96.

566. Fox, K.R., Page, A., Peters, D.M., Armstrong, N. and Kirby, B. (1994). Dietary restraint and fatness in early adolescent girls and boys. *Journal of Adolescence*, **17**, 149–61.

567. Fox, K., Peters, D., Armstrong, N., Sharpe, P. and Bell, M. (1993). Abdominal fat deposition in 11-year-old children. *International Journal of Obesity*, **17**, 11–16.

568. Foxdahl, P., Sjödin, B., Rudstam, H., Östman, C., Östman, B. and Hedenstierna, G.C. (1990). Lactate concentration differences in plasma, whole blood, capillary finger blood and erythrocytes during submaximal graded exercise in humans. *European Journal of Applied Physiology*, **61**, 218–22.

569. Frank, G.C., Farris, R.P., Ditmarsen, P., Voors, A.W. and Berenson, G.S. (1982). An approach to primary preventive treatment for children with high blood pressure in a total community. *Journal of the American College of Nutrition*, **1**, 357–74.

570. Fraser, G.E. (1986). *Preventive Cardiology*. New York, Oxford University Press.

571. Fraser, G.E., Phillips, R.L. and Harris, R. (1983). Physical fitness and blood pressure in schoolchildren. *Circulation*, **67**, 405–12.

572. Freedman, D.S., Newman, W.P., Tracy, R.E., Strong, J.P., Cresanta, J.L. and Berenson, G.S. (1987). Pathology of atherosclerosis in childhood. In B.J. Hetzel and G.S. Berenson (Eds.), *Cardiovascular Risk Factors in Childhood: Epidemiology and Prevention*. Amsterdam, Elsevier, pp. 83–100.

573. Freedson, P.S. (1989). Field monitoring of physical activity in children. *Pediatric Exercise Science*, **1**, 8–18.

574. Freedson, P.S. (1991). Electronic motion sensors and heart rate as measures of physical activity in children. *Journal of School Health*, **61**, 220–23.

575. Freedson, P.S. and Evenson, S. (1991). Familial aggregation in physical activity. *Research Quarterly for Exercise and Sport*, **62**, 384–9.

576. Freedson, P.S. and Rowland, T.W. (1992). Youth activity versus youth fitness: let's redirect our efforts. *Research Quarterly for Exercise and Sport*, **63**, 133–6.

577. Freedson, P.S., Ward, A. and Rippe, J.M. (1990. Resistance training for youth. In W.A. Grana, J.A. Lombardo, B.J. Sharkey and J.A. Stone (Eds.), *Advances in Sports Medicine and Fitness, Vol. 3*. Chicago, Year Book Medical Publishers, pp. 57–65.

578. Fried, L.P., Bateman, L., Stauch, T. and Pearson, T.A. (1986). Youthful predictors of physical activity level during middle age. *American Journal of Epidemiology*, **124**, 538.

579. Friedheim, L.C. and Town, G.P. (1989). Blood lactate methodologies compared. *Medicine and Science in Sports and Exercise*, **21** (Suppl.), S21.

580. Friedman, M.J. (1986). Injuries to the leg in athletes. In J.A. Nicholas and E.B. Hershman (Eds.), *The Lower Extremity and Spine in Sports Medicine*. St Louis, MO, C.V. Mosby Co., pp. 601–56.

581. Fripp, R.R. and Hodgson, J.L. (1987). Effect of resistive training on plasma lipid and lipoprotein levels in male adolescents. *Journal of Pediatrics*, **111**, 926–31.

582. Fripp, R.R., Hodgson, J.L., Kwiterovich, P.O., Werner, J.C., Schuler, H.G. and Whitman, V. (1985). Aerobic capacity, obesity and atherosclerotic risk factors in male adolescents. *Pediatrics*, **75**, 813–18.

583. Frisch, R.E., Gotz-Welbergen, A.V., MacArthur, J.W., Albright, T., Witschi, J., Bullen, B. *et al.* (1981). Delayed menarche and amenorrhea of college athletes in relation to age of onset of training. *Journal of the American Medical Association*, **246**, 1559–63.

584. Frisch, R.E. and McArthur, J.W. (1974). Menstrual cycles: fatness as a determinant of minimum weight for height necessary for their maintenance or onset. *Science*, **185**, 949–51.

585. Frisch, R.E. and Revelle, R. (1971). Height and weight at menarche and a hypothesis of critical body weights and adolescent events. *Science*, **169**, 397–9.

586. Frisch, R.E. and Revelle, R. (1971). Height and weight at menarche and a hypothesis of menarche. *Archives of Disease in Childhood*, **46**, 695–701.

587. Frisch, R.E. and Revelle, R. (1971). The height and weight of girls and boys at the time of initiation of the adolescent growth spurt in height and weight and the relationship to menarche. *Human Biology*, **43**, 140–59.

588. Frost, H.M. (1983). A determinant of bone architecture: the minimum effective strain. *Clinical and Orthopaedic Related Research*, **175**, 286–92.

589. Frost, H.M. (1987). Bone mass and the mechanostat: a proposal. *Anatomical Record*, **219**, 1–9.

590. Fuchs, R., Semmer, N.K., Lippert, P., Powell,K.E., Dwyer, J.H. and Hoffmeister, H. (1988). Patterns of physical activity among German adolescents: the Berlin-Bremen study. *Preventive Medicine*, **7**, 746–63.

591. Fukunaga, T. (1976). Die absolute Muskelkraft und das Krafttraining (Absolute muscle strength and strength training). *Sportarzt und Sportmedizin*, **27**, 255–66.

592. Fukunaga, T., Funato, K. and Ikegawa, S. (1992). The effects of resistance training on muscle area and strength in prepubescent age. *Annals of Physiological Anthropology*, **11**, 357–64.

593. Gadpaille, W.J., Sanborne, C.F. and Wagner, W.W. (1987). Athletic amenorrhea, major affective disorders and eating disorders. *American Journal of Psychology*, **144**, 939–42.

594. Gaesser, G.A. and Poole, D.C. (1986). Lactate and ventilatory thresholds: disparity in time course of adaptations to training. *Journal of Applied Physiology*, **61**, 999–1004.

595. Gaesser, G.A. and Rich, R.G. (1984). Effects of high and low intensity exercise training on aerobic capacity and blood lipids. *Medicine and Science in Sports and Exercise*, **16**, 269–74.

596. Gaisl, G. and Buchberger, J. (1977). The significance of stress acidosis in judging the physical working capacity of boys aged 11 to 15. In H. Lavallée and R.J. Shephard (Eds.), *Frontiers of Activity and Child Health*. Quebec, Pelican, pp. 161–8.

597. Gaisl, G. and Konig, H. (1985). The optimizationof endurance training in adolescent middle-distance runners. In R.A. Binkhorst, H.C.G. Kemper and W.H.M. Saris (Eds.), *Children and Exercise XI*. Champaign, IL, Human Kinetics, pp. 129–33.

598. Gaisl, G. and Weisspeiner, G. (1986). Training prescriptions for 9- to 17-year old figure skaters based on lactate assessment in the laboratory and on the ice. In J. Rutenfranz, R. Mocellin and F. Klimt (Eds.), *Children and Exercise XII*. Champaign, IL, Human Kinetics, pp. 59–66.

599. Galbo, H. (1988). Exercise and diabetes. *Scandinavian Journal of Sports Science*, **10**, 89–95.

600. Galdston, R. (1974). Mind over matter: observations on 50 patients hospitalized with anorexia nervosa. *Journal of the American Academy of Child Psychiatry*, **13**, 246–63.

601. Gallagher, S.S., Finison, K., Guyer, B. and Goodenough, S. (1984). The incidence of injuries among 87,000 Massachusetts children and adolescents: results of the 1980–81 Statewide Childhood Injury Prevention Program Surveillance System. *American Journal of Public Health*, **8**, 318–24.

602. Garfinkel, B.D., Froese, A. and Hood, J. (1982). Suicide attempts in children and adolescents. *American Journal of Psychiatry*, **139**, 1257–61.

603. Garg, A. (1994). Management of dyslipidemia in IDDM patients. *Diabetes Care*, **17**, 224–34.

604. Garner, D.M. and Garfinkel, P.E. (1980). Socio-cultural factors in the development of anorexia nervosa. *Psychological Medicine*, **10**, 647–56.

605. Garner, D.M., Garfinkel, P.E., Rockert, W. and Olmsted, M.P. (1987). A prospective study of eating disturbances in the ballet. *Psychotherapy and Psychosomatics*, **48**, 170–5.

606. Garrow, J.R. (1974). *Energy Balance and Obesity in Man*. Amsterdam, Elsevier, North Holland Publishers, pp. 47–92.

607. Garrow, J.S. (1988). *Obesity and Related Diseases*. London, Churchill Livingstone.

608. Gatch, W. and Byrd, R. (1979). Endurance training and cardiovascular function in 9 and 10 year old boys. *Archives of Physiology, Medicine and Rehabilitation*, **60**, 574–77.

609. Gatev, V., Stamatov, L. and Angelova, B. (1977). Contraction time in skeletal muscles of normal children. *Electromyography and Clinical Neurophysiology*, **17**, 441–51.

610. Gatev, V., Stefanova-Uzunova, M. and Stamatova, L. (1981). Influence of vertical posture development on the velocity properties of triceps surae muscle in normal children. *Journal of Neurological Sciences*, **52**, 85–90.

611. Geer, J.C., McGill, H.C., Robertson, W.B. and Strong, J.P. (1968). Histologic characteristics of coronary artery fatty streaks. *Laboratory Investigations*, **18**, 565–70.

612. Gentle, P.H., Caves, R., Armstrong, N., Balding,J. and Kirby, B. (1994). High and low exercisers among 14 and 15 year old British children. *Journal of Public Health Medicine*, **16**, 186–94.

613. Gilbey, H. and Gilbey, M. (1995). The physical activity of Singapore primary school children as estimated by heart rate monitoring. *Pediatric Exercise Science*, **7**, 26–35.

614. Gilliam, T.B. and Burke, M.B. (1978). Effect of exercise on serum lipids and lipoproteins in girls, ages 8 to 10 years. *Artery*, **4**, 203–13.

615. Gilliam, T.B. and Freedson, P.S. (1980). Effects of a 12 week school physical fitness program on peak VO_2, body composition and blood lipids in 7 to 9 year old children. *International Journal of Sports Medicine*, **1**, 73–8.

616. Gilliam, T.B., Freedson, P.S., Geenen, D.L. and Shahraray, B. (1981). Physical activity patterns determined by heart rate monitoring in 6–7 year old children. *Medicine and Science in Sports and Exercise*, **13**, 65–7.

617. Gilliam, T.B., Katch, V.L., Thorland, W. and Weltman, A. (1977). Prevalence of coronary heart disease risk factors in active children, 7 to 12 years of age. *Medicine and Science in Sports*, **9**, 21–5.

618. Gilliam, T.B. and MacConnie, S.E. (1984). Coronary heart disease in children and their physical activity patterns. In R.A. Boileau (Ed.), *Advances in Pediatric Sport Sciences, Vol. 1*. Champaign, IL, Human Kinetics, pp. 171–87.

619. Gilliam, T.B., MacConnie, S.E., Geenen, D.L., Pels, A.E. and Freedson, P.S. (1982). Exercise programs for children: a way to prevent heart disease. *The Physician and Sports Medicine*, **10**, 96–108.

620. Gilsanz, V., Gibbens, D.T. and Carlson, M. (1988). Peak trabecular vertebral density: a comparison of adolescent and adult females. *Calcified Tissue International*, **43**, 260–2.

621. Gilsanz, V., Gibbens, D.T., Roe, T.F., Carlson, M., Senac, M.O., Boechat, M.I. *et al.* (1988). Vertebral bone density in children: effect of puberty. *Radiology*, **166**, 847–50.

622. Glass, A.R., Deuster, P.A., Kyle, S.P., Yahiro, J.A., Vigersky, R.A. *et al.* (1987). Amenorrhoea in Olympic marathon runners. *Fertility and Sterility*, **48**, 740–5.

623. Glass, G., McGaw, B. and Smith, M. (1981). *Meta-Analysis in Social Research*. Beverly Hills, CA, Sage.

624. Glastre, C., Braillon, P., David, L., Cochat, P., Meunier, P.J. and Delmas, P.D. (1990). Measurement of bone mineral content of the lumbar spine by dual energy X-ray absorptiometry in normal children: correlations with growth parameters. *Journal of Clinical Endocrinology and Metabolism*, **70**, 1330–3.

625. Gleeson, N., Tancred, W. and Banks, M. (1989). Psycho-biological factors influencing habitual activities in male and female adolescents. *Physical Education Review*, **12**, 110–24.

626. Glenmark, B., Healberg, G. and Jansson, E. (1994). Prediction of physical activity level in adulthood by physical characteristics, physical performance and physical activity in adolescence: an 11-year follow-up study. *European Journal of Applied Physiology*, **69**, 530–8.

627. Godin, G. (1982). Multiples of the resting metabolic rate (METS) of physical activities. Cited by J.G. Ross, C.O. Dotson, G.G. Gilbert (1985), Are kids getting appropriate activity? National Children and Youth Fitness Survey. *Journal of Physical Education, Recreation and Dance*, **56**, 82–5.

628. Godin, G. and Shephard, R.J. (1984). Normative beliefs of schoolchildren concerning regular exercise. *Journal of School Health*, **54**, 443–5.

629. Godin, G. and Shephard, R.J. (1986). Psychosocial factors influencing intentions to exercise of young students from grades 7 to 9. *Research Quarterly for Exercise and Sport*, **57**, 41–52.

630. Godin, G., Shephard, R.J. and Colantonio, A. (1986). Children's perception of parental exercise: influence of age and sex. *Perceptual Motor Skills*, **62**, 511–16.

631. Goldberg, L. and Elliot, D.L. (1987). The effect of exercise on lipid metabolism in men and women. *Sports Medicine*, **4**, 307–21.

632. Goldberg, L., Elliot, D.L., Schutz, R.W. and Kloster, F.E. (1984). Changes in lipid and lipoprotein levels after weight training. *Journal of the American Medical Association*, **252**, 504–6.

633. Goldbloom, R.B. (1979). Obesity in childhood. In R.C. Goode and R. Volpe (Eds.), *The Child and Physical Activity*. Toronto, Ontario, Heart Foundation, pp. 55–70.

634. Goldstein, H. (1986). Efficient statistical modelling of longitudinal data. *Annals of Human Biology*, **13**, 129–41.

635. Gollnick, P.D., Armstrong, R.B., Saubert, C.W., Piehl, K. and Saltin, B. (1972). Enzyme activity and fibre composition in skeletal muscle of untrained and trained men. *Journal of Applied Physiology*, **33**, 312–19.

636. Goodman, D.S. (1988). Report of the National Cholesterol Education Program Expert Panel on detection, evaluation and treatment of high blood cholesterol in adults. *Annals of Internal Medicine*, **148**, 36–69.

637. Goran, M.I. (1994). Application of the doubly labelled water technique for studying total energy expenditure in young children: a review. *Pediatric Exercise Science*, **6**, 11–30.

638. Goran, M.I., Carpenter, W.H. and Poehlman, E.T. (1993). Total energy expenditure in 4 to 6 year old children. *American Journal of Physiology*, **246**, E706–E711.

639. Gordon, T., Castelli, W.P., Hjortland, M.C., Kannel, W.J. and Dawber, T.R. (1977). High density lipoprotein as a protective factor against coronary heart disease: the Framingham Study. *American Journal of Medicine*, **62**, 707–14.

640. Gortmaker, S.L., Dietz, W.H., Sobol, A.M. and Wehler, C.A. (1987). Increasing pediatric obesity in the United States. *American Journal of Diseases of Children*, **131**, 535–40.

641. Gottleib, N.H. and Baker, J.A. (1986). The relative influence of health beliefs, parental and peer behaviors and exercise program participation on smoking, alcohol use and physical activity. *Social Science and Medicine*, **22**, 915–27.

642. Gottleib, N.H. and Chen, M.-S. (1985). Sociocultural correlates of childhood sporting activities: their implications for heart health. *Social Science and Medicine*, **21**, 533–9.

643. Gotto, A.M. and Wittels, E.H. (1983). Diet, serum cholesterol, lipoproteins and coronary heart disease. In N.M. Kaplan and J.M. Stamler (Eds.), *Prevention of Coronary Heart Disease*. Philadelphia, PA, Saunders, pp. 33–50.

644. Graham, K.S. and McLellan, T.M. (1989). Variability of time to exhaustion and accumulated oxygen deficit in supramaximal exercise. *Australian Journal of Science and Medicine in Sport*, **21**, 11–14.

645. Graham, T.E. (1984). The measurement and interpretation of lactate. In H. Lollgen and H. Mellerowicz (Eds.), *Progress in Ergometry: Quality Control and Test Criteria*. Berlin, Springer, pp. 51–65.

646. Granhad, H., Jonson, R. and Hansson, T. (1987). The loads on the lumbar spine during extreme weight lifting. *Spine*, **12**, 146–9.

647. Gratas-Delamarche, A., Mercier, J., Ramonatxo, M., Dassonville, J. and Préfaut, C. (1993). Ventilatory response of prepubertal boys and adults to carbon dioxide at rest and during exercise. *European Journal of Applied Physiology*, **66**, 25–30.

648. Gray, B.F. (1981). On the surface law and basal metabolic rate. *Journal of Theoretical Biology*, **93**, 757–67.

649. Green, H.J., Hughson, R.L., Orr, G.W. and Ranney, D.A. (1983). Anaerobic threshold, blood lactate and muscle metabolites in progressive exercise. *Journal of Applied Physiology*, **53**, 1032–8.

650. Green, S. and Dawson, B. (1993). Measurement of anaerobic capacities in humans: definitions, limitations and unsolved problems. *Sports Medicine*, **15**, 312–27.

651. Greendorfer, S.L. and Ewing, M.E. (1981). Race and gender differences in children's socialization into sport. *Research Quarterly for Exercise and Sport*, **52**, 301–10.

652. Greene, J.A. (1939). Clinical study of the etiology of obesity. *Annals of Internal Medicine*, **12**, 1797–803.

653. Greenockle, K.M. (1988). *Physical activity patterns of high school students during a fitness unit*. Paper presented to AAHPERD National Convention, Kansas City, KS.

654. Greenockle, K.M., Lee, A.A. and Lomax, R. (1990). The relationship between selected student characteristics and activity patterns in a required

high school physical education class. *Research Quarterly for Exercise and Sport*, **61**, 59–69.

655. Greulich, W.W. and Pyle, I.S. (1959). *Radiographic Atlas of Skeletal Development of the Hand and Wrist*. Stanford University Press.

656. Griffin, J. (1991). Diet for children. In V. Grisogono (Ed.), *Children and Sport*. London, Murray, pp. 175–209.

657. Griffiths, M. and Payne, P. (1976). Energy expenditure in small children of obese and non-obese parents. *Nature*, **260**, 698–700.

658. Grimston, S., Morrison, K., Harder, J. and Hanley, D. (1992). Bone mineral density during puberty in Western Canadian children. *Bone Mineral*, **19**, 85–6.

659. Grimston, S.K., Willows, N.D. and Hanley, D.A. (1993). Mechanical loading regime and its relationship to bone mineral density in children. *Medicine and Science in Sports and Exercise*, **25**, 1203–10.

660. Grodjinovsky, A., Inbar, A.O., Dotan, R. and Bar-Or, O. (1980). Training effect on the anaerobic performance of children as measured by the Wingate Anaerobic test. In K. Berg and B. Eriksson (Eds.), *Children and Exercise IX*. Baltimore, MD, University Park Press, pp. 139–45.

661. Gruber, J.J. (1986). Physical activity and self-esteem development in children: a meta-analysis. In G.A. Stull and H.M. Eckert (Eds.), *Effects of Physical Activity on Children*. Champaign, IL, Human Kinetics, pp. 30–48.

662. Gullestad, R. (1977). Temperature regulation in children during exercise. *Acta Paediatrica Scandinavica*, **64**, 257–63.

663. Gumbs, V.L., Segal, D., Hallingan, J.B. and Lower, G. (1982). Bilateral distal radius and ulnar fracture in weight lifters. *American Journal of Sports Medicine*, **10**, 375–9.

664. Guo, S., Chumlea, W.C., Siervogel, R.M. and Roche, A.F. (1992). Tracking of body fatness from 9 to 21 years. *Medicine and Science in Sports and Exercise*, **24** (Suppl.), S189.

665. Gutin, B. and Kasper, M.J. (1992). Can vigorous exercise play a role in osteoporosis prevention? A review. *Osteoporosis International*, **2**, 55–69.

666. Gutin, B. and Manos, T.M. (1993). Physical activity in the prevention of childhood obesity. *Annals of the New York Academy of Sciences*, **699**, 115–26.

667. Hagan, R.D., Marks, J.F. and Warren, P.A. (1979). Physiologic responses of juvenile-onset diabetic boys to muscular work. *Diabetes*, **28**, 1114–19.

668. Hagberg, J.M. (1990). Exercise, fitness and hypertension. In C. Bouchard, R.J. Shephard, T. Stephens, J.R. Sutton and B.D. McPherson (Eds.), *Exercise, Fitness and Health*. Champaign, IL, Human Kinetics, pp. 455–66.

669. Hagberg, J.M., Coyle, E.F., Carroll, J.E., Miller, J.M., Martin, W.H. and Brooke, M.H. (1982). Exercise hyperventilation in patients with McArdle's disease. *Journal of Applied Physiology*, **52**, 991–4.

670. Hagberg, J.M., Ehsani, A.A., Goldring, D., Hernandez, A., Sinacore, D.R. and Holloszy, J.O. (1984). Effect of weight training on blood pressure and hemodynamics in hypertensive adolescents. *Journal of Pediatrics*, **104**, 147–51.

671. Hagberg, J.M., Goldring, D., Ehsani, A.A., Heath, G.W., Hernandez, A., Schechtman, K. *et al.* (1983). Effects of exercise training on the blood

pressure and hemodynamics of adolescent hypertensives. *American Journal of Cardiology*, **52**, 763–8.

672. Hagberg, J.M., Goldring, D., Heath, G.W., Ehsani, A.A., Hernandez, A. and Holloszy, J.O. (1984). Effect of exercise training on plasma catecholamines and haemodynamics of adolescent hypertensives during rest, submaximal exercise and orthostatic stress. *Clinical Physiology*, **4**, 117–24.

673. Hagberg, J.M., Nagle, F.J. and Carlson, J.L. (1978). Transient O₂ uptake response at the onset of exercise. *Journal of Applied Physiology*, **44**, 90–2.

674. Hale, R.W. (1989). Oligomenorrhea during athletic training. In N.J. Smith (Ed.), *Common Problems in Pediatric Sports Medicine*. Chicago, Year Book Medical Publishers, pp. 65–9.

675. Hale, T., Armstrong, N., Hardman, A., Jakeman, P., Sharp, C. and Winter, E. (1989). *Position Statement on the Physiological Assessment of the Elite Competitor*. Leeds, British Association of Sports Sciences.

676. Haliouia, L. and Anderson, J.J.B. (1989). Lifetime calcium intake and physical activity habits: independent and combined effects on the radial bone of healthy premenopausal Caucasian women. *American Journal of Clinical Nutrition*, **49**, 534–41.

677. Halmi, K., Goldberg, S.C., Eckert, E., Casper, R. and Davis, J.M. (1977). Pretreatment evaluation in anorexia nervosa. In R.Vigersky (Ed.), *Anorexia Nervosa*. New York, Raven Press, pp. 34–54.

678. Hamel, P., Simoneau, J.A., Lortie, G., Boulay, M.R. and Bouchard, C. (1986). Heredity and muscle adaptation to endurance training. *Medicine and Science in Sports and Exercise*, **18**, 690–6.

679. Hamill, B.P. (1994). Relative safety of weightlifting and weight training. *Journal of Strength and Conditioning Research*, **8**, 53–7.

680. Hamilton, P. and Andrew, G.M. (1976). Influence of growth and athletic training on heart and lung function. *European Journal of Applied Physiology*, **36**, 27–38.

681. Hamsten, A., Walldius, G., Szamosi, A., Dahlen, G. and de Faire, U. (1986). Relationship of angiographically defined coronary disease to serum lipoproteins and apolipoproteins in young survivors of myocardial infarction. *Circulation*, **73**, 1097–110.

682. Hansen, H.S., Froberg, K., Hydlebrandt, N. and Nielsen, J.R. (1991). A controlled study of eight months of physical training and reduction of blood pressure in children: the Odense schoolchild study. *British Medical Journal*, **303**, 682–5.

683. Haralambie, G. (1982). Enzyme activities in skeletal muscle of 13–15 years old adolescents. *Bulletin Européen Physiopathologie Respiratoire*, **18**, 65–74.

684. Harlan, W.R., Landis, J.R., Flegal, K.M., Davis, C.S. and Miller, M.E. (1988). Trends in body mass in the United States, 1969–1980. *American Journal of Epidemiology*, **128**, 1065–74.

685. Harris, D.V. (1970). Physical activity history and attitudes of middle aged men. *Medicine and Science in Sports*, **2**, 203–8.

686. Harris, J. (1994). Health-related exercise in the National Curriculum: results of a pilot study in secondary schools. *British Journal of Physical Education Research Supplement*, **14**, 6–11.

687. Harrison, J.E. and Chow, R. (1990). Discussion: exercise, fitness, osteoarthritis and osteoporosis. In C. Bouchard, R.J. Shephard, T. Stephens, J.R. Sutton and B.D. McPherson (Eds.), *Exercise, Fitness, and Health*. Champaign, IL, Human Kinetics, pp. 529–32.

688. Harsha, D.Q., Frerichs, R.R. and Berenson, G.S. (1978). Densitometry and anthropometry of black and white children. *Human Biology*, **50**, 261–80.

689. Hartley, G.A. (1988). A comparative view of talent selection for sport in two socialist states – the USSR and the GDR – with particular reference to gymnasts. In *The Growing Child and Competitive Sport*. Leeds, National Coaching Foundation, pp. 50–6.

690. Hartung, G.H., Foreyt, J.P., Mitchell, R.E., Vlasek, I. and Gotto, A.M. (1980). Relation of diet to high intensity lipoprotein cholesterol in middle aged marathon runners, joggers and inactive men. *New England Journal of Medicine*, **302**, 357–61.

691. Harvey, J.S. (1982). Overuse syndromes in young athletes. *Pediatric Clinics of North America*, **29**, 1369–81.

692. Hassan, S.E.A. (1991). Die Trainierbarkeit der Maximalkraft bei 7- bis 13-jährigen Kindern. *Leistungssport*, **5**, 17–24.

693. Haverty, M., Kenny, W.L. and Hodgson, J.L. (1988). Lactate and gas exchange responses to incremental and steady state running. *British Journal of Sports Medicine*, **2**, 51–4.

694. Hawkins, D.B. and Gruber, J.J. (1982). Little league baseball and players' self-esteem. *Perceptual and Motor Skills*, **55**, 1335–40.

695. Hawley, R.M. (1985). The outcome of anorexia nervosa in younger subjects. *British Journal of Psychology*, **146**, 657–60.

696. Hawton, K. and Fagg, J. (1992). Deliberate self-poisoning and self-injury in adolescents. A study of characteristics and trends in Oxford, 1976–89. *British Journal of Psychiatry*, **161**, 816–23.

697. Hayashi, T., Fujino, M., Shindo, M., Hiroki, T. and Arakawa, K. (1987). Echocardiographic and electrocardiographic measures in obese children after an exercise program. *International Journal of Obesity*, **11**, 465–72.

698. Hayward, K.A. (1991). The role of physical education in the development of active lifestyles. *Research Quarterly for Exercise and Sport*, **62**, 151–6.

699. Heald, F.P. and Hollander, R.J. (1965). The relationship between obesity in early adolescence and early growth. *Journal of Pediatrics*, **67**, 35.

700. Heaney, R. (1991). The effect of calcium on skeletal development, bone loss, and risk of fractures. *American Journal of Medicine*, **91** (Suppl. 5B), 23S–28S.

701. Heartbeat Wales (1986). *Welsh Youth Health Survey 1986*. (Heartbeat Report No. 5), Cardiff, Heartbeat Wales.

702. Heartbeat Wales (1987). *Exercise for Health*. (Heartbeat Report No. 23), Cardiff, Heartbeat Wales.

703. Heath, G.W., Pratt, M., Warner, C.W. and Kann, L. (1994). Physical activity patterns in American high school students. *Archives of Pediatric and Adolescent Medicine*, **148**, 1131–6.

704. Heck, H., Mader, A., Hess, G., Mucke, S., Muller, R. and Hollman, W. (1985). Justification of the 4 mmol·L^{-1} lactate threshold. *International Journal of Sports Medicine*, **6**, 117–30.

705. Hejna, W.F., Rosenberg, A., Buturusis, D.J. and Krieger, A. (1982).The prevention of sports injuries in high school students through strength training. *National Strength and Conditioning Association Journal*, **4**, 28–31.

706. Henderson, R., Kemp, G. and Campion, H. (1992). Residual bone-mineral density and muscle strength after fractures of the tibia and femur in children. *Journal of Bone and Joint Surgery*, **74**, 211–18.

707. Hendry, L. (1978). *School Sport and Leisure*. London, Lepus Books.

708. Henritze, J., Weltman, A., Schurrer, R.L. and Barlow, L. (1985). Effects of training at and above the lactate threshold on the lactate threshold and maximal oxygen uptake. *European Journal of Applied Physiology*, **54**, 84–8.

709. Hermanson, L. (1979). Effect of acidosis on skeletal muscle performance during maximal exercise in man. *Bulletin Européen de Physiopathologie Respiratoire*, **15**, 229–38.

710. Hermanson, L. and Medbø, J.I. (1984). The relative significance of aerobic and anaerobic processes during maximal exercise of short duration. In P. Marconnet, J. Poortmans and L. Hermanson (Eds.), *Physiological Chemistry of Training and Detraining*. Basel, Karger, pp. 56–7.

711. Herzog, D.B. and Copeland, P.M. (1985). Eating disorders. *New England Journal of Medicine*, **313**, 295–303.

712. Hettinger, T.H. (1958). Die Trainerbarkeit menschlicher Muskeln in Abhängigkeit vom Alter und Geschlecht. *Internationale Zeitschrift für Angewandte Physiologie Einschliesslich Arbeitphysiologie*, **17**, 371–7.

713. Heuneman, R.L., Shapiro, L.R., Hampton, M.C. and Mitchell, B.W. (1966). A longitudinal study of gross body composition and body conformation and their association with food and activity in a teenage population. *American Journal of Clinical Nutrition*, **18**, 325–38.

714. Heusner, A.A. (1982). Energy metabolism and body size. I. Is the 0.75 mass exponent of Kleiber's equation a statistical artifact? *Respiration Physiology*, **48**, 1–12.

715. Heusner, A.A. (1987). What does the power function reveal about structure and function in animals of different size? *Annual Reviews in Physiology*, **49**, 121–33.

716. Hickie, J.B., Sutton, J., Russo, P. and Ruys, J. (1974). Serum cholesterol and serum triglyceride levels in adolescent males. *Medical Journal of Australia*, **1**, 825–8.

717. Hicks, A.L., MacDougall, J.D. and Muckle, T.J. (1987). Acute changes in high-density lipoprotein cholesterol with exercise of different intensities. *Journal of Applied Physiology*, **63**, 1956–60.

718. Hickson, R.C., Bomze, H.A. and Holloszy, J.O. (1978). Faster adjustment of O_2 uptake to the energy requirement of exercise in the trained state. *Journal of Applied Physiology*, **44**, 877–81.

719. Highet, R. (1989). Athletic amenorrhea: an update on etiology, complications and management. *Sports Medicine*, **7**, 82–108.

720. Hill, A.V. (1925). *Muscular Activity*. London, Ballière, Tindall and Cox.

721. Hill, A.V., London, C.N.H. and Lupton, H. (1924). Muscular exercise, lactic acid and the supply and utilization of oxygen. Parts IV–VIII. *Proceedings of the Royal Society of London*, **B97**, 84–138, 155–76.

722. Hillman, M. (Ed.) (1993). *Children, Transport and the Quality of Life.* London, Policy Studies Institute.

723. Hillman, M. (1993). One false move ... an overview of the findings and issues they raise. In M. Hillman (Ed.), *Children, Transport and the Quality of Life.* London, Policy Studies Institute, pp. 7–14.

724. Hillman, M., Adams, J. and Whitelegg, J. (1990). *One False Move.* London, Policy Studies Institute.

725. Hilyer, J.C., Wilson, D.G., Dillon, C., Caro, L., Jenkins, C., Spencer, W.A. *et al.* (1982). Physical fitness training and counselling as treatment for youth offenders. *Journal of Counselling Psychology,* **29**, 292–303.

726. Hislop, H.J. and Perrine, J.J. (1967). Isokinetic concept of exercise. *Physical Therapy,* **47**, 114–17.

727. Hoes, M., Binkhorst, R.A., Smeekes-Kuyl, A. and Vissurs, A.C. (1968). Measurement of forces exerted on a pedal crank during work on the bicycle ergometer at different loads. *Internationale Zeitschift fur Angewandte Physiologie,* **26**, 33–42.

728. Hoffmans, M.D.A.F., Krohout, D. and de Lezenne Coulander, C. (1988). The impact of body mass index of 78,612 18-year old Dutch men on 32-year mortality from all causes. *Journal of Clinical Epidemiology,* **41**, 749–56.

729. Hohorst, H.J. (1965). L-(+) Lactate determination with lactic dehydro-genase and DPN. In H.V. Bergmeyer (Ed.), *Methods of Enzymatic Analysis, 2nd edition.* New York, Academic Press, pp. 226–70.

730. Holloway, J.B., Beuter, A. and Duda, J.L. (1988). Self-efficacy and training for strength in adolescent girls. *Journal of Applied Social Psychology,* **18**, 699–719.

731. Holman, R.L., McGill, H.C., Strong, J.P. and Geer, J.C. (1958). The natural history of atherosclerosis: the early aortic lesions as seen in New Orleans in the middle of the 20th century. *American Journal of Pathology,* **34**, 209–35.

732. Horton, E.S. (1989). Exercise and diabetes in youth. In C.V. Gisolfi and D.R. Lamb (Eds.), *Perspectives in Exercise Science and Sports Medicine, Vol. 2, Youth, Exercise, and Sport.* Indianapolis, IN, Benchmark Press, pp. 539–74.

733. Horton, E.S. (1995). Diabetes mellitus. In B. Goldberg (Ed.), *Sports and Exercise for Children with Chronic Health Conditions.* Champaign, IL, Human Kinetics, pp. 355–73.

734. Houmard, J.A., Israel, R.G., McCammon, M.R., O'Brien, K.P., Omer, J. and Zamora, B.S. (1991). Validity of a near-infrared device for estimating body composition in a college football team. *Journal of Applied Sport Science Research,* **5**, 53–9.

735. Houmard, J.A., Smith, R. and Jendrasiak, G.L. (1995). Relationship between MRI relaxation time and muscle fibre composition. *Journal of Applied Physiology,* **78**, 807–9.

736. Houtkooper, L.B., Going, S.B., Lohman, T.G., Roche, A.F. and Van Loan, M. (1992). Bioelectrical impedance estimation of fat-free body mass in children and youth: a cross-validation study. *Journal of Applied Physiology,* **72**, 366–73.

737. Houtkooper, L.B., Lohman, T.G., Going, S.B. and Hall, M.C. (1989). Validity of bioelectrical impedance for body composition assessment in children. *Journal of Applied Physiology*, **66**, 814–21.

738. Hovell, M.F., Bursick, J.H., Sharkey, R. and McClure, J. (1978). An evaluation of elementary students' voluntary physical activity during recess. *Research Quarterly*, **49**, 460–74.

739. Howell, M.L. and MacNab, R.LB.J. (1968). *The Physical Work Capacity of Canadian Children Aged 7 to 17*. Toronto, Ontario, Canadian Association for Health, Physical Education and Recreation.

740. Hui, S.L., Johnston, C.C. and Mazess, R.B. (1985). Bone mass in normal children and young adults. *Growth*, **49**, 34–43.

741. Hui, S.L., Slemenda, C.W., Johnston, P.H. and Johnston, C.C. (1989). Baseline measurement of bone mass predicts fracture in white women. *Annals of Internal Medicine*, **111**, 355–61.

742. Hulkko, A. and Orava, S. (1987). Stress fractures in athletes. *International Journal of Sports Medicine*, **8**, 221–6.

743. Hulley, S.B., Rosenham, R.H., Bawol, R.D. and Brand, R.J. (1980). Epidemiology as a guide to clinical decisions: the association between triglyceride and coronary heart disease. *New England Journal of Medicine*, **302**, 1383–9.

744. Hunt, J.F. and White, J.R. (1980). Effects of ten weeks of vigorous daily exercise on serum lipids and lipoproteins in teenage males. *Medicine and Science in Sports*, **12**, 93.

745. Hurley, B.F., Hagberg, J.M., Seals, D.R., Goldberg, A.P. and Holloszy, J.O. (1986). Circuit weight training reduces coronary artery disease risk factors independent of changes in VO_2 max. *Medicine and Science in Sports and Exercise*, **18**, 568–9.

746. Huttunen, N.P., Lankela, S.L., Knip, M., Lautala, P., Kaar, M.L., Laasonen, K. *et al.* (1989). Effect of once-a-week training program on physical fitness and metabolic control in children with IDDM. *Diabetes Care*, **12**, 737–40.

747. Ilmarinen, J. and Rutenfranz, J. (1980). Longitudinal studies of the changes in habitual physical activity of schoolchildren and working adolescents. In K. Berg and B.O. Eriksson (Eds.), *Children and Exercise IX*. Baltimore, MD, University Park Press, pp. 149–59.

748. Inbar, O. and Bar-Or, O. (1977). Relationships of anerobic and aerobic arm and leg capacities to swimming performance of 8–12 year old children. In R.J. Shephard and H. Lavallée (Eds.), *Frontiers of Activity and Child Health*. Quebec, Pelican, pp. 283–93.

749. Inbar, O., Dotan, R. and Bar-Or, O. (1986). Aerobic and anerobic characteristics in male children and adolescents. *Medicine and Science in Sports and Exercise*, **18**, 264–9.

750. Inbar, O., Dotan, R., Bar-Or, O. and Gutin, B. (1985). Passive versus active exposures to dry heat as methods of heat acclimatization in young children. In R.A. Binkhorst, H.C.G. Kemper and W.H.M. Saris (Eds.), *Children and Exercise XI*. Champaign, IL, Human Kinetics, pp. 329–40.

751. Inbar, O., Kaiser, P. and Tesch, P. (1981). Relationship between leg muscle fibre type distribution and leg exercise performance. *International Journal of Sports Medicine*, **2**, 154–9.

752. Ivy, J.L., Withers, R.T., Van Handel, P.J., Elger, D.H. and Costill, D.L. (1980). Muscle respiratory capacity and fiber type as determinants of the lactate threshold. *Journal of Applied Physiology*, **48**, 523–7.

753. Izumi, I. and Ishiko, T. (1984). Lactate threshold in pubescent boys. *Japanese Journal of Physical Education*, **28**, 309–14.

754. Jackson, R.L. and Kelly, H.G. (1948). A study of physical activity in juvenile diabetic patients. *Journal of Pediatrics*, **33**, 155–66.

755. Jacobs, B.W. and Isaac, S. (1986). Pre-pubertal anorexia: a retrospective controlled study. *Journal of Child Psychology and Psychiatry*, **27**, 237–50.

756. Jacobs, I., Tesch, P.A., Bar-Or, O., Karlsson, J. and Dotan, R. (1983). Lactate in human skeletal muscle after 10s and 30s of supramaximal exercise. *Journal of Applied Physiology*, **55**, 365–8.

757. Jacobsson, B. (1986). Sports accidents among children and teenagers: a 1-year study of incidence and severity in a Swedish rural municipality. *Scandinavian Journal of Sports Sciences*, **8**, 75–9.

758. Janz, K.F., Golden, J.C., Hansen, J.R. and Mahoney, L.T. (1992). Heart rate monitoring of physical activity in children and adolescents: the Muscatine study. *Pediatrics*, **89**, 256–61.

759. Janz, K.F., Neilsen, D.H., Cassady, S.L., Cook, J.S., Wu, Y.-T. and Hansen, J.R. (1993). Cross-validation of the Slaughter skinfold equations for children and adolescents. *Medicine and Science in Sports and Exercise*, **25**, 1070–6.

760. Janz, K.F., Witt, J. and Mahoney, L.T. (1995). The stability of children's physical activity as measured by accelerometry and self-report. *Medicine and Science in Sports and Exercise*, **27**, 1326–32.

761. Jauhianen, M., Laitinen, M., Penttila, I., Nousioanen, U. and Ahonen, E. (1985). Lipids and apolipoproteins A-I, B and C-II and different weight loss programs (weight lifters, wrestlers, boxers and judokas). *International Journal of Biochemistry*, **17**, 167–74.

762. Jetté, M., Barry, W. and Pearlman, L. (1977). The effects of an extra curricular physical activity program on obese adolescents. *Canadian Journal of Public Health*, **68**, 39–42.

763. Johansson, C. (1980). The diabetic's own view on physical exercise as a part of life. *Acta Paediatrica Scandinavica*, **283** (Suppl.), 117–19.

764. Johnson, C., Miller, J., Slemenda, C., Reister, T.K., Hui, S., Christian, J.C. *et al.* (1992). Calcium supplementation and increases in bone mineral density in children. *New England Journal of Medicine*, **327**, 82–7.

765. Johnson, M.D., Jay, M.S., Shoup, B. and Rickert, V.I. (1988). Anabolic steroid use in adolescent males. *Journal of Adolescent Health Care*, **9**, 263.

766. Johnson, M.L., Burke, B.S. and Mayer, J. (1956). Relative importance of inactivity and overeating in the energy balance of obese high school girls. *American Journal of Clinical Nutrition*, **4**, 37–44.

767. Jones, C. (1996). Physical education at key stage 3. In N. Armstrong (Ed.), *New Directions in Physical Education, Vol. 3, Change and Innovation*. London, Cassell, pp. 48–61.

768. Jones, D.A. and Mills, M.E. (1995). Muscle strength and training in children. In N. Maffulli (Ed.), *Colour Atlas of Sports Medicine in Childhood and Adolescence*. London, Mosby-Wolfe, pp. 101–8.

769. Jones, P.J.H. and Leatherdale, S.T. (1991). Stable isotopes in clinical research: safety re-affirmed. *Clinical Science*, **80**, 277–80.

770. Jones, P.L., Winthrop, A.L., Schoeller, D.A., Swyer, P.R., Smith, J., Filler, R.M. *et al.* (1987). Validation of doubly labelled water for assessing energy expenditure in infants. *Pediatric Research*, **21**, 242–6.

771. Jones, P.R.M. and Pearson, J. (1969). Anthropometric determination of leg fat and muscle plus bone volumes in young male and female adults. *Journal of Physiology*, **204**, 63P–66P.

772. Joslin, E.P. (1959). The treatment of diabetes mellitus. In E.P. Joslin, H.F. Root, P. White and A. Marble (Eds.), *Treatment of Diabetes Mellitus*. Philadelphia, PA, Lea and Febiger, pp. 243–300.

773. Kackowski, W., Montgomery, D.L., Taylor, A.W. and Klissouras, V. (1982). The relationship between muscle fibre composition and maximal anaerobic power and capacity. *Journal of Sports Medicine and Physical Fitness*, **22**, 407–13.

774. Kaiserauer, S., Snyder, A.C., Sleeper, M. and Sierath, J. (1989). Nutritional, physiological, and menstrual status of distance runners. *Medicine and Science in Sports and Exercise*, **21**, 120–5.

775. Kanaley, J.A. and Boileau, R.A. (1988). The onset of the anaerobic threshold at three stages of physical maturity. *Journal of Sports Medicine and Physical Fitness*, **28**, 367–74.

776. Kanders, B., Dempster, D.W. and Lindsay, R. (1983). Interaction of calcium nutrition and physical activity on bone mass in young women. *Journal of Bone Mineral Research*, **3**, 145–9.

777. Kanis, J.A. and Pitt, F.A. (1992). Epidemiology of osteoporosis. *Bone*, **31** (Suppl. 1), 7–15.

778. Kannel, W.B. (1983). An overview of the risk factors for cardiovascular disease. In N.M. Kaplan and J. Stamler (Eds.), *Prevention of Coronary Heart Disease*. Philadelphia, PA, W.B. Saunders, pp. 1–19.

779. Kannel, W.B., Castelli, W.P. and Gordon, T. (1979). Cholesterol in the prediction of atherosclerotic disease. New perspectives based on the Framingham Study. *Annals of Internal Medicine*, **90**, 85–91.

780. Kannel, W.B., Castelli, W.P., Gordon, T. and McNamara, P.M. (1971). Serum cholesterol, lipoproteins and the risk of coronary heart disease. *Annals of Internal Medicine*, **74**, 1–12.

781. Kannel, W.B., Castelli, W.P., McNamara, P.M., McKee, P.A. and Feinleib, M. (1972). Role of blood pressure in the development of congestive heart failure. The Framingham Study. *New England Journal of Medicine*, **287**, 781–7.

782. Kannel, W.B. and Dawber, T.R. (1972). Atherosclerosis as a pediatric problem. *Journal of Pediatrics*, **80**, 544–54.

783. Kannel, W.B., Dawber, T.R. and McGee, D.L. (1980). Perspectives on systolic hypertension. The Framingham Study. *Circulation*, **61**, 1179–82.

784. Kannel, W.B., Doyle, S.T., Ostfield, A.M., Jenkins, C.D., Kuller, L., Podell, R.N. *et al.* (1984). Original resources for primary prevention of atherosclerotic diseases. *Circulation*, **70**, 157A–205A.

785. Kaplan, N. (1986). *Clinical Hypertension*. Baltimore, MD, Williams and Wilkins.

786. Kaplan, N.M. (1989). The deadly quartet: upper-body obesity, glucose intolerance, hypertriglyceridemia and hypertension. *Annals of Internal Medicine*, **149**, 1514–20.

787. Kappagoda, C., Linden, R. and Newell, J. (1979). Effects of the Canadian Air Force Training Program on a submaximal exercise test. *Quarterly Journal of Experimental Physiology*, **64**, 185–204.

788. Karlsson, J. (1971). Lactate and phosphagen concentration in working muscle of man with special reference to oxygen deficit at the onset of work. *Acta Physiologica Scandinavica*, **358** (Suppl.), 1–72.

789. Karlsson, J., Holmgren, A., Linnarson, D. and Astrom, H. (1984). OBLA exercise stress testing in health and disease. In H. Lollgen and H. Mellerowicz (Eds.), *Progress in Ergometry: Quality Control and Test Criteria*. Berlin, Springer, pp. 66–91.

790. Karvonen, M.J., Cwalbinska-Moneto, J. and Synajakangas, S. (1984). Comparison of heart rates measured by ECG and microcomputer. *The Physician and Sports Medicine*, **12**, 65–9.

791. Karvonen, M.J. and Vuorimaa, T. (1988). Heart rate and exercise intensity during sports activities. *Sports Medicine*, **5**, 303–12.

792. Katch, F.I., Girandola, F.N. and Katch, V.L. (1971). The relationship of body weight to maximum oxygen uptake and heavy work endurance capacity on the bicycle ergometer. *Medicine and Science in Sports*, **3**, 101–6.

793. Katch, V.L. (1972). Correlational and ratio adjustments of body weight in exercise-oxygen studies. *Ergonomics*, **15**, 671–80.

794. Katch, V.L. (1973). Use of the oxygen/body weight ratio in correlational analyses: spurious correlations and statistical considerations. *Medicine and Science in Sports*, **5**, 252–7.

795. Katch, V.L. (1983). Physical conditioning of children. *Journal of Adolescent Health Care*, **3**, 241–6.

796. Katch, V.L. and Katch, F.I. (1974). Use of weight-adjusted oxygen uptake scores that avoid spurious correlation. *Research Quarterly*, **45**, 447–51.

797. Katzman, D.K., Bachrach, L.K., Carter, D.R. and Marcus, R. (1991). Clinical and anthropometric correlates of bone mineral acquisition in healthy adolescent girls. *Journal of Clinical Endocrinology and Metabolism*, **73**, 1332–9.

798. Kavanagh, T. (1987). Exercise for the post-coronary patient. In *Exercise Heart Health*. London, Coronary Prevention Group, pp. 47–56.

799. Kay, C. and Shephard, R.J. (1969). On muscle strength and the threshold of anaerobic work. *Internationale Zeitschift für Angewandte Physiologie*, **27**, 311–28.

800. Kellet, D.W., Willan, P.L.T. and Bagnall, K.J. (1978). A study of potential Olympic swimmers: part 2. Changes due to three months of intensive training. *British Journal of Sports Medicine*, **12**, 87–92.

801. Kemmer, F.W. and Berger, M. (1983). Exercise and diabetes mellitus: Physical activity as a part of daily life and its role in the treatment of diabetic patients. *International Journal of Sports Medicine*, **4**, 77–88.

802. Kemmer, F.W., Berchtold, P., Berger, M., Starke, A., Cuppers, H.-J., Gries, F.A. *et al.* (1979). Exercise-induced fall of blood glucose in insulin-treated

diabetics unrelated to alteration of insulin mobilization. *Diabetes*, **28**, 1131–7.

803. Kemper, H.C.G. (Ed.) (1985). Growth, health and fitness of teenagers. *Medicine and Sport Science*, **20**, 1–202.

804. Kemper, H.C.G. (1994). Is leg muscle mass decisive in reaching a plateau in oxygen uptake during maximal treadmill running? Analysis of data from the Amsterdam Growth and Health Study. *American Journal of Human Biology*, **6**, 437–44.

805. Kemper, H.C.G. (1995). *The Amsterdam Growth Study*. Champaign, IL, Human Kinetics.

806. Kemper, H.C.G. and Coudert, J. (Eds.) (1994). Physical health and fitness of Bolivian boys. *International Journal of Sports Medicine*, **15** (Suppl. 2), S71–S114.

807. Kemper, H.C.G., Dekker, H.J.P., Ootjers, M.G., Post, B., Snel, J., Splinter, P.G. *et al.* (1983). Growth and health of teenagers in the Netherlands: survey of multi-disciplinary longitudinal studies and comparison to recent results of a Dutch study. *International Journal of Sports Medicine*, **4**, 202–14.

808. Kemper, H.C.G. and Niemeyer, C. (1995). The importance of a physically active lifestyle during youth for peak bone mass. In C.J.R. Blimkie and O. Bar-Or (Eds.), *New Horizons in Pediatric Exercise Science*. Champaign, IL, Human Kinetics, pp. 77–96.

809. Kemper, H.C.G. and Verschuur, R. (1981). Maximal aerobic power in 13- and 14-year-old teenagers in relation to biologic age. *International Journal of Sports Medicine*, **2**, 97–100.

810. Kemper, H.C.G. and Verschuur, R. (1985). Maximal aerobic power. *Medicine and Sport Science*, **20**, 107–26.

811. Kemper, H.C.G., Verschuur, R. and de Mey, L. (1989). Longitudinal changes of aerobic fitness in youth ages 12 to 23. *Pediatric Exercise Science*, **1**, 257–70.

812. Kerr, J.H. and Rodgers, M.M. (1981). Primary school physical education: non-specialist teacher preparation and attitudes. *Bulletin of Physical Education*, **17**, 13–20.

813. Keul, J., Doll, E. and Keppler, D. (1972). Energy metabolism of human muscles. *Medicine and Sport*. Basel, Karger.

814. Keul, J., Kindermann, W. and Simon, G. (1978). Die aerobe und anaerobe Kapazität als Grundlage für die Leistungsdiagnostik. *Leistungssport*, **8**, 22–32.

815. Keys, A. (1975). Coronary heart disease – the global picture. *Atherosclerosis*, **22**, 149–92.

816. Keys, A., Aravanis, C., Blackburn, H., van Buchem, F.S.P., Buzina, R., Djordjevic, B.S. *et al.* (1966). Epidemiological studies related to coronary heart disease: characteristics of men aged 40–59 in seven countries. *Acta Medica Scandinavica*, **460**, 1–392.

817. Kibler, W.B. and Chandler, T.J. (1993). Musculoskeletal adaptations and injuries associated with intensive participation in youth sports. In B.R. Cahill and A.J. Pearl (Eds.), *Intensive Participation in Children's Sports*. Champaign, IL, Human Kinetics, pp. 203–16.

818. Kindermann, W., Simon, G. and Keul, J. (1979). The significance of the aerobic-anaerobic transition for the determination of work load intensities during endurance training. *European Journal of Applied Physiology*, **42**, 25–34.

819. King, A.C. (1991). Community intervention for promotion of physical activity and fitness. *Exercise and Sport Sciences Reviews*, **19**, 211–49.

820. King, A.J.C. and Coles, B. (1992). *The Health of Canada's Youth*. Canada, Ottawa, Ministry of Health and Welfare.

821. Kirby, B., McManus, A., Welsman, J., Harwood, C., Balding, J., Gentle, P. *et al.* (1993). Aerobic fitness, physical activity and apolipoproteins in children. *Pediatric Exercise Science*, **5**, 434.

822. Kirkendall, D.R. (1986). Effects of physical activity on intellectual development and academic performance. In G.A. Stull and H.M. Eckert (Eds.), *Effects of Physical Activity on Children*. Champaign, IL, Human Kinetics, pp. 49–63.

823. Kirsten, G. (1963). Der Einfluss isometrischen Muskeltrainings auf die Entwicklung der Muskelkraft. *Internationale Zeitschrift für Angewandte Physiologie Einschliesslich Arbeitsphysiologie*, **19**, 387–402.

824. Klausen, K., Rasmussen, B. and Schibye, B. (1985). Evaluation of the physical activity of school children during a physical education lesson. In J. Rutenfranz, R. Mocellin and F. Klimt (Eds.), *Children and Exercise XII*. Champaign, IL, Human Kinetics, pp. 93–101.

825. Kleiber, M. (1932). Body size and metabolism. *Hilgardia*, **6**, 315–53.

826. Kleiber, M. (1950). Physiological meaning of regression equations. *Journal of Applied Physiology*, **2**, 417–23.

827. Klesges, L.M. and Klesges, R.C. (1987). The assessment of children's physical activity: a comparison of methods. *Medicine and Science in Sports and Exercise*, **19**, 511–17.

828. Klesges, R.C., Coates, T.J., Moldenhauer-Klesges, L.M., Holzer, B., Gustavson, J. and Barnes, J. (1984). The FATS: an observational system for assessing physical activity in children and associated parent behaviour. *Behavioural Assessment*, **6**, 333–45.

829. Klesges, R.C., Eck, L.H., Hanson, C.L., Haddock, C.K. and Klesges, L.M. (1990). Effects of obesity, social interactions, and physical environment on physical activity in preschoolers. *Health Psychology*, **9**, 435–49.

830. Klesges, R.C., Haddock, C.K. and Eck, L.H. (1990). A multimethod approach to the measurement of childhood physical activity and its relationship to blood pressure and body weight. *Journal of Pediatrics*, **116**, 888–93.

831. Klesges, R.C., Klesges, L.M., Swenson, A.M. and Pheley, A.M. (1985). A validation of two motion sensors in the prediction of child and adult physical activity levels. *American Journal of Epidemiology*, **122**, 400–10.

832. Klesges, R.C., Mallot, J.M., Boschee, P.F. and Weber, J.M. (1986). The effects of parental influences on children's food intake, physical activity, and relative weight. *International Journal of Eating Disorders*, **5**, 335–46.

833. Knittle, J.L. (1972). Obesity in childhood: a problem in adipose tissue cellular development. *Pediatrics*, **81**, 1048–59.

834. Kobayashi, K., Kitamura, K., Miura, M., Sodeyama, H., Murase, Y., Miyashita, M. *et al.* (1978). Aerobic power as related to body growth and training in Japanese boys: a longitudinal study. *Journal of Applied Physiology*, **44**, 666–72.

835. Koch, G. (1980). Aerobic power, lung dimensions, ventilatory capacity and muscle blood flow in 12–16 year old boys with high physical activity. In K. Berg and B.O. Eriksson (Eds.), *Children and Exercise IX*. Baltimore, MD, University Park Press, pp. 99–108.

836. Koch, G. (1980). Adrenergic activity at rest and during exercise in normotensive boys and young adults and in hypertensive patients. In K. Berg and B.O. Eriksson (Eds.), *Children and Exercise IX*. Baltimore, MD, University Park Press, pp. 375–83.

837. Koch, G. and Eriksson, B.O. (1973). Effect of physical training on anatomical R-L shunt at rest and pulmonary diffusing capacity during near-maximal exercise in boys 11 to 13 years old. *Scandinavian Journal of Clinical and Laboratory Investigations*, **31**, 95–105.

838. Koch, G. and Fransson, L. (1986). Essential cardiovascular and respiratory determinants of physical performance at age 12–17 years during intensive physical training. In J. Rutenfranz, R. Mocellin and F. Klimt (Eds.), *Children and Exercise XII*. Champaign, IL, Human Kinetics, pp. 75–292.

839. Koch, G. and Rocker, L. (1980). Total amount of hemoglobin, plasma and blood volumes, and intravascular protein masses in trained boys. In K. Berg and B.O. Eriksson (Eds.), *Children and Exercise IX*. Baltimore, MD, University Park Press, pp. 109–15.

840. Kofsky, P.R., Goode, R.C. and Romet, T.T. (1983). Effects of a short period of intense activity on schoolchildren. *Australian Journal of Sports Medicine*, **3**, 19–21.

841. Koivisto, V. and Felig, P. (1978). Effects of leg exercise on insulin absorption in diabetic patients. *New England Journal of Medicine*, **298**, 77–83.

842. Kokkinos, P.F. and Hurley, B.F. (1990). Strength training and lipoprotein-lipid profiles. *Sports Medicine*, **9**, 266–72.

843. Komi, P.V. (1986). Training of muscle strength and power: interaction of neuromotoric, hypertrophic and mechanical factors. *International Journal of Sports Medicine*, **7** (Suppl.), 10–15.

844. Komi, P.V. and Karlsson, J. (1979). Physical performance, skeletal muscle enzyme activities, and fibre types in monozygous and dizygous twins of both sexes. *Acta Physiologica Scandinavica*, **462** (Suppl.), 1–28.

845. Koocher, G.P. (1971). Swimming competence and personality change. *Journal of Personality and Social Psychology*, **18**, 275–8.

846. Krabbe, S., Christiansen, C., Rodbro, P. and Transbol, I. (1979). Effects of puberty on rates of bone growth and mineralisation. *Archives of Disease in Childhood*, **54**, 950–3.

847. Kraemer, W.J., Fry, A.C., Frykman, P.N., Conroy, B. and Hoffman, J. (1989). Resistance training and youth. *Pediatric Exercise Science*, **1**, 336–50.

848. Kraft, R.E. (1989). Children at play. *Journal of Physical Education, Recreation and Dance*, **60**, 21–4.

849. Krahenbuhl, G.S. and Pangrazi, R.P. (1983). Characteristics associated with running performance in young boys. *Medicine and Science in Sports and Exercise*, **15**, 486–90.

850. Krahenbuhl, G.S., Pangrazi, R.P., Stone, W.J., Morgan, D.W. and Williams, T. (1989). Fractional utilization of maximal aerobic capacity in children 6 to 8 years of age. *Pediatric Exercise Science*, **1**, 271–7.

851. Krahenbuhl, G.S., Skinner, J.S. and Kohrt, W.M. (1985). Developmental aspects of maximal aerobic power in children. *Exercise and Sport Sciences Reviews*, **13**, 503–38.

852. Kriska, A.M., Blair, S.N. and Pereira, M.A. (1994). The potential role of physical activity in the prevention of non-insulin-dependent diabetes mellitus: the epidemiological evidence. *Exercise and Sport Sciences Reviews*, **22**, 121–43.

853. Kriska, A., Sandler, R., Cauley, J., LaPorte, R., Horn, D. and Pambianco, G. (1988). The assessment of historical physical activity and its relation to adult bone parameters. *American Journal of Epidemiology*, **127**, 1053–63.

854. Kristiansen, B. (1983). Associated football injuries in school boys. *Scandinavian Journal of Sports Sciences*, **5**, 1–2.

855. Kroger, H., Kotaniemi, A., Vainio, P. and Alhava, E. (1992). Bone densitometry of the spine and femur in children by dual-energy X-ray absorptiometry. *Bone Mineral*, **17**, 75–85.

856. Kromhout, D., Obermann-de-Boer, G.L. and DeLezenne Coulander, C.L. (1981). Major CHD risk indicators in Dutch schoolchildren aged 10–14 years. The Zutphen Schoolchildren Study. *Preventive Medicine*, **10**, 195–210.

857. Krotkiewski, M., Bjorntorp, P., Sjostrom, L. and Smith, U. (1983). Impact of obesity on metabolism in men and women. Importance of regional adipose tissue distribution. *Journal of Clinical Investigation*, **72**, 1150–62.

858. Krotkiewski, M., Kral, J.G. and Karlsson, J. (1980). Effects of castration and testosterone substitution on body composition and muscle metabolism in rats. *Acta Physiologica Scandinavica*, **109**, 233–7.

859. Krowchuck, D.P., Anglin, T.M., Goodfellow, D.B., Stancin, T., Williams, P. and Zimet, G.D. (1989). High school athletes and the use of ergogenic aids. *American Journal of Diseases of Children*, **143**, 486–9.

860. Kucera, M. (1985). Spontaneous physical activity in preschool children. In R.A. Binkhorst, H.C.G. Kemper and W.H.M. Saris (Eds.), *Children and Exercise XI*. Champaign, IL, Human Kinetics, pp. 175–82.

861. Kuczmarski, R.J., Flegal, K.M., Campbell, S.M. and Johnson, C.L. (1994). Increasing prevalence of overweight among US adults: the National Health and Nutrition Examination Surveys 1960 to 1991. *Journal of the American Medical Association*, **272**, 205–11.

862. Kuh, D.J.L. and Cooper, C. (1992). Physical activity at 36 years: patterns and childhood predictors in a longitudinal study. *Journal of Epidemiology and Community Health*, **46**, 114–19.

863. Kujala, U.M., Kvist, M. and Heinonen, O. (1985). Osgood-Schlatter's disease in adolescent athletes: retrospective study of incidence and duration. *American Journal of Sports Medicine*, **13**, 236–41.

864. Kuno, S., Katsuta, S., Inouye, T., Anno, I., Matsumoto, K. and Akisada, M. (1988). Relationship between MR relaxation time and muscle fiber composition. *Radiology*, **169**, 657–68.

865. Kunze, D. (1983). Reference values and tracking of blood lipid levels in childhood. *Preventive Medicine*, **12**, 806–9.

866. Kushner, R.F., Schoeller, D.A., Fjeld, C.R. and Danford, L. (1992). Is the impedance index (ht²/R) significant in predicting total body water? *American Journal of Clinical Nutrition*, **56**, 835–9.

867. Kusinitz, I. and Keeney, C.E. (1958). Effects of progressive weight training on health and physical fitness of adolescent boys. *Research Quarterly*, **29**, 294–301.

868. Kvist, H., Chowchuny, B., Grangard, B., Tylen, U. and Sjostrom, L. (1988). Total and visceral adipose-tissue volumes derived from measurements with computed tomography in adult men and women: predictive equations. *American Journal of Clinical Nutrition*, **48**, 1351–61.

869. Kwee, A. and Wilmore, J.H. (1990). Cardiorespiratory fitness and risk factors for coronary artery disease in 8- to 15-year-old boys. *Pediatric Exercise Science*, **2**, 372–83.

870. Laasko, L., Rimpela, M. and Telema, R. (1979). Relationship between physical activity and some health habits of Finnish youth. *Schriftenreihe des Bundestinstituts für Sportwissenschaft*, **36**, 76–81.

871. Lac, G., Duché, P., Falgairette, G. and Robert, A. (1992). Adrenal androgens profiles in saliva throughout puberty in both sexes. In J. Coudert and E. Van Praagh (Eds.), *Pediatric Work Physiology*. Paris, Masson, pp. 221–3.

872. Laird, W.P., Fixler, D.E. and Swanborm, C.D. (1979). Effect of chronic weight lifting on the blood pressure in hypertensive adolescents. *Preventive Medicine*, **8**, 184.

873. Lamb, K.L. and Brodie, D.A. (1990). The assessment of physical activity by leisure-time physical activity questionnaire. *Sports Medicine*, **10**, 159–80.

874. Landt, K.W., Campaigne, B.N., James, F.W. and Sperling, M.A. (1985). Effects of exercise training on insulin sensitivity in adolescents with type I diabetes. *Diabetes Care*, **8**, 461–5.

875. LaPorte, R.E., Cauley, J.A., Kinsey, C.M., Corbett, W., Robertson, R., Black-Saunder, R. *et al.* (1982). The epidemiology of physical activity in children, college students, middle-aged men, menopausal females, and monkeys. *Journal of Chronic Diseases*, **35**, 787–95.

876. LaPorte, R.E., Dearwater, S., Cauley, J.A., Slemenda, C. and Cook, T. (1985). Physical activity or cardiovascular fitness: which is more important for health? *The Physician and Sports Medicine*, **13**, 145–50.

877. LaPorte, R.E., Kuller, L.H., Kupfer, D.J., McPartland, R.M., Mathews, G. and Casperson, C. (1979). An objective measure of physical activity for epidemiological research. *American Journal of Epidemiology*, **109**, 158–68.

878. Larsson, Y., Persson, B., Sterky, G. and Thoren, C. (1964). Functional adaptation to rigorous training and exercise in diabetic and nondiabetic adolescents. *Journal of Applied Physiology*, **19**, 629–35.

879. Larsson, Y., Sterky, G., Persson, B. and Thoren, C. (1964). Effect of exercise on blood-lipids in juvenile diabetes. *Lancet*, **i**, 350–5.

880. Laskarewski, P., Morrison, J.A., de Groot, I., Kelly, K.A., Mellies, M.J., Khoury, P. *et al.* (1979). Lipid and lipoprotein tracking in 108 children over a four year period. *Pediatrics*, **64**, 584–91.

881. Lau, E.M.C. (1993). Hip fracture in Asia: trends, risk factors and prevention. In C. Christiansen and B. Riis (Eds.), *Proceedings of the 4th International Symposium on Osteoporosis*. Aalborg, Handelstrykkeriet, pp. 58–61.

882. Lauer, R.M., Burns, T.L., Mahoney, L.T. and Tipton, C.M. (1989). Blood pressure in children. In C.V. Gisolfi and D.R. Lamb (Eds.), *Perspectives in Exercise Science and Sports Medicine, Vol. 2, Youth, Exercise and Sport.* Indianapolis, IN, Benchmark Press, pp. 431–59.

883. Lauer, R.M., Connor, W.E. and Leaverton, P.E. (1975). Coronary heart disease risk factors in school children: the Muscatine Study. *Journal of Pediatrics*, **86**, 697–706.

884. Lauer, R.M., Lee, J. and Clarke, W.R. (1988). Factors affecting the relationship between childhood and adult cholesterol levels: the Muscatine Study. *Pediatrics*, **82**, 309–18.

885. Lauer, R.M., Lee, J. and Clarke, W.R. (1989). Predicting adult cholesterol levels from measurements in childhood and adolescence: the Muscatine Study. *Bulletin of the New York Academy of Medicine*, **65**, 1127–42.

886. Lauer, R.M. and Shekelle, R.B. (1980). *Childhood Prevention of Atherosclerosis and Hypertension.* New York, Raven Press.

887. Laughlin, G.A., Loucks, A.B. and Yen, S.S.C. (1991). Marked augmentation of nocturnal melatonin secretion in amenorrheic athletes but not in cycling athletes: unaltered by opioidergic or dopaminergic blockade. *Journal of Clinical Endocrinology and Metabolism*, **73**, 1321–6.

888. Lauritzen, T., Frost-Larsen, K., Larsen, H.-W. and Deckert, T. (1983). Steno Study Group. Effect of 1 year near-normal blood glucose levels on retinopathy in insulin-dependent diabetics. *Lancet*, **i**, 200–4.

889. Lauter, S. (1926). Zur Genese der Fettsucht. *Dtsch. Arch. Klin.*, **150**, 315–65. Cited by H.J. Montoye and H.L. Taylor (1984). Measurement of physical activity in population studies. A review. *Human Biology*, **56**, 195–216.

890. Lawrence, M. (1984). *The Anorexic Experience.* London, The Women's Press.

891. LeBlanc, J.A. (1967). Use of heart rate as an index of work output. *Journal of Applied Physiology*, **10**, 275–80.

892. Lee, C.J. (1978). Nutritional status of selected teenagers in Kentucky. *American Journal of Clinical Nutrition*, **3**, 1453–64.

893. Léger, L. and Thivierge, M. (1988). Heart rate monitors: validity, stability, and functionality. *The Physician and Sports Medicine*, **16**, 143–51.

894. Legius, E., Proesmans, W., Eggermont, E., Vandamme-Lombaerts, R., Bouillon, R. and Smet, M. (1989). Rickets due to dietary calcium deficiency. *European Journal of Pediatrics*, **148**, 784–5.

895. Lehmann, M., Keul, J., Huber, G. and DaPrada, M. (1981). Plasma catecholamines in trained and untrained volunteers during graduated exercise. *International Journal of Sports Medicine*, **2**, 143–7.

896. Lehmann, M., Keul, J. and Korsten-Reck, U. (1981). Einfluss einer stufenweisen Laufbändergeometrie bei Kindern und Erwachsenen auf die

Plasmacatecholamine, die aerobe und anaerobe Kapazität. (The influence of graduated treadmill exercise on plasma catecholamines, aerobic and anaerobic capacity in boys and adults). *European Journal of Applied Physiology*, **47**, 301–11.

897. Lengyel, M. and Gyarfas, I. (1979). The importance of echocardiography in the assessment of left ventricular hypertrophy in trained and untrained schoolchildren. *Acta Cardiologica*, **34**, 63–9.

898. Leon, G.R. (1991). Eating disorders in female athletes. *Sports Medicine*, **12**, 219–27.

899. Leon, G.R., Perry, C.L., Mangelsdorf, C. and Tell, G.J. (1989). Adolescent nutritional and psychological patterns and risk for the development of an eating disorder. *Journal of Youth and Adolescence*, **18**, 273–82.

900. Lewko, J.H. and Greendorfer, S.L. (1982). Family influences and sex differences in children's socialization into sport: a review. In F.L. Smoll, R.A. Magill and M.J. Ash (Eds.), *Children in Sport, 3rd edition*. Champaign, IL, Human Kinetics, pp. 265–86.

901. Li, X.J. and Dunham, P. (1993). Fitness load and exercise time in secondary physical education classes. *Journal of Teaching in Physical Education*, **12**, 180–7.

902. Liang, M.T.C. and Norris, S. (1993). Effects of skin blood flow and temperature on bioelectric impedance after exercise. *Medicine and Science in Sports and Exercise*, **25**, 1231–9.

903. Lifson, N., Gordon, G.B. and McClintock, R. (1955). Measurement of total carbon dioxide production by means of $D_2{}^{18}O$. *Journal of Applied Physiology*, **7**, 704–10.

904. Lifson, N., Little, W.S., Levitt, D.G. and Henderson, R.M. (1975). $D_2{}^{18}O$ (deuterium oxide) method for CO_2 output in small mammals and economic feasibility in man. *Journal of Applied Physiology*, **39**, 657–64.

905. Lindberg, J.S., Fears, W.B., Hunt, M.M., Powell, M.R., Boll, D. and Wade, C.E. (1984). Exercise induced amenorrhea and bone density. *Annals of Internal Medicine*, **101**, 647–8.

906. Linder, C.W. and DuRant, R.H. (1982). Exercise, serum lipids and cardiovascular disease – risk factors in children. *Pediatric Clinics of North America*, **29**, 1341–54.

907. Linder, C.W., DuRant, R.H. and Mahoney, O.M. (1983). The effect of physical conditioning on serum lipids and lipoproteins in white male adolescents. *Medicine and Science in Sports and Exercise*, **15**, 232–6.

908. Linder, C.W., DuRant, R.H., Gray, R.G. and Harkness, J.W. (1979). The effect of exercise in serum lipid levels in children. *Clinical Research*, **27**, 297.

909. Lippert, P., Hoffmeister, H., Thefeld, W., Lopez, H. and Eichberg, H. (1981). Cardiovascular and pulmonary risk factors in Berlin (West) schoolchildren. Findings of an exploratory study. *Preventive Medicine*, **10**, 159–72.

910. Livingstone, M.B.E. (1994). Energy expenditure and physical activity in relation to fitness in children. *Proceedings of the Nutrition Society*, **53**, 207–21.

911. Livingstone, M.B.E., Coward, A.W., Prentice, A.M., Davies, P.S.W., Strain, J.J., McKenna, P.G. *et al.* (1992). Daily energy expenditure in free-living

children: comparison of heart rate monitoring with the doubly labelled water ($^2H_2^{18}O$) method. *American Journal of Clinical Nutrition*, **56**, 343–52.

912. Lloyd, T., Andon, M.B., Rollings, N., Martel, J.K., Landis, R., Demers, L.M. *et al.* (1993). Calcium supplementation and bone mineral density in adolescent girls. *Journal of the American Medical Association*, **270**, 841–4.

913. Lloyd, T., Myers, K., Buchanan, J.R. and Demers, L.M. (1988). Collegiate women athletes with irregular menses during adolescence have decreased bone density. *Obstetrics and Gynaecology*, **72**, 639–42.

914. Lohman, T.G. (1982). Measurements of body composition in children. *Journal of Physical Education, Recreation and Dance*, **53**, 67–70.

915. Lohman, T.G. (1984). Research progress in validation of laboratory methods of assessing body composition. *Medicine and Science in Sports and Exercise*, **16**, 596–603.

916. Lohman, T.G. (1986). Applicability of body composition techniques and constants for children and youth. *Exercise and Sport Sciences Reviews*, **14**, 325–57.

917. Lohman, T.G. (1987). The use of skinfolds to estimate body fatness in children and youth. *Journal of Physical Education, Recreation and Dance*, **58**, 98–102.

918. Lohman, T.G. (1989). Assessment of body composition in children. *Pediatric Exercise Science*, **1**, 19–30.

919. Lohman, T.G. (1992). *Advances in Body Composition Assessment*. Champaign, IL, Human Kinetics.

920. Lohman, T.G., Boileau, R.A. and Slaughter, M.H. (1984). Body composition in children and youth. In R.A. Boileau (Ed.), *Advances in Pediatric Sports Science*. Champaign, IL, Human Kinetics, pp. 229–57.

921. Lohman, T.G., Roche, A.F. and Martorell, R. (1988). *Anthropometric Standardization Reference Manual*. Champaign, IL, Human Kinetics.

922. Lokey, E.A. and Tran, Z.V. (1989). Effects of exercise training on serum lipid and lipoprotein concentrations in women: a meta-analysis. *International Journal of Sports Medicine*, **10**, 424–9.

923. Lombardo, J.A. (1990). Drugs and ergogenic aids. In J.A. Sullivan and W.A. Grana (Eds.), *The Pediatric Athlete*. Park Ridge, IL, American Academy of Orthopaedic Surgeons, pp. 45–52.

924. Lombardo, J.A. (1993). The efficacy and mechanisms of action of anabolic steroids. In C.E. Yesalis (Ed.), *Anabolic Steroids in Sport and Exercise*. Champaign, IL, Human Kinetics, pp. 89–106.

925. Lopez, R. and Pruett, D.M. (1982). The child runner. *Journal of Physical Education, Recreation and Dance*, **53**, 78–81.

926. Loucks, A.B. (1988). Osteoporosis prevention begins in childhood. In E.W. Brown and C.F. Branta (Eds.), *Competitive Sports for Children and Youth*. Champaign, IL, Human Kinetics, pp. 213–23.

927. Loucks, A.B. (1989). Athletics and menstrual dysfunction in young women. In C.V. Gisolfi and D.R. Lamb (Eds.), *Perspectives in Exercise Science and Sports Medicine, Vol. 2, Youth, Exercise, and Sport*. Indianapolis, IN, Benchmark Press, pp. 513–38.

928. Loucks, A.B. (1995). The reproductive system and physical activity in adolescents. In C.J.R. Blimkie and O. Bar-Or (Eds.), *New Horizons in Pediatric Exercise Science*. Champaign, IL, Human Kinetics, pp. 27–38.

929. Loucks, A.B., Vaitukaitis, J., Cameron, J.L., Rogol, A.D., Skrinar, G., Warren, M.P. *et al.* (1992). The reproductive system and exercise in women. *Medicine and Science in Sports and Exercise*, **24**, S288–S293.

930. Luke, M.D. and Sinclair, G.D. (1991). Gender differences in adolescents' attitudes toward school physical education. *Journal of Teaching in Physical Education*, **11**, 31–46.

931. Lussier, L. and Buskirk, E.R. (1977). Effects of an endurance training regimen on assessment of work capacity in prepubertal children. *Annals of the New York Academy of Science*, **30**, 734–47.

932. Lutter, J.M. and Cushman, S. (1982). Menstrual patterns in female runners. *The Physician and Sportsmedicine*, **10**, 60–72.

933. MacConnie, S.E., Gilliam, T.B., Geenen, D.L. and Peles, A.E. (1982). Daily physical activity patterns of prepubertal children involved in a vigorous exercise program. *International Journal of Sports Medicine*, **3**, 302–7.

934. MacDonald, M.J. (1987). Postexercise late-onset hypoglycemia in insulin-dependent diabetic patients. *Diabetes Care*, **10**, 584–8.

935. MacDougall, J.D. and Wenger, H.A. (1991). The purpose of physiological testing. In J.D. MacDougall, H.A. Wenger and H.J. Green (Eds.), *Physiological Testing of the High-Performance Athlete*. Champaign, IL, Human Kinetics, pp. 1–6.

936. MacDougall, J.D., Wenger H.A. and Green, H.J. (Eds.) (1991). *Physiological Testing of the High-Performance Athlete*. Champaign, IL, Human Kinetics.

937. Macek, M. (1986). Aerobic and anaerobic energy output in children. In J. Rutenfranz, R. Mocellin and F. Klimt (Eds.), *Children and Exercise XII*. Champaign, IL, Human Kinetics, pp. 3–9.

938. Macek, M., Bell, D., Rutenfranz, J., Vavra, J., Masopust, J., Niedhart, B. *et al.* (1989). A comparison of coronary risk factors in groups of trained and untrained adolescents. *European Journal of Applied Physiology*, **58**, 577–82.

939. Macek, M., Rutenfranz, J., Lange Andersen, K., Masopust, J., Vavra, J., Klimmer, F. *et al.* (1985). Favourable levels of cardiovascular health and risk indicators during childhood and adolescence. *European Journal of Pediatrics*, **144**, 360–7.

940. Macek, M. and Vavra, J. (1977). Relation between aerobic and anaerobic energy supply during maximal exercise in boys. In H. Lavallée and R.J. Shephard (Eds.), *Frontiers of Activity and Child Health*. Quebec, Editions du Pelican, pp. 157–9.

941. Macek, M. and Vavra, J. (1980). The adjustment of oxygen uptake at the onset of exercise: a comparison between prepubertal boys and young adults. *International Journal of Sports Medicine*, **1**, 75–7.

942. Macek, M., Vavra, J., Benesova, H. and Radvansky, J. (1984). The adjustment of oxygen uptake at the onset of exercise: relation to age and to workload. In J. Ilmarinen and I. Valimaki (Eds.), *Children and Sport*. Berlin, Springer, pp. 129–34.

943. Macek, M., Vavra, J. and Novosadova, J. (1976). Prolonged exercise in prepubertal boys. I. Cardiovascular and metabolic adjustment. II. Changes in plasma volume and in some blood constituents. *European Journal of Applied Physiology*, **35**, 291–303.

944. Maciejko, J.J., Holmes, D.R., Kottke, B.A., Zinsmeister, A.R., Dinh, D.M. and Mao, S.J.T. (1983). Apolipoprotein A-1 as a marker for angiographically assessed coronary artery disease. *New England Journal of Medicine*, **309**, 385–9.

945. Maffeis, C., Schena, F., Zaffanello, M., Zoccante, L., Schutz, Y. and Pinelli, L. (1994). Maximal aerobic power during running and cycling in obese and non-obese children. *Acta Paediatrica*, **83**, 113–16.

946. Maffulli, N. (1990). Intensive training in young athletes. The orthopaedic surgeon's viewpoint. *Sports Medicine*, **9**, 229–43.

947. Maffulli, N. and Helms, P. (1988). Controversies about intensive training in young athletes. *Archives of Disease in Childhood*, **63**, 1405–7.

948. Mahon, A.D. and Vaccaro, P. (1990). The effects of exercise training on submaximal and maximal blood lactate concentrations in children. *Pediatric Exercise Science*, **3**, 80–1.

949. Malina, R.M. (1969). Quantification of fat, muscle and bone in man. *Clinical Orthopaedics and Related Research*, **65**, 9–38.

950. Malina, R.M. (1975). Anthropometric correlates of performance. *Exercise and Sport Sciences Reviews*, **3**, 249–74.

951. Malina, R.M. (1980). Physical activity, growth and functional capacity. In R.E. Johnson, A.F. Roche and C. Susanne (Eds.), *Human Physical Growth and Maturation*. New York, Plenum Press, pp. 303–27.

952. Malina, R.M. (1982). Physical growth and maturity characteristics of young athletes. In R.A. Magill, M.J. Ash and F.L. Smoll (Eds.), *Children in Sport*. Champaign, IL, Human Kinetics, pp. 73–96.

953. Malina, R.M. (1983). Human growth, maturation, and regular physical activity. *Acta Medica Auxologica*, **15**, 5–27.

954. Malina, R.M. (1983). Menarche in athletes: a synthesis and hypothesis. *Annals of Human Biology*, **10**, 1–24.

955. Malina, R.M. (1984). Human growth, maturation and regular physical activity. In R.A. Boileau (Ed.), *Advances in Pediatric Sports Science, Vol. 1*. Champaign, IL, Human Kinetics, pp. 59–83.

956. Malina, R.M. (1986). Genetics of motor development and performance. In R.M. Malina and C. Bouchard (Eds.), *Sport and Human Genetics*. Champaign, IL, Human Kinetics, pp. 23–58.

957. Malina, R.M. (1986). Growth of muscle tissue and muscle mass. In F. Falkner and J.M. Tanner (Eds.), *Human Growth, Vol. 2, Postnatal Growth*. New York, Plenum Press, pp. 77–99.

958. Malina, R.M. (1988). Biological maturity status of young athletes. In R.M. Malina (Ed.), *Young Athletes*. Champaign, IL, Human Kinetics, pp. 121–40.

959. Malina, R.M. (1988). Competitive youth sports and biological maturation. In E.W. Brown and C.F. Branta (Eds.), *Competitive Sports for Children and Youth*. Champaign, IL, Human Kinetics, pp. 227–46.

960. Malina, R.M. (1989). Growth and maturation: normal variation and effect of training. In C.V. Gisolfi and D.R. Lamb (Eds.), *Perspectives in Exercise Science and Sports Medicine, Vol. 2, Youth, Exercise, and Sport*. Indianapolis, IN, Benchmark Press, pp. 223–65.

961. Malina, R.M. (1989). Tracking of physical fitness and performance during growth. In G. Beunen, J. Ghesquiere, R. Reybrouck and A.L. Claessens (Eds.), *Children and Exercise XIV*. Stuttgart, Enke, pp. 1–10.

962. Malina, R.M. (1994). Attained size and growth rate of female volleyball players between 9 and 13 years of age. *Pediatric Exercise Science*, **6**, 257–66.

963. Malina, R.M. (1994). Physical activity and training: effects on stature and the adolescent growth spurt. *Medicine and Science in Sports and Exercise*, **26**, 759–66.

964. Malina, R.M. (1994). Physical growth and biological maturation of young athletes. *Exercise and Sport Sciences Reviews*, **22**, 389–433.

965. Malina, R.M. and Bielicki, T. (1992). Growth and maturation of boys active in sports: longitudinal observations from the Wroclaw Growth Study. *Pediatric Exercise Science*, **4**, 68–77.

966. Malina, R.M. and Bouchard, C. (1986). *Sport and Human Genetics* Champaign, IL, Human Kinetics.

967. Malina, R.M. and Bouchard, C. (1991). *Growth, Maturation and Physical Activity*. Champaign, IL, Human Kinetics.

968. Malina, R.M., Bouchard, C. and Beunen, G. (1988). Human growth: selected aspects of current research on well-nourished children. *Annual Review of Anthropology*, **17**, 187–219.

969. Malina, R.M., Meleski, B.W. and Shoup, R.F. (1982). Anthropometric, body composition, and maturity characteristics of selected school-age athletes. *Pediatric Clinics of North America*, **29**, 1305–23.

970. Maliszewski, A.F., Freedson, P.S., Ebbeling, C.J., Crussemeyer, J. and Kastango, K.B. (1991). Validity of the Caltrac accelerometer in estimating energy expenditure and activity in children and adults. *Pediatric Exercise Science*, **3**, 141–51.

971. Mallick, M.J., Whipple, T.W. and Huerta, E. (1987). Behavioural and psychological traits of weight-conscious teenagers. *Adolescence*, **22**, 157–67.

972. Maquet, P. and Furlong, R. (1986). *The Laws of Bone Remodelling. Julius Wolff*. Berlin, Springer.

973. Marcus, R., Cann, C., Madvid, P., Minkoff, J., Goddard, M., Bayer, M. *et al.* (1985). Menstrual function and bone mass in elite women distance runners. *Annals of Internal Medicine*, **102**, 158–63.

974. Marella, M., Colli, R. and Faina, M. (1986). Evaluation de l'aptitude physique: Eurofit, batterie experimentagle. *Romes Scuola Dello Sport*. Cited by W. Tuxworth (1988), The fitness and physical activity of adolescents. *The Medical Journal of Australia*, **148**, 513–21.

975. Margaria, R., Aghemo, P. and Rovelli, E. (1966). Measurement of muscular power (anaerobic) in man. *Journal of Applied Physiology*, **21**, 1662–4.

976. Margolis, S. and Dobs, A.S. (1989). Nutritional management of plasma lipid disorders. *Journal of the American College of Nutrition*, **8** (Suppl.), 33S–45S.

977. Margonato, A., Gerundini, P., Videcomini, G., Gilardi, M.C., Pozza, G. and Fazio, F. (1986). Abnormal cardiovascular response to exercise in young asymptomatic diabetic patients with retinopathy. *American Heart Journal*, **112**, 554–60.

978. Marker, K. (1981). Influence of athletic training on the maturity process of girls. In J. Borms, M. Hebbelinck and A. Venerando (Eds.), *The Female Athlete: A Socio-psychological and Kinanthropometric Approach*. Basel, Karger, pp. 117–26.

979. Marshall, W.A. and Tanner, J.M. (1986). Puberty. In F. Falkner and J.M. Tanner (Eds.), *Human Growth*. London, Plenum Press, pp. 171–209.

980. Marti, B. and Vartiainen, E. (1989). Relation between leisure time exercise and cardiovascular risk factors among 15-year-olds in eastern Finland. *Journal of Epidemiology and Community Health*, **43**, 228–33.

981. Martinez, L.R. and Haymes, E.M. (1992). Substrate utilization during tread-mill running in prepubertal girls and women. *Medicine and Science in Sports and Exercise*, **24**, 975–83.

982. Martinsen, E.W. (1990). Benefits of exercise for the treatment of depression. *Sports Medicine*, **9**, 380–9.

983. Massicotte, D.R. and Macnab, R.B.J. (1974). Cardiorespiratory adaptations to training at specified intensities in children. *Medicine and Science in Sports*, **6**, 242–6.

984. Matkovic, V., Fontana, D., Tominac, C., Goel, P. and Chestnut, C.H. (1990). Factors that influence peak bone mass formation: a study of calcium balance and the inheritance of bone mass in adolescent females. *American Journal of Clinical Nutrition*, **52**, 878–88.

985. Matkovic, V. and Heaney, R.P. (1992). Calcium balance during human growth: evidence for threshold behaviour. *American Journal of Clinical Nutrition*, **55**, 992–6.

986. Matkovic, V., Kostial, K., Siminovic, I., Buzina, R., Brodarec, A. and Nordin, B. (1979). Bone status and fracture rates in two regions of Yugoslavia. *American Journal of Clinical Nutrition*, **52**, 878–88.

987. Matsusaki, M., Ikeda, M., Tashiro, E., Koga, M., Miura, S., Ideishi, M. *et al.* (1992). Influence of workload on the antihypertensive effect of exercise. *Clinical Experiments in Pharmacological Physiology*, **19**, 471–9.

988. Mayer, J. (1975). Obesity during childhood. In M. Winick (Ed.), *Childhood Obesity*. New York, Wiley, pp. 73–80.

989. Mayers, N. and Gutin, B. (1979). Physiological characteristics of elite prepubertal cross-country runners. *Medicine and Science in Sports*, **11**, 172–6.

990. Mazess, R.B. (1982). On aging bone loss. *Clinical Orthopaedics*, **165**, 239–52.

991. McCloskey, D. and Streatfield, K. (1975). Muscular reflex stimuli to the cardiovascular system during isometric contraction of muscle groups of different mass. *Journal of Physiology*, **230**, 431–41.

992. McComas, A.J., Sica, R.E.P. and Petito, P. (1973). Muscle strength in boys of different ages. *Journal of Neurology, Neurosurgery and Psychiatry*, **36**, 171–3.

993. McCulloch, R.G., Bailey, D.A., Houston, C.S. and Dodd, B.L. (1990). Effects of physical activity, dietary calcium intake and selected lifestyle factors on bone density in young women. *Canadian Medical Association Journal*, **142**, 221–7.

994. McCulloch, R.G., Bailey, D.A., Whalen, R.L., Houston, C.S., Faulkner, R.A. and Craven, B.R. (1992). Bone density and bone mineral content of adolescent soccer athletes and competitive swimmers. *Pediatric Exercise Science*, **4**, 319–30.

995. McCusker, J. (1985). Involvement of 15–19-year-olds in sport and physical activity. In L. Haywood and I. Henry (Eds.), *Leisure and Youth*, London, Leisure Studies Association Conference Report No. 17. Cited by B. Dickenson (1987). *A Survey of the Activity Patterns of Young People and their Attitudes and Perceptions of Physical Activity and Physical Education in an English Local Education Authority*. Unpublished MPhil thesis, Loughborough University of Technology.

996. McGill, H.C. (1968). *The Geographic Pathology of Atherosclerosis*. Baltimore, MD, Williams and Wilkins.

997. McGill, H.C. (1974). The lesion. In R. Paoletti and M. Gotto (Eds.), *Atherosclerosis III*. Berlin, Springer, pp. 27–38.

998. McGill, H.C. (1984). Persistent problems in the pathogenesis of atheroscerosis. *Arteriosclerosis*, **4**, 443–51.

999. McGovern, M.B. (1984). Effects of circuit weight training on the physical fitness of prepubescent children. *Dissertation Abstracts International*, **45**, 452A–453A.

1000. McGowen, R.W., Jarman, B.O. and Pedersen, D.M. (1974). Effects of a competitive endurance training program on self-concept and peer approval. *Journal of Psychology*, **86**, 57–60.

1001. McGuire, R.T. and Cook, D.L. (1986). The influence of others and the decision to participate in youth sports. *Journal of Sport Behaviour*, **6**, 9–16.

1002. McKeag, D.B., Fuller, R. and Bakker-Arkema, F.W. (1978). Cardiorespiratory performance testing in children and adolescent competitive swimmers: a demographic study. In F. Landry and W.A.R. Orban (Eds.), *Physical Activity and Human Well-Being*. Miami, FL, Symposia Specialists, pp. 415–24.

1003. McKenzie, T.L. (1991). Observational measures of children's physical activity. *Journal of School Health*, **61**, 224–7.

1004. McKenzie, T.L. and Carlson, B.R. (1989). Systematic observation and computer technology. In P. Darst, D. Zakrajsek and V. Mancini (Eds.), *Analyzing Physical Education and Sport Instruction*. Champaign, IL, Human Kinetics, pp. 81–9.

1005. McKenzie, T.L., Buono, M. and Nelson, J. (1984). Modification of coronary heart disease risk factors in obese boys through diet and exercise. *American Corrective Therapy Journal*, **38**, 35–7.

1006. McKenzie, T.L., Feldman, H., Woods, S.E., Romero, K.A., Dahlstrom, V., Stone, E.J. *et al.* (1995). Children's activity levels and lesson context during third-grade physical education. *Research Quarterly for Exercise and Sport*, **66**, 184–93.

1007. McLain, L.G. (1989). Anabolic steroids and high school students. *Medicine and Science in Sports and Exercise*, **21** (Suppl.), S25.

1008. McLean, K.P. and Skinner, J.S. (1992). Validity of Futrex-5000 for body composition determination. *Medicine and Science in Sports and Exercise*, **24**, 253–8.

1009. McLellan, T. (1987). The anaerobic threshold: concept and controversy. *Australian Journal of Science and Medicine in Sport*, **19**, 3–8.

1010. McMahon, J.R. and Gross, R.T. (1987). Physical and psychological effects of aerobic exercise in boys with learning disabilities. *Developmental and Behavioural Pediatrics*, **8**, 274–7.

1011. McMahon, J.R. and Gross, R.T. (1988). Physical and psychological effects of aerobic exercise in delinquent adolescent males. *Sports Medicine*, **142**, 1361–6.

1012. McMahon, T. (1973). Size and shape in biology. Elastic criteria impose limits on biological proportions, and consequently on metabolic rates. *Science*, **174**, 1201–4.

1013. McManus, A. and Armstrong, N. (1995). Patterns of physical activity among primary schoolchildren. In F.J. Ring (Ed.), *Children in Sport*. Bath, University Press, pp. 17–23.

1014. McManus, A. and Armstrong, N. (1996). The physical inactivity of girls – a school issue? *British Journal of Physical Education*, **27**, 34–5.

1015. McManus, A. and Armstrong, N. (in press). Physical activity patterns of Hong Kong Chinese primary schoolchildren. *Pediatric Exercise Science*, **8**, 179–80.

1016. McManus, A., Armstrong, N. and Williams, C. (manuscript under review). The effect of two different training programmes on the peak $\dot{V}O_2$ of prepubescent girls.

1017. McMiken, D.F. (1976). Maximum aerobic power and physical dimensions of children. *Annals of Human Biology*, **3**, 141–7.

1018. McNamara, J.J., Molot, M.A., Stremple, J.F. and Catting, R.T. (1971). Coronary artery disease in combat casualties in Vietnam. *Journal of the American Medical Association*, **216**, 1185–7.

1019. McNaught-Davis, P. (1991). *Flexibility*. London, Partridge Press.

1020. Medbø, J.I., Mohn, A.C., Tabata, I., Bahr, R., Vaage, O. and Sejersted, O.M. (1988). Anaerobic capacity determined by maximal accumulated O_2 deficit. *Journal of Applied Physiology*, **64**, 50–60.

1021. Medelli, J. (1985). Etude de la transition aérobie-anaérobie lors des épreuves d'effort chez l'enfant. *Cinesiology*, **24**, 431–6.

1022. Meijer, G.A., Westerterp, K.R., Koper, H. and Ten Hoor, F. (1989). Assessment of energy expenditure by recording heart rate and body acceleration. *Medicine and Science in Sports and Exercise*, **21**, 343–7.

1023. Melton, L.J., O'Fallon, W.M. and Riggs, B.L. (1987). Secular trends in the incidence of hip fractures. *Calciferous Tissue International*, **41**, 57–64.

1024. Mendoza, S., Nucete, H., Zerpa, A., Prado, E., Somoza, B., Morrison, J.A. *et al.* (1980). Lipids and lipoproteins in 13–18-year-old Venezuelan and American schoolchildren. *Atherosclerosis*, **37**, 219–29.

1025. Mercier, B., Mercier, J., Granier, P., Le Gallais, D. and Préfaut, C. (1992). Maximal anaerobic power: relationship to anthropometric characteristics during growth. *International Journal of Sports Medicine*, **13**, 21–6.

1026. Mercier, J., Varray, A., Ramonatxo, Mercier, B. and Préfaut, C. (1991). Influence of anthropometric characteristics on changes in maximal exercise ventilation and breathing pattern during growth in boys. *European Journal of Applied Physiology*, **63**, 235–41.

1027. Mero, A. (1988). Blood lactate production and recovery from anaerobic exercise in trained and untrained boys. *European Journal of Applied Physiology*, **57**, 660–6.

1028. Mero, A., Kauhanen, H., Peltola, E. and Vuorimaa, T. (1988). Changes in endurance, strength and speed capacity of different prepubescent athletic groups during one year of training. *Journal of Human Movement Studies*, **14**, 219–39.

1029. Mero, A., Kauhaner, H., Peltola, E. and Vuorimaa, T. (1989). Transfer from prepuberty to puberty: effects of three years of training. *Journal of Human Movement Studies*, **16**, 267–78.

1030. Mersch, F. and Stoboy, H. (1989). Strength training and muscle hypertrophy in children. In S. Oseid and K.-H. Carlsen (Eds.), *Children and Exercise XIII*. Champaign, IL, Human Kinetics, pp. 165–82.

1031. Michael, E., Evert, J. and Jeffers, K. (1972). Physiological changes of teenage girls during months of detraining. *Medicine and Science in Sports*, **4**, 214–18.

1032. Micheli, L.J. (1983). Overuse injuries in children's sport: the growth factor. *Orthopedic Clinics of North America*, **14**, 337–60.

1033. Micheli, L.J. (1986). Lower extremity overuse injuries. *Acta Medica Scandinavica*, **711** (Suppl.), 171–7.

1034. Micheli, L.J. (1986). Pediatric and adolescent sports injury. Recent trends. *Exercise and Sport Sciences Reviews*, **14**, 359–74.

1035. Micheli, L.J. (1988). Strength training in the young athlete. In E.W. Brown and C.F. Branta (Eds.), *Competitive Sports for Children and Youth*. Champaign, IL, Human Kinetics, pp. 99–105.

1036. Micheli, L.J. and Ireland, M.L. (1987). Prevention and management of calcaneal apophysitis in children: an overuse syndrome. *Journal of Pediatric Orthopedics*, **7**, 34–8.

1037. Miller, J., Kimes, T., Hui, S., Andon, M.B. and Johnston, C.C. (1991). Nutrient intake variability in a pediatric population: implications for study design. *Journal of Nutrition*, **121**, 265–74.

1038. Miller, N.E., Hammett, F., Saltissi, S., Rao, S. and Van Zeller, H. (1981). Relation of angiographically defined coronary artery disease to plasma lipoprotein subfractions and apolipoproteins. *British Medical Journal*, **282**, 1741–4.

1039. Miller, N.E., Weinstein, D.B., Carew, T.E., Koschinsky, T. and Steinberg, D. (1977). Interaction between high density and low density lipoprotein uptake and degradation by cultured human fibroblasts. *Journal of Clinical Investigation*, **60**, 78–88.

1040. Miller, N.E., Weinstein, D.B. and Steinberg, D. (1977). Binding, internalization and degradation of high density lipoprotein by cultured human fibroblasts. *Journal of Lipid Research*, **18**, 438–50.

1041. Mirwald, R.L. and Bailey, D.A. (1986). *Maximal Aerobic Power*. London, Ontario, Sports Dynamics.

1042. Mirwald, R.L., Bailey, D.A., Cameron, N. and Rasmussen, R.L. (1981). Longitudinal comparison of aerobic power in active and inactive boys aged 7.0 to 17.0 years. *Annals of Human Biology*, **8**, 405–14.

1043. Mitchell, J., Armstrong, N., Balding, J., Gentle, P. and Kirby, B. (1991). The association of selected coronary risk factors between family members. *Journal of Sport Sciences*, **9**, 424–5.

1044. Mitchell, J.E. (1989). Bulimia nervosa. *Contemporary Nutrition*, **14**, 1–2.

1045. Mitchell, J.H., Sproule, B.J. and Chapman, C.B. (1958). The physiological meaning of the maximum oxygen intake test. *Journal of Clinical Investigation*, **37**, 538–47.

1046. Mitchell, T.H., Abraham, G., Schiffrin, A., Leiter, L.A. and Marliss, E.B. (1988). Hyperglycemia after intensive exercise in IDDM subjects during continuous subcutaneous insulin infusion. *Diabetes Care*, **11**, 311–17.

1047. Mocellin, R., Heusgen, M. and Gildein, H.P. (1991). Anaerobic threshold and maximal steady-state blood lactate in prepubertal boys. *European Journal of Applied Physiology*, **62**, 56–60.

1048. Mocellin, R., Heusgen, M. and Korsten-Reck, U. (1990). Maximal steady state blood lactate levels in 11-year-old boys. *European Journal of Pediatrics*, **149**, 771–3.

1049. Mocellin, R. and Wasmund, U. (1973). Investigations on the influence of a running-training program on the cardiovascular and motor performance capacity in 53 boys and girls of a second and third primary class. In O. Bar-Or (Ed.), *Pediatric Work Physiology*. Natanya, Israel, Wingate Institute, pp. 279–85.

1050. Molnar, G.E., Alexander, J. and Gutfeld, N. (1979). Reliability of quantitative strength measurements in children. *Archives of Physical Medicine and Rehabilitation*, **60**, 218–21.

1051. Montenegro, M.R. and Eggen, D.A. (1968). Topography of atherosclerosis in the coronary arteries. *Laboratory Investigations*, **8**, 586–93.

1052. Montoye, H.J. (1982). Age and oxygen utilization during submaximal treadmill exercise in males. *Journal of Gerontology*, **37**, 396–402.

1053. Montoye, H.J. (1986). Physical activity, physical fitness and heart disease risk factors in children. In American Academy of Physical Education, *Effects of Physical Activity on Children*. Champaign, IL, Human Kinetics, pp. 127–52.

1054. Montoye, H.J. (1990). Discussion: assessment of physical activity during leisure and work. In C. Bouchard, R.J. Shephard, T. Stephens, J.R. Sutton and B.D. McPherson (Eds.), *Exercise, Fitness and Health*. Champaign, IL, Human Kinetics, pp. 71–4.

1055. Montoye, H.J., Block, W.D. and Gayle, R. (1978). Maximal oxygen uptake and blood lipids. *Journal of Chronic Diseases*, **31**, 111–18.

1056. Montoye, H.J. and Lamphier, D.E. (1977). Grip and arm strength in males and females, age 10 to 69. *Research Quarterly*, **48**, 109–20.

1057. Montoye, H.J., Metzner, H.L., Keller, J.B., Johnson, B.C. and Epstein, F.H. (1972). Habitual physical activity and blood pressure. *Medicine and Science in Sports*, **4**, 175–81.

1058. Montoye, H.J. and Taylor, H.L. (1984). Measurement of physical activity in population studies: a review. *Human Biology*, **56**, 195–216.

1059. Montoye, H.J., Van Huss, W. and Zuidema, M. (1959). Sports activities of athletes and non-athletes in later life. *Physical Education*, **16**, 48–51.

1060. Montoye, H.J., Washburn, R., Servais, S., Ertl, A., Webster, J. and Nagle, F. (1983). Estimation of energy expenditure by a portable accelerometer. *Medicine and Science in Sports and Exercise*, **15**, 403–7.

1061. Moody, D.L., Wilmore, J.H., Girandola, R.N. and Royce, J.P. (1972). The effects of a jogging program on the body composition of normal and obese high school girls. *Medicine and Science in Sports*, **4**, 210–13.

1062. Moore, D.C. (1988). Body image and eating behaviours in adolescent girls. *American Journal of Diseases of Children*, **142**, 1114–18.

1063. Moore, L.L., Lombardi, D.A., White, M.J., Campbell, J.L., Oliveria, S.A. and Ellison, R.C. (1991). Influence of parents' physical activity levels on activity levels of young children. *Journal of Pediatrics*, **118**, 215–19.

1064. Morgan, W.P. (1985). Psychogenic factors and exercise metabolism. A review. *Medicine and Science in Sports and Exercise*, **17**, 309–16.

1065. Morgan, W.P. and Goldston, S.E. (1987). *Exercise and Mental Health*. Washington, DC, Hemisphere Publishing.

1066. Morgan, W.P. and O'Connor, P.J. (1988). Exercise and mental health. In R.K. Dishman (Ed.), *Exercise Adherence*. Champaign, IL, Human Kinetics, pp. 91–122.

1067. Morgan, W.P., Brown, D.R., Raglin, J.J., O'Connor, P.J. and Ellickson, K.A. (1987). Psychological monitoring of overtraining and staleness. *British Journal of Sports Medicine*, **21**, 107–14.

1068. Morris, J.N., Heady, J.A. and Raffle, P.A. (1956). Physique of London busmen: epidemiology of uniforms. *Lancet*, **ii**, 569–70.

1069. Morris, J.N., Heady, J., Raffle, P., Roberts, C. and Parks, J. (1953). Coronary heart disease and physical activity of work. *Lancet*, **ii**, 1053–7, 1111–20.

1070. Morrow, J.R. and Freedson, P.S. (1994). Relationship between habitual physical activity and aerobic fitness in adolescents. *Pediatric Exercise Science*, **6**, 315–29.

1071. Morse, M., Schlutz, F.W. and Cassels, D.E. (1949). Relation of age to physiological responses of the older boy to exercise. *Journal of Applied Physiology*, **1**, 683–709.

1072. Mosher, R.E., Rhodes, E.C., Filsinger, B. and Wenger, H.A. (1985). Interval training: the effects of a 12-week program on elite, pre-pubertal male soccer players. *Journal of Sports Medicine and Physical Fitness*, **25**, 5–9.

1073. Mota, J. (1994). Children's physical education activity, assessed by telemetry. *Journal of Human Movement Studies*, **27**, 245–50.

1074. Mueller, W.H. (1982). The changes with age of the anatomical distribution of fat. *Social Science and Medicine*, **16**, 191–6.

1075. Mukeshi, M., Gutin, B., Anderson, W., Zybert, P. and Basch, C. (1990). Validation of the Caltrac movement sensor using direct observation in young children. *Pediatric Exercise Science*, **2**, 249–54.

1076. Mullen, W.H., Churchouse, F.H., Keedy, F.H. and Vadgama, P.M. (1986). Enzyme electrode for the measurement of lactate in undiluted blood. *Clinica Chimica Acta*, **157**, 191–8.

1077. Murase, Y., Kobayashi, K., Kamei, S. and Matsui, H. (1981). Longitudinal study of aerobic power in superior junior athletes. *Medicine and Science in Sports and Exercise*, **13**, 180–4.

1078. Murphy, J.K., Alpert, B.S., Christman, J.V. and Willey, E.S. (1988). Physical fitness in children: a survey method based on parental report. *American Journal of Public Health*, **78**, 708–10.

1079. Must, A., Jacques, P.F., Dallal, G.E., Bajema, C.J. and Dietz, W.H. (1992). Long-term morbidity and mortality of overweight adolescents. *New England Journal of Medicine*, **327**, 1350–5.

1080. Myers, J., Walsh, D., Sullivan, M. and Froelicher, V. (1990). Effect of sampling on variability and plateau in oxygen uptake. *Journal of Applied Physiology*, **68**, 404–10.

1081. Myerson, M., Gutin, B., Warren, M.P., May, M.T., Contento, I., Lee, M. *et al.* (1991). Resting metabolic rate and energy balance in amenorrheic and eumenorrheic runners. *Medicine and Science in Sports and Exercise*, **23**, 15–22.

1082. Myerson, M., Gutin, B., Warren, M.P., Wang, J., Lichtman, S. and Pierson, R.N. Jr. (1992). Total body bone density in amenorrheic runners. *Obstetrics and Gynecology*, **79**, 973–8.

1083. Nagawa, A. and Ishiko, T. (1970). Assessment of aerobic capacity with special reference to sex and age of junior and senior high school students in Japan. *Japanese Journal of Physiology*, **20**, 118–29.

1084. Nakamura, Y., Mutoh, Y. and Myashita, M. (1985). Determination of the peak power output during maximal brief pedalling bouts. *Journal of Sports Sciences*, **2**, 181–7.

1085. Narcici, M.V., Roi, G.S., Landoni, L., Minetti, A.E. and Cerretteli, P. (1989). Changes in force, cross-sectional area and neural activation during strength training and detraining of the human quadriceps. *European Journal of Applied Physiology*, **59**, 310–19.

1086. National Academy of Sciences, Food and Nutrition Board (1995). Summary: weighing the options – criteria for evaluating weight management programmes. *Journal of the American Dietetic Association*, **95**, 96–105.

1087. National Research Council of the United States of America (1989). *Diet and Health: implications for reducing chronic risk*. Washington, DC, National Academic Press.

1088. National Strength and Conditioning Association (1985). Position paper on prepubescent strength training. *National Strength and Conditioning Association Journal*, **7**, 27–31.

1089. Nau, K.L., Katch, V.L., Beckman, R.H. and Dick, M. (1990). Acute intra-arterial blood pressure response to bench press weight lifting in children. *Pediatric Exercise Science*, **2**, 37–45.

1090. Neinstein, L.S. (1982). Adolescent self-assessment of sexual maturation. *Clinical Pediatrics*, **21**, 482–4.

1091. Nelson, L., Jennings, G.L., Esler, M.D. and Korner, P.I. (1986). Effect of changing levels of physical activity on blood pressure and haemodynamics in essential hypertension. *Lancet*, **i**, 473–6.

1092. Nelson, M.A. (1991). The role of physical education and children's activity in the Public Health. *Research Quarterly for Exercise and Sport*, **62**, 148–50.

1093. Nelson, M.E., Fisher, E.C., Catsos, P.D., Meredith, C.N., Turksoy, R.N. and Evans, W.J. (1986). Diet and bone status in amenorrheic runners. *American Journal of Clinical Nutrition*, **43**, 910–16.

1094. Nevill, A.M. (1994). Evidence of an increasing proportion of leg muscle mass to body mass in male adolescents and its implication on performance. *Journal of Sports Science*, **12**, 163–4.

1095. Nevill, A. (1994). The need to scale for differences in body size *and* mass: an explanation of Kleiber's 0.75 mass exponent. *Journal of Applied Physiology*, **77**, 2870–3.

1096. Nevill, A.M. and Holder, R.L. (1995). Scaling, normalizing and per ratio standards: an allometric modeling approach. *Journal of Applied Physiology*, **79**, 1027–31.

1097. Nevill, A.M., Lakomy, H.K.A. and Lakomy, J. (1992). Rowing ergometer performance and maximum oxygen uptake of the 1992 Cambridge University boat crews. *Journal of Sports Sciences*, **10**, 574.

1098. Nevill, A., Ramsbottom, R. and Williams, C. (1992). Scaling physiological measurements for individuals of different body size. *European Journal of Applied Physiology*, **65**, 110–17.

1099. Newman, M. (1986). *Michigan consortium of schools student survey*. Minneapolis, MN, Hazelden Research Services.

1100. Newman, W.P., Freedman, D.S., Voors, A.W., Gard, P.D., Srinivasan, S.R., Cresanta, J.L. *et al.* (1986). Relation of serum lipoprotein levels and systolic blood pressure to early atherosclerosis: the Bogalusa Heart Study. *New England Journal of Medicine*, **314**, 138–44.

1101. Newsholme, E.A. and Leech, A.R. (1983). *Biochemistry for the Medical Sciences*. Chichester, Wiley.

1102. Newton, J.L. and Robinson, S. (1965). The distribution of blood lactate and pyruvate during work and recovery. *Federation Proceedings*, **24**, 590.

1103. Nicholls, J.G. (1992). The general and the specific in the development and expression of achievement motivation. In G. Roberts (Ed.), *Motivation in Sports and Exercise*. Champaign, IL, Human Kinetics, pp. 31–56.

1104. Nichols, J.F., Spindler, A.A., La Fave, K.L. and Sartoris, D.J. (1995). A comparison of bone mineral density and hormone status of preadolescent gymnasts, swimmers and controls. *Medicine, Exercise, Nutrition and Health*, **4**, 101–6.

1105. Nielsen, B., Nielsen, K., Behrendt-Hansen, M. and Asmussen, E. (1980). Training of functional muscular strength in girls 7–19 years old. In K. Berg and B.O. Eriksson (Eds.), *Children and Exercise IX*. Champaign, IL, Human Kinetics, pp. 69–78.

1106. Nindl, B.C., Mahar, M.T., Harman, E. and Patton, J.F. (1995). Lower and upper body anaerobic performance in male and female adolescent athletes. *Medicine and Science in Sports and Exercise*, **27**, 235–41.

1107. Nizankowska-Blaz, T. and Abramowicz, T. (1983). Effects of intensive physical training on serum lipids and lipoprotein. *Acta Paediatrica Scandinavica*, **72**, 357–9.

1108. Noakes, T.D. (1988). Implications of exercise testing for prediction of athletic performance: a contemporary perspective. *Medicine and Science in Sports and Exercise*, **20**, 319–30.

1109. Noland, M., Danner, F., Dwalt, K., McFadden, M. and Kotchen, J.M. (1990). The measurement of physical activity in young children. *Research Quarterly for Exercise and Sport*, **61**, 146–53.

1110. Norris, R., Carroll, D. and Cochrane, R. (1991). The effects of physical activity and exercise training on psychological stress and well-being in an adolescent population. *Journal of Clinical Psychology*, **36**, 55–65.

1111. North, C.T., McCullagh, P. and Tran, Z.V. (1990). Effect of exercise on depression. *Exercise and Sport Sciences Reviews*, **18**, 379–415.

1112. Nylander, I. (1971). The feeling of being fat and dieting in a school population. *Acta Sociomedica Scandinavica*, **1**, 17–26.

1113. O'Connell, J.K., Price, J.H., Roberts, S.M., Jurs, S.G. and McKinley, R. (1985). Utilizing the health belief model to predict dieting and exercise behaviour of obese and nonobese adolescents. *Health Education Quarterly*, **12**, 343–51.

1114. O'Hara, N.M., Baranowski, T., Simons-Morton, B.G., Wilson, B.S. and Parcel, G.S. (1989). Validity of the observation of children's physical activity. *Research Quarterly for Exercise and Sport*, **60**, 42–7.

1115. Oakes, R. (1984). Sex patterns in DSM-III: bias or basis for theory development. *American Psychologist*, **39**, 1320–2.

1116. Oberhansli, I., Pometta, D., Micheli, H., Raymond, L. and Suenran, A. (1982). Lipid, lipoprotein and APO-A and APO-B lipoprotein distribution in Italian and Swiss schoolchildren. The Geneva Survey. *Pediatric Research*, **16**, 665–9.

1117. Office of Population Censuses and Surveys (1993). *Health Survey for England 1991*. London, Her Majesty's Stationery Office.

1118. Orava, S. and Puranen, J. (1978). Exertion injuries in adolescent athletes. *British Journal of Sports Medicine*, **12**, 4–10.

1119. Orchard, T.J., Donahue, R.P., Kuller, L.H., Hodges, P.N. and Drash, A.L. (1983). Cholesterol screening in childhood: does it predict adult hypercholesterolaemia? The Beaver County experience. *Journal of Pediatrics*, **103**, 687–91.

1120. Orchard, T.J., Rodgers, M., Hedley, A.J. and Mitchell, J.R.A. (1980). Changes in blood lipids and blood pressure during adolescence. *British Medical Journal*, **280**, 1563–7.

1121. Oscai, L.B. (1989). Exercise and obesity: Emphasis on animal models. In C.V. Gisolfi and D.R. Lamb (Eds.), *Perspectives in Exercise Science and Sports Medicine, Vol. 2, Youth, Exercise, and Sport*. Indianapolis, IN, Benchmark Press, pp. 273–93.

1122. Oseid, S. and Hermansen, L. (1971). Hormonal and metabolic changes during and after prolonged work in pre-pubertal boys. *Acta Paediatrica Scandinavica*, **217** (Suppl.), 147–53.

1123. Oseid, S., Horde, R., Osnes, J.B. and Hermansen, L. (1969). Circulatory responses to prolonged exercise in pre-pubertal boys. *Acta Physiologica Scandinavica*, **310** (Suppl.), 90.

1124. Oswald, J. (1980). Sleep as a restorative process: human clues. In P.S. McConnell, G.J. Boer, H.J. Romijin, N.E. van de Poll and M.A. Corner (Eds.), *Adaptive Capabilities of the Nervous System*. New York, Elsevier, pp. 279–88.

1125. Ozmun, J.C., Mikesky, A.E. and Surburg, P.R. (1991). Neuromuscular adaptations during prepubescent strength training. *Medicine and Science in Sports and Exercise*, **23**, S32.

1126. Paffenbarger, R.S. Jr. and Wing, A.L. (1967). Chronic disease in former college students: X. The effects of single and multiple characteristics on risk of fatal coronary heart disease. *American Journal of Epidemiology*, **90**, 527–35.

1127. Palgi, Y., Gutin, B., Young, J. and Alejandro, D. (1984). Physiologic and anthropometric factors underlying endurance performance in children. *International Journal of Sports Medicine*, **5**, 67–73.

1128. Panico, S., Celentano, E., Krogh, V., Jossa, F., Farinaro, E., Trevisan, M. *et al.* (1987). Physical activity and its relationship to blood pressure in schoolchildren. *Journal of Chronic Diseases*, **40**, 925–30.

1129. Párizková, J. (1961). Total fat and skinfold thickness in children. *Metabolism*, **10**, 794–807.

1130. Párizková, J. (1974). Particularities of lean body mass and fat development in growing boys as related to their motor activity. *Acta Paediatrica Belgica*, **28**, 233–42.

1131. Párizková, J. (1982). Physical training in weight reduction of obese adolescents. *Annals of Clinical Research*, **14**, 63–8.

1132. Parker, D.F. and Bar-Or, O. (1991). Juvenile obesity. *The Physician and Sports Medicine*, **19**, 113–25.

1133. Parker, D.F., Round, J.M., Sacco, P. and Jones, D.A. (1990). A cross-sectional survey of upper and lower limb strength in boys and girls during childhood and adolescence. *Annals of Human Biology*, **17**, 199–211.

1134. Parkkola, R., Alanen, A., Kalimo, H., Lillsunde, I., Komu, M. and Kormano, M. (1993). MR relaxation times and fiber type predominance of the psoas and multifidus muscle. *Acta Radiologica*, **34**, 16–19.

1135. Passmore, R. and Durnin, J.V.G.A. (1955). Human energy expenditure. *Physiological Reviews*, **35**, 801–40.

1136. Pate, R.R. (1988). The evolving definition of physical fitness. *Quest*, **40**, 174–9.

1137. Pate, R.R. (1993). Physical activity assessment in children and adolescents. *Critical Reviews in Food Science and Nutrition*, **33**, 321–6.

1138. Pate, R.R., Dowda, M. and Ross, J.G. (1990). Associations between physical activity and physical fitness in American children. *American Journal of Diseases of Children*, **144**, 1123–9.

1139. Pate, R.R., Long, B.J. and Heath, G. (1994). Descriptive epidemiology of physical activity in adolescents. *Pediatric Exercise Science*, **6**, 434–47.

1140. Pate, R.R. and Ross, J.G. (1987). Factors associated with health-related fitness. *Journal of Physical Education, Recreation and Dance*, **58**, 93–6.

1141. Pate, R.R. and Shephard, R.J. (1989). Characteristics of physical fitness in youth. In C.V. Gisolfi and D.R. Lamb (Eds.), *Perspectives in Exercise Science and Sports Medicine, Vol. 2, Youth, Exercise, and Sport*. Indianapolis, IN, Benchmark Press, pp. 1–46.

1142. Pate, R.R. and Ward, D.S. (1990). Endurance exercise trainability in children and youth. In W.A. Grana, J.A. Lombardo, B.J. Sharkey and J.A.

Stone (Eds.), *Advances in Sports Medicine and Fitness, Vol. 3.* Chicago, IL, Year Book Medical Publishers, pp. 37–55.

1143. Paterson, D.H. and Cunningham, D.A. (1985). Development of anaerobic capacity in early and late maturing boys. In R.A. Binkhorst, H.C. G. Kemper and W.H.M. Saris (Eds.), *Children and Exercise XI.* Champaign, IL, Human Kinetics, pp. 119–28.

1144. Paterson, D.H., Cunningham, D.A. and Bonk, J.M. (1980). Anaerobic capacity of athletic males aged 10, 15 and 21 years. *International Symposium: Growth and Development of the Child.* Trois-Rivières, Quebec.

1145. Paterson, D.H., Cunningham, D.A. and Bumstead, L.A. (1981). Development of anaerobic capacity in boys aged 11 to 15 years. *Canadian Journal of Applied Sports Sciences,* **6**, 134.

1146. Paterson, D.H., Cunningham, D.A. and Donner, A. (1981). The effect of different treadmill speeds on the variability of $\dot{V}O_2$ max in children. *European Journal of Applied Physiology,* **47**, 113–22.

1147. Paterson, D.H., McLellan, T.M., Stella, R.S. and Cunningham, D.A. (1987). Longitudinal study of ventilation threshold and maximal O_2 uptake in athletic boys. *Journal of Applied Physiology,* **62**, 2051–7.

1148. Patton, J.F., Murphy, M.M. and Frederick, F.A. (1985). Maximal power outputs during the Wingate anaerobic test. *International Journal of Sports Medicine,* **6**, 82–5.

1149. Payne, V.G. and Morrow, J.R. (1993). Exercise and $\dot{V}O_2$ max: a meta analysis. *Research Quarterly for Exercise and Sport,* **64**, 305–13.

1150. Peacock, M. (1991). Calcium absorption efficiency and calcium requirements in children and adolescents. *American Journal of Clinical Nutrition,* **54**, 251S–265S.

1151. Pearl, P.M. (1987). The effects of exercise on the development and function of the coronary collateral circulation. *Sports Medicine,* **4**, 86–94.

1152. Pedley, F.G. (1942). Coronary heart disease and occupation. *Canadian Medical Association Journal,* **46**, 147–51.

1153. Peiris, A.N., Sothman, M.N., Hoffmann, G., Hennes, M.L., Wilson, C.R., Gustafson, A.B. *et al.* (1989). Adiposity, fat distribution and cardiovascular risk. *Annals of Internal Medicine,* **110**, 867–72.

1154. Peltenburg, A.L., Erich, W.B.M., Zonderland, M.L., Bernink, M.J.E., van den Brande, J.L. and Huisveld, I.A. (1984). A retrospective growth study of female gymnasts and girl swimmers. *International Journal of Sports Medicine,* **5**, 262–7.

1155. Peltonen, P., Marnierni, J., Hietanen, E., Vuori, I. and Ehnholm, C. (1981). Changes in serum lipids, lipoproteins and heparin releasable lipolytic enzymes during moderate physical training in man: a longitudinal study. *Metabolism,* **30**, 518–20.

1156. Pendergast, D.R., Shindell, D., Cerretelli, P. and Rennie, D.W. (1980). Role of central and peripheral circulatory adjustments in oxygen transport at the onset of exercise. *International Journal of Sports Medicine,* **1**, 160–70.

1157. Perrine, J.J. (1968). Isokinetic exercise and the mechanical energy potentials of muscle. *Journal of Health, Physical Education and Recreation,* **39**, 40–4.

1158. Persson, B. and Thoren, C. (1980). Prolonged exercise in adolescent boys with juvenile diabetes mellitus. *Acta Paediatrica Scandinavica*, **283** (Suppl.), 61–9.

1159. Perusse, L., LeBlanc, C. and Bouchard, C. (1988). Familial resemblance in lifelong components: results from the Canada Fitness Survey. *Canadian Journal of Public Health*, **79**, 201–5.

1160. Perusse, L., Tremblay, A., LeBlanc, C. and Bouchard, C. (1989). Genetic and environmental influences on level of physical activity and exercise participation. *American Journal of Epidemiology*, **129**, 1012–22.

1161. Peters, D., Fox, K., Armstrong, N., Sharpe, P. and Bell, M. (1994). Estimation of body fat and body fat distribution in 11-year-old children using magnetic resonance imaging and hydrostatic weighing, skinfolds, and anthropometry. *American Journal of Human Biology*, **6**, 237–43.

1162. Petrie, J.C., O'Brien, E.T., Littler, W.A. and deSwiet, M. (1986). Recommendations on blood pressure measurement. *British Medical Journal*, **293**, 611–15.

1163. Petrofsky, J.S. and Phillips, C.A. (1986). The physiology of static exercise. *Exercise and Sport Sciences Reviews*, **14**, 1–44.

1164. Petruzello, S.J., Landers, D.M., Hartfield, B.D., Kubitz, K.A. and Salazar, W. (1991). A meta-analysis on the anxiety reducing effects of acute and chronic exercise: outcomes and mechanisms. *Sports Medicine*, **11**, 143–82.

1165. Petterson, F., Fries, H. and Nillius, S.J. (1973). Epidemiology of secondary amenorrhea. I. Incidence and prevalance rates. *American Journal of Obstetrics and Gynecology*, **117**, 80–6.

1166. Pfeiffer, R.D. and Francis, R.S. (1986). Effects of strength training on muscle development in prepubescent, pubescent, and postpubescent males. *The Physician and Sports Medicine*, **14**, 134–43.

1167. Physical Education Association (1987). *A Commission of Enquiry: Physical Education in Schools*. London, Ling Publishers.

1168. Physical Education Association (1987). Health-related fitness testing and monitoring in schools. A position statement. *British Journal of Physical Education*, **18**, 141–2.

1169. Piekarski, C., Morfeld, B., Kampmann, R., Illmarinen, and Wenzel, H.G. (1986). Heat-stress reactions of the growing child. In J. Rutenfranz, R. Mocellin and F. Klimt (Eds.), *Children and Exercise XII*. Champaign, IL, Human Kinetics, pp. 403–12.

1170. Pirnay, F. and Crielaard, J.M. (1980). Anaerobic power in children and adolescents. *Conference Proceedings of the 2nd European Seminar on Testing Physical Fitness*. University of Birmingham, pp. 39–44.

1171. Plowman, S.A. (1989). Maturation and exercise training in children. *Pediatric Exercise Science*, **1**, 303–12.

1172. Pocock, N.A., Eisman, J.A., Hopper, J.L., Yeates, M.G., Sambrook, P.N. and Eben, S. (1987). Genetic determinants of bone mass in adults: a twin study. *Journal of Clinical Investigations*, **80**, 706–10.

1173. Pollock, M.L. (1973). The quantification of endurance training programs. *Exercise and Sport Sciences Reviews*, **1**, 158–88.

1174. Poortmans, J.R., Bossche, J.D.V. and LeClerq, R. (1978). Lactate uptake by inactive forearm during progressive leg exercise. *Journal of Applied Physiology*, **45**, 835–9.

1175. Poortmans, J.R., Saerens, P., Edelman, R., Vertongen, F. and Dorchy, H. (1986). Influence of the degree of metabolic control on physical fitness in type I diabetic adolescents. *International Journal of Sports Medicine*, **7**, 232–5.

1176. Powell, K.E. and Dysinger, W. (1987). Childhood participation in organised school sports and physical education as precursors of adult physical activity. *American Journal of Preventive Medicine*, **3**, 276–81.

1177. Powell, K.E., Thompson, P.D., Casperson, C.J. and Kendrick, J.S. (1987). Physical activity and the incidence of coronary heart disease. *Annual Reviews of Public Health*, **8**, 253–87.

1178. Preece, M.A. (1986). Prepubertal and pubertal endocrinology. In F. Falkner and J.M. Tanner (Eds.), *Human Growth, Vol. 2, Postnatal Growth*. London, Plenum Press, pp. 211–24.

1179. Prentice, A.M. (1990). *The Doubly-Labelled Water Method for Measuring Energy Expenditure: Technical Recommendations for use in Humans. A Consensus Report by the IDECG Working Group*. Vienna, International Atomic Energy Agency.

1180. Prentice, A.M. and Jebb, S. (1995). Obesity in Britain: gluttony or sloth? *British Medical Journal*, **311**, 437–9.

1181. Prentice, A.M., Parsons, T.J. and Cole, T.J. (1994). Uncritical use of bone mineral density in absorptiometry may lead to size-related artifacts in the identification of bone mineral determinants. *American Journal of Clinical Nutrition*, **60**, 837–42.

1182. Prior, J.C., Ho Yuen, B., Clement, P., Bowie, L. and Thomas, J. (1982). Reversible luteal phase changes and infertility associated with marathon training. *Lancet*, July 31, 269–70.

1183. Prior, J.C., Vigna, Y.M. and McKay, D.W. (1992). Reproduction for the athletic woman: new understandings of physiology and management. *Sports Medicine*, **14**, 190–9.

1184. Prud'Homme, D., Bouchard, C., Leblanc, C., Landry, F. and Fontaine, E. (1984). Sensitivity of maximal aerobic power to training is genotype-dependent. *Medicine and Science in Sports and Exercise*, **16**, 489–93.

1185. Pugliese, M.T., Lifshitz, G., Grad, P., Fort, P. and Marks-Katz, M. (1983). Fear of obesity. A cause of short stature and delayed puberty. *New England Journal of Medicine*, **309**, 513–18.

1186. Puhl, J.L. (1989). Energy expenditure among children: implications for childhood obesity I: resting and dietary energy expenditure. *Pediatric Exercise Science*, **1**, 212–29.

1187. Puhl, J.L., Greaves, K., Hoyt, M. and Baranowski, T. (1990). Children's activity rating scale (CARS): description and calibration. *Research Quarterly for Exercise and Sport*, **61**, 26–36.

1188. Puska, P., Vartiainen, E., Pallonen, U., Routsalainen, P., Tuomilehto, J., Koskela, K. *et al.* (1981). The North Karelia youth project. *Preventive Medicine*, **10**, 133–48.

1189. Pyle, R.L., Halvorson, P.A., Neuman, P.A. and Mitchell, J.E. (1986). The increasing prevalence of bulimia in freshman college students. *International Journal of Eating Disorders*, **5**, 631–47.

1190. Raglin, J.S. (1990). Exercise and mental health: beneficial and detrimental effects. *Sports Medicine*, **9**, 323–9.

1191. Rahn, B.A. (1982). Bone healing: histologic and physiologic concepts. In G. Sumener-Smith (Ed.), *Bone in Clinical Orthopaedics*. Philadelphia, PA, Saunders, pp. 335–41.

1192. Raitakari, O.T., Porkka, K.V.K., Rasenen, L., Ronnemaa, T. and Viikari, J.S.A. (1994). Clustering and six-year cluster-tracking of serum total cholesterol, HDL-cholesterol and diastolic blood pressure in children and young adults. *Journal of Clinical Epidemiology*, **47**, 1085–93.

1193. Raitakari, O.T., Porkka, K.V.K., Taimelo, S., Telema, R., Rasenen, L. and Viikari, J.S.A. (1994). Effects of persistent physical activity and inactivity on coronary risk factors in children and young adults. *American Journal of Epidemiology*, **140**, 195–205.

1194. Ramsay, J.A., Blimkie, C.J.R., Smith, K., Garner, S., MacDougall, J.D. and Sale, D.G. (1990). Strength training effects in prepubescent boys. *Medicine and Science in Sports and Exercise*, **22**, 605–14.

1195. Rape, R.N. (1987). Running and depression. *Perceptual and Motor Skills*, **64**, 1303–10.

1196. Rarick, G.L. (1978). Competitive sports in childhood and adolescence. In R.A. Magill, M.J. Ash and F.L. Smoll (Eds.), *Children in Sport*. Champaign, IL, Human Kinetics, pp. 113–28.

1197. Raven, P.B. and Hagan, R.D. (1994). Cardiovascular responses to exercise and training. In M. Harries, C. Williams, W.D. Stanish and L.J. Micheli (Eds.), *Oxford Textbook of Sports Medicine*. Oxford University Press, pp. 161–72.

1198. Recker, R. (1987). Bone mass and calcium nutrition. *Nutrition Research*, **11**, 19–21.

1199. Recker, R.R., Davies, K.M., Hinders, S.M., Heaney, R.P., Stegman, R.P. and Kimmel, D.B. (1992). Bone gain in young adult women. *Journal of the American Medical Association*, **268**, 2403–8.

1200. Reilly, T. (1978). Some observations on weight-training. *British Journal of Sports Medicine*, **12**, 45–7.

1201. Reybrouck, T., Weymans, M., Ghesquiere, J., Van Gervan, D. and Stijns, H. (1982). Ventilatory threshold in kindergarten children during treadmill exercise. *European Journal of Applied Physiology*, **50**, 79–86.

1202. Reynolds, K.D., Killen, J.D., Bryson, S.W., Maron, D.J., Barr Taylor, C., Maccoby, N. *et al.* (1990). Psychosocial predictors of physical activity in adolescents. *Preventive Medicine*, **19**, 541–51.

1203. Rians, C.B., Weltman, A., Cahill, B.R., Janney, C.A., Tippett, S.R. and Katch, F.I. (1987). Strength training for prepubescent males: is it safe? *American Journal of Sports Medicine*, **15**, 483–9.

1204. Richter, E., Ruderman, N., Gavras, H., Belur, E. and Galbo, H. (1982). Muscle glycogenolysis during exercise: dual control by epinephrine and contractions. *American Journal of Physiology*, **242** (Endocrinology and Metabolism 5), E25–E32.

1205. Riddoch, C. (1990). *Northern Ireland Health and Fitness Survey.* Belfast, Sports Council for Northern Ireland and Department of Health and Social Services.

1206. Riddoch, C.J. and Boreham, C.A.G. (1995). The health-related physical activity of children. *Sports Medicine*, **19**, 86–102.

1207. Riddoch, C., Mahoney, C., Murphy, N., Boreham, C. and Cran, G. (1991). The physical activity patterns of Northern Irish schoolchildren ages 11 to 16 years. *Pediatric Exercise Science*, **3**, 300–9.

1208. Riddoch, C., Savage, J.M., Murphy, N., Cran, G.W. and Boreham, C. (1991). Long-term health implications of fitness and physical activity patterns. *Archives of Disease in Childhood*, **66**, 1426–33.

1209. Riggs, B.L. and Melton, L.J. (1988). *Osteoporosis. Etiology, Diagnosis and Management.* New York, Raven Press.

1210. Riis, B.J., Krabbe, S., Christiansen, C., Catherwood, B.D. and Deftos, L.J. (1985). Bone turnover in male puberty: a longitudinal study. *Calcified Tissue International*, **37**, 213–17.

1211. Rimm, I.J. and Rimm, A.A. (1976). Association between juvenile onset obesity and severe adult obesity in 73,532 women. *American Journal of Public Health*, **6**, 479–81.

1212. Ritmeester, J.W., Kemper, H.C.G. and Verschuur, R. (1985). Is a levelling-off criterion in oxygen uptake a prerequisite for a maximal performance in teenagers? In R.A. Binkhorst, H.C.G. Kemper and W.H.M. Saris (Eds.), *Children and Exercise XI.* Champaign, IL, Human Kinetics, pp. 161–9.

1213. Rivera, M.A., Metz, K.F. and Robertson, R. (1980). Competitive female swimmers' metabolic and performance responses to anaerobic threshold and high intensity training. *International Congress on Women and Sport*, Rome.

1214. Rivera-Brown, A.M., Rivera, M.A. and Frontera, W.R. (1992). Applicability of criteria for $\dot{V}O_2$ max in active adolescents. *Pediatric Exercise Science*, **4**, 331–9.

1215. Rivera-Brown, A.M., Rivera, M.A. and Frontera, W.R. (1994). Achievement of $\dot{V}O_2$ max criteria in adolescent runners: effects of testing protocol. *Pediatric Exercise Science*, **6**, 236–45.

1216. Rivera-Brown, A.M., Rivera, M.A. and Frontera, W.R. (1995). Reliability of $\dot{V}O_2$ max in adolescent runners: a comparison between plateau achievers and nonachievers. *Pediatric Exercise Science*, **7**, 203–10.

1217. Roberts, S.B., Coward, W.A., Schlingenseipen, K.H., Norhria, V. and Lucas, A. (1986). Comparison of the doubly labelled water ($^2H_2^{18}O$) method with indirect calorimetry and a nutrient-balance study for simultaneous determination of energy expenditure, water intake, and metabolizable energy intake in preterm infants. *American Journal of Clinical Nutrition*, **54**, 499–505.

1218. Robins, L.N., Helzer, J.E. and Weissman, M.M. (1984). Lifetime prevalence of specific psychiatric disorders in three sites. *Archives of General Psychiatry*, **41**, 949–58.

1219. Robinson, S. (1938). Experimental studies of physical fitness in relation to age. *Arbeitsphysiologie*, **10**, 251–323.

1220. Robinson, T.N., Hammer, L.D., Killen, J.D., Kraemer, H.C., Wilson, D.M., Hayward, C. *et al.* (1993). Does television viewing increase obesity and reduce physical activity? Cross-sectional and longitudinal analyses among adolescent girls. *Pediatrics*, **91**, 273–80.

1221. Rocchini, A.P., Katch, V., Anderson, J., Hinderliter, J., Becque, D., Martin, M. *et al.* (1988). Blood pressure in obese adolescents: effect of weight loss. *Pediatrics*, **82**, 16–23.

1222. Roche, A.F., Chumlea, W.C. and Thissen, D. (1988). *Assessing the Skeletal Maturity of the Hand-Wrist: Fels Method.* Springfield, IL, Thomas.

1223. Roche, A.F., Siervogel, R.M., Chumlea, W.C. and Webb, P. (1981). Grading fatness from limited anthropometric data. *American Journal of Clinical Nutrition*, **34**, 2831–8.

1224. Roche, A.F., Wainer, H. and Thissen, D. (1975). *Skeletal Maturity: Knee Joint as a Biological Indicator.* New York, Plenum Press.

1225. Rode, A., Bar-Or, O. and Shephard, R.J. (1973). Cardiac output and oxygen conductance. A comparison of Canadian Eskimo and city dwellers. In O. Bar-Or (Ed.), *Proceedings of Pediatric Work Physiology*. Natanya, Israel, Wingate Institute, pp. 45–7.

1226. Roemmich, J.N. and Rogol, A.D. (1995). Physiology of growth and development. *Clinics in Sports Medicine*, **14**, 483–502.

1227. Rogers, D.M., Turley, K.R., Kujawa, K.I., Harper, K.M. and Wilmore, J.H. (1995). Allometric scaling factors for oxygen uptake during exercise in children. *Pediatric Exercise Science*, **7**, 12–25.

1228. Rogol, A.D. (1988). Pubertal development in endurance-trained female athletes. In E.W. Brown and C.F. Branta (Eds.), *Competitive Sports for Children and Youth.* Champaign, IL, Human Kinetics, pp. 173–93.

1229. Rogol, A.D. (1994). Growth at puberty: interaction of adrogens and growth hormone. *Medicine and Science in Sports and Exercise*, **26**, 767–70.

1230. Rogol, A.D. (1995). Growth and growth hormone secretion at puberty in males. In C.J.R. Blimkie and O. Bar-Or (Eds.), *New Horizons in Pediatric Exercise Science.* Champaign, IL, Human Kinetics, pp. 39–54.

1231. Rogol, A.D., Weltman, A., Weltman, J.Y., Seip, R.L., Snead, D.B., Levine, S. *et al.* (1992). Durability of the reproductive axis in eumenorrheic women during 1 yr of endurance training. *Journal of Applied Physiology*, **72**, 1571–80.

1232. Rolland-Cachera, M.-F., Bellisle, F., Deheeger, M., Pequignot, F. and Sempe, M. (1990). Influence of body fat distribution during childhood on body fat distribution in adulthood: a two-decade follow-up study. *International Journal of Obesity*, **14**, 473–81.

1233. Rolland-Cachera, M.-F., Cole, T.J., Skempe, M., Tichet, J., Rossignol, C. and Charraud, A. (1991). Body mass index variations: centiles from birth to 87 years. *European Journal of Clinical Nutrition*, **45**, 13–21.

1234. Rose, H.E. and Mayer, J. (1968). Activity, caloric intake and the energy balance of infants. *Pediatrics*, **41**, 18–29.

1235. Ross, J.G., Dotson, C.O. and Gilbert, G.G. (1985). Are kids getting appropriate activity? *Journal of Physical Education, Recreation and Dance*, **56**, 82–5.

1236. Ross, J.G., Dotson, C.O. and Gilbert, G.G. (1985). Youth fitness revisited Part III. *Parks and Recreation*, 81–7.

1237. Ross, J.G., Dotson, C.O., Gilbert, G.G. and Katz, S.J. (1985). After physical education … physical activity outside of school physical education programmes. *Journal of Physical Education, Recreation and Dance*, **56**, 77–81.

1238. Ross, J.G., Dotson, C.O., Gilbert, G.G. and Katz, S.J. (1985). What are kids doing in school physical education? *Journal of Physical Education, Recreation and Dance*, **56**, 73–6.

1239. Ross, J.G. and Gilbert, G.G. (1985). The National Children and Youth Fitness Study. A summary of findings. *Journal of Physical Education, Recreation and Dance*, **56**, 45–50.

1240. Ross, J.G. and Pate,R.R. (1987). The National Children and Youth Fitness Study II: a summary of findings. *Journal of Physical Education, Recreation and Dance*, **58**, 51–6.

1241. Ross, J.G., Pate, R.R., Casperson, C.J., Damberg, C.L. and Svilar, M. (1987). Home and community in children's exercise habits. *Journal of Physical Education, Recreation and Dance*, **58**, 85–92.

1242. Ross, J.G., Pate, R.R., Corbin, C.B., Delpy, L.A. and Gold, R.S. (1987). What is going on in the elementary physical education programme? *Journal of Physical Education, Recreation and Dance*, **58**, 78–84.

1243. Ross, J.G., Pate, R.R., Lohman, T.G. and Christenson, G.M. (1987). Changes in the body composition of children. *Journal of Physical Education, Recreation and Dance*, **58**, 74–7.

1244. Ross, K.D., and Reese, G. (1964). Smoking and high school performance. *Pediatrics*, **107**, 117–21.

1245. Ross, R., Leger, L., Morris, D., de Guise, J. and Guardo, R. (1992). Quantification of adipose tissue by MRI: relationship with anthropometric variables. *Journal of Applied Physiology*, **72**, 787–95.

1246. Ross, W.D., Bailey, D.A., Mirwald, R.L., Faulkner, R.A., Rasmussen, R., Kerr, D.A. *et al.* (1991). Allometric relationship of estimated muscle mass and maximal oxygen uptake in boys studied longitudinally age 8 to 16 years. In R. Frenkl and I. Szmodis (Eds.), *Children and Exercise, Pediatric Work Physiology XV*. Budapest, National Institute for Health Promotion, pp. 135–42.

1247. Ross, W.D. and Marfell-Jones, M.J. (1982). Kinanthropometry. In J.D. MacDougall, H.A. Wenger and H.J. Geen (Eds.), *Physiological Testing of the High-Performance Athlete*. Champaign, IL, Human Kinetics, pp. 223–308.

1248. Rotstein, A., Dotan, R., Bar-Or, O. and Tenebaum, G. (1986). Effect of training on anaerobic threshold, maximal aerobic power and anaerobic performance of preadolescent boys. *International Journal of Sports Medicine*, **7**, 281–6.

1249. Round, J.M., Nevill, A.M., Honour, J. and Jones, D.A. (1996). Testosterone and the developmental differences in strength between boys and girls. *Journal of Physiology*, **491**, 79.

1250. Routh, D.K., Walton, M.D. and Padan-Belkin, E. (1978). Development of activity level in children revisited: effects of mother presence. *Developmental Psychology*, **14**, 571–81.

1251. Rowe, F.A. (1933). Growth comparisons of athletes and non-athletes. *Research Quarterly*, **4**, 108–16.

1252. Rowe, R.A. (1979). Cartilage fracture due to weight lifting. *British Journal of Sports Medicine*, **13**, 130–1.

1253. Rowland, T.W. (1985). Aerobic response to endurance training in pre-pubescent children: a critical analysis. *Medicine and Science in Sports and Exercise*, **17**, 493–7.

1254. Rowland, T.W. (1987). Serum testosterone response to training in adolescent runners. *American Journal of Diseases of Children*, **141**, 881–3.

1255. Rowland, T.W. (1989). Ethical considerations in pediatric research: how much is too much? *Pediatric Exercise Science*, **1**, 93–5.

1256. Rowland, T.W. (1989). Oxygen uptake and endurance fitness in children: a developmental perspective. *Pediatric Exercise Science*, **1**, 313–28.

1257. Rowland, T.W. (1990). Developmental aspects of physiological function relating to aerobic exercise in children. *Sports Medicine*, **10**, 255–66.

1258. Rowland, T.W. (1990). *Exercise and Children's Health*. Champaign, IL, Human Kinetics.

1259. Rowland, T.W. (1992). Aerobic responses to physical training in children. In R.J. Shephard and P.O. Astrand (Eds.), *Endurance in Sport*. London, Blackwell Scientific, pp. 377–84.

1260. Rowland, T.W. (1992). Exercise, nutrition, and the prevention of cardio-vascular disease: a pediatric perspective. *Medicine, Exercise, Nutrition and Health*, **1**, 34–41.

1261. Rowland, T.W. (1992). Trainability of cardiorespiratory system during childhood. *Canadian Journal of Sports Science*, **17**, 259–63.

1262. Rowland, T.W. (1993). Aerobic exercise testing protocols. In T.W. Rowland (Ed.), *Pediatric Laboratory Exercise Testing*. Champaign, IL, Human Kinetics, pp. 19–42.

1263. Rowland, T.W. (1993). Does peak $\dot{V}O_2$ reflect $\dot{V}O_2$ max in children? Evidence from supramaximal testing. *Medicine and Science in Sports and Exercise*, **25**, 689–93.

1264. Rowland, T.W. (1993). The physiological impact of intensive training on the prepubertal athlete. In B.R. Cahill and A.J. Pearl (Eds.), *Intensive Participation in Children's Sports*. Champaign, IL, Human Kinetics, pp. 167–94.

1265. Rowland, T.W. (1994). Effect of prolonged inactivity on aerobic fitness of children. *Journal of Sports Medicine and Physical Fitness*, **34**, 147–55.

1266. Rowland, T.W. (1995). The horse is dead; let's dismount. *Pediatric Exercise Science*, **7**, 117–20.

1267. Rowland, T.W., Auchinachie, J.A., Keenan, T.J. and Green, G.M. (1987). Physiologic responses to treadmill running in adult and prepubertal males. *International Journal of Sports Medicine*, **8**, 292–7.

1268. Rowland, T.W. and Freedson, P.S. (1994). Physical activity, fitness and health in children: a close look. *Pediatrics*, **93**, 669–72.

1269. Rowland, T.W. and Green, G.M. (1988). Physiological responses to treadmill exercise in females: adult-child differences. *Medicine and Science in Sports and Exercise*, **20**, 474–8.

1270. Rowland, T.W., Marth, P.M. Jr., Reiter, E.O. and Cunningham, L.N. (1992). The influence of diabetes mellitus on cardiovascular function in children and adolescents. *International Journal of Sports Medicine*, **13**, 431–5.

1271. Rowland, T.W., Staab, J.S., Unnithan, V.B., Rambusch, J.M. and Siconolfi, S.F. (1990). Mechanical efficiency during cycling in prepubertal and adult males. *International Journal of Sports Medicine*, **11**, 452–5.

1272. Rowland, T.W., Swadba, L.A., Biggs, D.E., Burke, E.J. and Reiter, E.O. (1985). Glycemic control with physical training in insulin-dependent diabetes mellitus. *Sports Medicine*, **139**, 307–10.

1273. Rowland, T.W., Varzeas, M.R. and Walsh, C.A. (1991). Aerobic responses to walking training in sedentary adolescents. *Journal of Adolescent Health*, **12**, 30–4.

1274. Roy, S., Caine, D. and Singer, K.M. (1985). Stress changes of the distal radial epiphysis in young gymnasts: a report of twenty-one cases and a review of the literature. *American Journal of Sports Medicine*, **13**, 301–8.

1275. Royal College of Physicians of London (1983). Obesity. *Journal of the Royal College of Physicians*, **17**, 3–58.

1276. Royal College of Physicians of London (1991). *Medical Aspects of Exercise: Benefits and Risks*. London, Royal College of Physicians.

1277. Rubin, C.T. and Lanyon, L.E. (1984). Regulation of bone formation by applied dynamic loads. *Journal of Bone and Joint Surgery*, **66**, 397–402.

1278. Rubin, C.T. and Lanyon, L.E. (1985). Regulation of bone mass by mechanical strain magnitude. *Calcified Tissue International*, **38**, 411–17.

1279. Ruffin, M.T.I., Hunter, R.E. and Arendt, E.A. (1990). Exercise and secondary amenorrhea linked through endogenous opioids. *Sports Medicine*, **10**, 65–71.

1280. Rutenfranz, J., Andersen, K.L., Seliger, V., Ilmarinen, J., Klimmer, F., Kylian, H. *et al.* (1982). Maximal aerobic power affected by maturation and body growth during childhood and adolescence. *European Journal of Pediatrics*, **139**, 106–12.

1281. Rutenfranz, J., Andersen, K.L., Seliger, V., Klimmer, F., Ilmarinen, J., Ruppel, M. *et al.* (1981). Exercise ventilation during the growth spurt period: comparison between two European countries. *European Journal of Pediatrics*, **136**, 135–42.

1282. Rutenfranz, J., Berndt, I. and Knauth, P. (1974). Daily physical activity investigated by time budget studies and physical performance capacity of schoolboys. *Acta Paediatrica Belgica*, **28**, 79–86.

1283. Rutter, M., Graham, P., Chadwick, O. and Yule, W. (1976). Adolescent turmoil: fact or fiction? *Journal of Child Psychology and Psychiatry*, **17**, 35–56.

1284. Ryan, A.J. (1984). Exercise and health: lessons from the past. In H.M. Eckert and H.J. Montoye (Eds.), *Exercise and Health*. Champaign, IL, Human Kinetics, pp. 3–13.

1285. Ryan, J.R. and Salcicciolo, G.C. (1976). Fracture of the distal radial epiphysis in adolescent weight-lifters. *American Journal of Sports Medicine*, **4**, 26–7.

1286. Rychtecky, A. (1994). Contributions of school physical education to lifelong activity. *International Council of Health Physical Education and Recreation Journal*, **30**, 39–45.

1287. Ryle, J.A. and Russel, W.T. (1949). The natural history of coronary disease: clinical and epidemiological study. *British Heart Journal*, **11**, 370–89.
1288. Saavedra, C., Lagassé, P., Bouchard, C. and Simoneau, J.A. (1991). Maximal anaerobic performance of the knee extensor muscles during growth. *Medicine and Science in Sports and Exercise*, **23**, 1083–9.
1289. Sady, S.P. (1981). Transient oxygen uptake and heart rate response at the onset of relative endurance exercise in pre-pubertal boys and adult men. *International Journal of Sports Medicine*, **2**, 240–4.
1290. Sady, S.P. (1986). Cardiorespiratory exercise training in children. *Clinics in Sports Medicine*, **5**, 493–514.
1291. Sady, S.P., Katch, V.L., Villanacci, J.F. and Gilliam, T.B. (1983). Children-adult comparisons of oxygen uptake and heart rate kinetics during submaximum exercise. *Research Quarterly for Exercise and Sport*, **54**, 55–9.
1292. Sady, S.P., Thomson, W.H., Berg, K. and Savage, M. (1984). Physiological characteristics of high ability pre-pubescent wrestlers. *Medicine and Science in Sports and Exercise*, **16**, 72–6.
1293. Sailors, M. and Berg, K. (1987). Comparison of responses to weight training in pubescent boys and men. *Journal of Sports Medicine and Physical Fitness*, **27**, 30–6.
1294. Salber, E.J., Reed, R.B. and Harrison, S.U. (1963). Smoking behaviour, recreational activities and attitudes towards smoking among Newton secondary school children. *Pediatrics*, **22**, 911–18.
1295. Sale, D.G. (1987). Influence of exercise and training on motor unit activation. *Exercise and Sport Sciences Reviews*, **15**, 95–151.
1296. Sale, D.G. (1989). Strength training in children. In C.V. Gisolfi and D.R. Lamb (Eds.), *Perspectives in Exercise Science and Sports Medicine, Vol. 2, Youth, Exercise and Sport*. Indianapolis, IN, Benchmark Press, pp. 165–216.
1297. Sale, D.G. (1990). Testing strength and power. In J.D. MacDougall, H.A. Wenger and H.J. Green (Eds.), *Physiological Testing of the High-Performance Athlete*. Champaign, IL, Human Kinetics, pp. 21–106.
1298. Sallis, J.F. (1987). A commentary on children and fitness: a public health perspective. *Research Quarterly for Exercise and Sport*, **58**, 326–30.
1299. Sallis, J.F. (1991). Self-report measures of children's physical activity. *Journal of School Health*, **61**, 215–19.
1300. Sallis, J.F. (1993). Epidemiology of physical activity and fitness in children and adolescents. *Critical Reviews of Food Science and Nutrition*, **33**, 403–8.
1301. Sallis, J.F. (1994). Determinants of physical activity behaviour in children. In R.R. Pate and R.C. Hohn (Eds.), *Health and Fitness Through Physical Education*. Champaign, IL, Human Kinetics, pp. 31–43.
1302. Sallis, J.F. (1994). Physical activity guidelines for adolescents. *Pediatric Exercise Science*, **6**, 299–463.
1303. Sallis, J.F. (1995). A behavioural perspective on children's physical activity. In L.W.Y. Cheung and J.B. Richmond (Eds.), *Child Health, Nutrition, and Physical Activity*. Champaign, IL, Human Kinetics, pp. 125–38.
1304. Sallis, J.F., Buono, M.J. and Freedson, P.S. (1991). Bias in estimating caloric expenditure from physical activity in children. *Sports Medicine*, **11**, 203–9.

1305. Sallis, J.F., Buono, M.J., Roby, J.J., Carlsen, D. and Nelson, J.A. (1990). The Caltrac accelerometer as a physical activity monitor for school-age children. *Medicine and Science in Sports and Exercise*, **22**, 698–703.

1306. Sallis, J.F., Buono, M.J., Roby, J.J., Micale, F.G. and Nelson, J.A. (1993). Seven-day recall and other physical activity self-reports in children and adolescents. *Medicine and Science in Sports and Exercise*, **25**, 99–108.

1307. Sallis, J.F. and McKenzie, T.L. (1991). Physical education's role in public health. *Research Quarterly for Exercise and Sport*, **62**, 124–37.

1308. Sallis, J.F., McKenzie, T.L. and Alcaraz, J.E. (1993). Habitual physical activity and health-related physical fitness in fourth-grade children. *American Journal of Diseases of Children*, **147**, 890–5.

1309. Sallis, J.F. and Patrick, K. (1994). Physical activity guidelines for adolescents: a consensus statement. *Pediatric Exercise Science*, **6**, 302–14.

1310. Sallis, J.F., Patterson, T.L., Buono, M.J., Atkins, C.J. and Nader, P.R. (1988). Aggregation of physical activity habits in Mexican-American and Anglo families. *Journal of Behavioural Medicine*, **11**, 31–41.

1311. Sallis, J.F., Patterson, T.L., Buono, M.J. and Nader, P.R. (1988). Relation of cardiovascular fitness and physical activity to cardiovascular disease risk factors in children and adults. *American Journal of Epidemiology*, **127**, 933–41.

1312. Sallis, J.F., Patterson, T.L., McKenzie, T.L. and Nader, P.R. (1988). Family variables and physical activity in preschool children. *Journal of Developmental and Behavioural Pediatrics*, **9**, 57–61.

1313. Sallis, J.F., Simons-Morton, B.G., Stone, E.J., Corbin, C.B., Epstein, L.H., Faucette, N. *et al.* (1992). Determinants of physical activity and interventions in youth. *Medicine and Science in Sports and Exercise*, **24**, S248–S257.

1314. Salonen, J.T. and Lakka, T. (1987). Assessment of physical activity in population studies – validity and consistency of the methods in the Kuopio ischemic heart disease risk factor study. *Scandinavian Journal of Sports Sciences*, **9**, 89–95.

1315. Saltin, B. (1990). Anaerobic capacity: past, present and prospective. In A.W. Taylor (Ed.), *Biochemistry of Exercise VII*. Champaign, IL, Human Kinetics, pp. 387–412.

1316. Saltin, B. (1990). Cardiovascular and pulmonary adaptation to physical activity. In C. Bouchard, R.J. Shephard, T. Stephens, J.R. Sutton and B.D. McPherson (Eds.), *Exercise, Fitness and Health*. Champaign, IL, Human Kinetics, pp. 187–204.

1317. Saltin, B., Blomqvist, G., Mitchell, J.H., Johnson, R.L. Jr., Wildenthal, K. and Chapman, C. (1968). Response to exercise after bedrest and after training. *Circulation*, **38** (Suppl. 7), 1–78.

1318. Saltykov, S. (1915). Jugendliche und beginnende Atherosclerose, *Korrespondenzblatt für Schweizer Aertze Basel*, XLV, 1057. Cited by R.D. Voller and W.B. Strong (1981). Pediatric aspects of atherosclerosis. *American Heart Journal*, **101**, 815–36.

1319. Salva, P.D. and Bacon, G.E. (1989). Anabolic steroids and growth hormone in the Texas Panhandle. *Texas Medicine*, **85**, 43–4.

1320. Sandler, R.B., Slemenda, C.W., LaPorte, R.E., Cauley, J.A., Schramm, M.M., Barresi, M.L. *et al.* (1985). Postmenopausal bone density and milk consumption in childhood and adolescence. *American Journal of Clinical Nutrition*, **42**, 270–4.

1321. Sangi, H. and Mueller, W.H. (1991). Which measure of body fat distribution is best for epidemiologic research among adolescents? *American Journal of Epidemiology*, **133**, 870–83.

1322. Sannika, R., Terho, P., Suominen, J. and Santti, R. (1983). Testosterone concentrations in human seminal plasma and saliva and its correlation with non-protein bound and total testosterone levels in serum. *International Journal of Andrology*, **6**, 319–30.

1323. Sapega, A.A., Sokolow, D.P., Graham, T.J. and Chance, B. (1987). Phosporus nuclear magnetic resonance: a non-invasive technique for the study of muscle bioenergetics during exercise. *Medicine and Science in Sports and Exercise*, **19**, 410–20.

1324. Saris, W.H.M. (1982). *Aerobic Power and Daily Physical Activity in Children*. Meppel, Netherlands, Kripps Repro.

1325. Saris, W.H.M. (1985). The assessment and evaluation of daily physical activity in children: a review. *Acta Paediatrica Scandinavica*, **318**, 37–48.

1326. Saris, W.H.M. (1986). Habitual physical activity in children: methodology and findings in health and disease. *Medicine and Science in Sports and Exercise*, **18**, 253–63.

1327. Saris, W.H.M. (1992). New developments in the assessment of physical activity in children. In J. Coudert and E. Van Praagh (Eds.), *Pediatric Work Physiology*. Paris, Masson, pp. 107–14.

1328. Saris, W.H.M. and Binkhorst, R.A. (1977). The use of pedometer and acto-meter in studying daily physical activity in man. Part I: reliability of pedo-meter and actometer. *European Journal of Applied Physiology*, **37**, 219–28.

1329. Saris, W.H.M. and Binkhorst, R.A. (1977). The use of pedometer and actometer in studying daily physical activity in man. Part II: validity of pedometer and actometer measuring the daily physical activity. *European Journal of Applied Physiology*, **37**, 229–35.

1330. Saris, W.H.M., Binkhorst, R.A., Cramwinckel, A.B., van Waes Berghe, F. and van der Veen-Hezemans, A.M. (1980). The relationship between working performance, daily physical activity, fatness, blood lipids, and nutrition in schoolchildren. In K. Berg and B.O. Eriksson (Eds.), *Children and Exercise IX*. Baltimore, MD, University Park Press, pp. 166–74.

1331. Saris, W.H.M., Elvers, J.W.H., Van't Hof, M.A. and Binkhorst, R.A. (1986). Changes in physical activity of children aged 6 to 12 years. In J. Rutenfranz, R. Mocellin and F. Klimt (Eds.), *Children and Exercise XII*. Champaign, IL, Human Kinetics, pp. 121–30.

1332. Saris, W.H.M., Noordeloos, A.M., Ringnalda, B.E.M., Van't Hof, M.A. and Binkhorst, R.A. (1985). Reference values for aerobic power of healthy 4 to 18 year old Dutch children: preliminary results. In R.A. Binkhorst, H.C.G. Kemper and W.H.M. Saris (Eds.), *Children and Exercise XI*. Champaign, IL, Human Kinetics, pp. 151–60.

1333. Sarma, J.S.M., Tschurtschenthaler, G.V. and Bing, R.J. (1978). Effect of high density lipoproteins on the cholesterol uptake by isolated pig coronary arteries. *Artery*, **4**, 214–23.

1334. Sasaki, J., Shindo, M., Tanaka, H., Ando, M. and Arakawa, K. (1987). A long-term aerobic exercise program decreases the obesity index and increases the high density lipoprotein cholesterol concentration in obese children. *International Journal of Obesity*, **11**, 339–45.

1335. Sato, Y., Iguchi, A. and Sakamoto, N. (1984). Biochemical determination of training effects using insulin clamp technique. *Hormone and Metabolic Research*, **16**, 483–6.

1336. Savage, M.P., Petratis, M.M., Thomson, W.H., Berg, K., Smith, J.L. and Sady, S.P. (1986). Exercise training effects on serum lipids of prepubescent boys and adult men. *Medicine and Science in Sports and Exercise*, **18**, 197–204.

1337. Scanlon, R.K. and Passer, M.W. (1978). Factors related to competitive stress among male youth sport participants. *Medicine and Science in Sports*, **10**, 103–8.

1338. Scanu, A.M. (1978). Plasma lipoproteins and coronary heart disease. *Annals of Clinical Laboratory Science*, **8**, 79–83.

1339. Scarr, S. (1966). Genetic factors in activity motivation. *Child Development*, **37**, 663–71.

1340. Schmidt-Nielsen, K. (1984). *Scaling: Why is Animal Size so Important?*. Cambridge University Press.

1341. Schmucker, B. and Hollman, W. (1974). The aerobic capacity of trained athletes from 6 to 7 years of age. *Acta Paediatrica Belgica*, **28** (Suppl.), 92–104.

1342. Schoeller, D.A. (1988). Measurement of energy expenditure in free-living humans by using doubly labeled water. *Journal of Nutrition*, **118**, 1278–89.

1343. Schoeller, D.A. and Fjeld, C.R. (1991). Human energy metabolism: what have we learned from the doubly labelled water method? *Annual Reviews of Nutrition*, **11**, 355–73.

1344. Schoeller, D.A. and Webb, P. (1984). Five day comparison of the doubly labelled water method with respiratory gas exchange. *American Journal of Clinical Nutrition*, **40**, 153–8.

1345. School Sport Forum (1988). *Sport and Young People*. London, Sports Council.

1346. Schulman, J.L. and Reisman, J.M. (1959). An objective measure of hyperactivity. *American Journal of Mental Deficiency*, **64**, 455–6.

1347. Schulman, J.L., Stevens, T.M. and Kupst, M.J. (1977). The biomotometer: a new device for the measurement and remediation of hyperactivity. *Child Development*, **48**, 1152–4.

1348. Schwab, R.S. (1953). Motivation in measurements of fatigue. In W.F. Floyd and A.T. Welford (Eds.), *Symposium on Fatigue*. London, Lewis, p. 245.

1349. Schwane, J.A. and Cundiff, D.E. (1979). Relationships among cardio-respiratory fitness, regular physical activity and plasma lipids in young adults. *Metabolism*, **28**, 771–6.

1350. Schwartz, L., Britten, E.H. and Thompson, L.R. (1928). Studies in physical development and posture I. The effect of exercise in the physical condition and development of adolescent boys. *Public Health Bulletin*, **179**, 1–38.

1351. Scow, R.O., Blanchette-Mackie, E.J. and Smith, L.C. (1980). Transport of lipid across capillary endothelium. *Federation Proceedings*, **39**, 2610–17.

1352. Seals, D.R. and Hagberg, J.M. (1984). The effect of exercise training on human hypertension: a review. *Medicine and Science in Sports and Exercise*, **16**, 207–15.

1353. Secher, N., Vaage, O., Jensen, K. and Jackson, R.C. (1983). Maximal aerobic power in oarsmen. *European Journal of Applied Physiology*, **51**, 155–62.

1354. Secondary Heads Association (1991). *Enquiry into the Provision of Physical Education in Secondary Schools*. Aylesbury, Secondary Heads Association.

1355. Secondary Heads Association (1994). *Enquiry into the Provision of Physical Education in Schools*. Aylesbury, Secondary Heads Association.

1356. Seefeldt, V., Haubenstricker, J., Branta, C.F. and Evans, S. (1988). Physical characteristics of elite young distance runners. In E.W. Brown and C.F. Branta (Eds.), *Competitive Sports for Children and Youth*. Champaign, IL, Human Kinetics, pp. 247–58.

1357. Segal, K.R., Van Loan, M., Fitzgerald, P.I., Hodgson, J.A. and Van Itallie, T.B. (1988). Lean body mass estimation by bioelectrical impedance analysis: a four-site cross-validation study. *American Journal of Clinical Nutrition*, **47**, 7–14.

1358. Seidell, J.C., Bakker, C.J.G. and van der Kooy, K. (1990). Imaging techniques for measuring adipose-tissue distribution: A comparison between computed tomography and 1.5-T magnetic resonance. *American Journal of Clinical Nutrition*, **51**, 953–7.

1359. Seidell, J.C., Bjorntorp, P., Sjostrom, L., Sannerstedt, R., Krokiewski, M. and Kvist, H. (1989). Regional distribution of muscle and fat mass in men: new insight into the risk of abdominal obesity using computer tomography. *International Journal of Obesity*, **13**, 289–303.

1360. Seidell, J.C., Oosterlee, A., Deurenberg, P., Hautvast, J.G.A. and Ruijs, J.H. (1988). Abdominal fat depots measured with computed tomography: effects of degree of obesity, sex and age. *European Journal of Clinical Nutrition*, **42**, 805–15.

1361. Seidell, J.C., Oosterlee, A. and Thjissen, M.A.O. (1987). Assessment of intra-abdominal and subcutaneous abdominal fat: relation between anthropometry and computed tomography. *American Journal of Clinical Nutrition*, **45**, 7–13.

1362. Seliger, V.S., Trefny, S., Bartenkova, S. and Pauer, M. (1974). The habitual physical activity and fitness of 12-year-old boys. *Acta Paediatrica Belgica*, **28**, 54–9.

1363. Seltzer, C.C. and Mayer, J. (1970). An effective weight control program in a public school system. *American Journal of Public Health*, **60**, 679–89.

1364. Sengupta, A., Saka, D., Muklonadhyay, S. and Gosivamn, P. (1979). Relationship between pulse rate and energy expenditure during graded work at different temperatures. *Ergonomics*, **22**, 1207–15.

1365. Sentipal, J.M., Wardlaw, G.M., Mahan, J. and Matkovic, V. (1991). Influence of calcium intake and growth indexes on vertebral bone mineral density in young females. *American Journal of Clinical Nutrition*, **54**, 425–8.

1366. Seresse, O., Lortie, G., Bouchard, C. and Boulay, M.R. (1987). Estimation of the contribution of the various energy systems during maximal work of short duration. *International Journal of Sports Medicine*, **9**, 456–60.

1367. Sewall, L. and Micheli, L.J. (1986). Strength training for children. *Journal of Pediatric Orthopedics*, **6**, 143–6.

1368. Shangold, M.M. (1984). Exercise and the adult female: hormonal and endocrine effects. *Exercise and Sport Sciences Reviews*, **12**, 53–79.

1369. Shapiro, S., Skinner, E.A. and Kessler, L.G. (1984). Utilization of health and mental health services. *Archives of General Psychiatry*, **41**, 971–8.

1370. Sharp, C. (1991). The exercise physiology of children. In V. Grisogono (Ed.), *Children and Sport*. London, Murray, pp. 32–71.

1371. Sharp, M.W. and Reilley, R.R. (1975). The relationship of aerobic physical fitness to selected personality traits. *Journal of Clinical Psychology*, **31**, 428–32.

1372. Shasby, G.B. and Hagerman, F.C. (1975). The effects of conditioning on cardiorespiratory function in adolescent boys. *Journal of Sports Medicine and Physical Fitness*, **15**, 97–107.

1373. Shauer, L.G. (1972). Comparison of physical fitness scores of high school girl smokers and non-smokers. *American Corrective Therapy Journal*, **26**, 174–7.

1374. Sheehan, J.M., Rowland, T.W. and Burke, E.J. (1987). A comparison of four treadmill protocols for determination of maximal oxygen uptake in 10 to 12 year old boys. *International Journal of Sports Medicine*, **8**, 31–4.

1375. Shephard, R.J. (1971). The working capacity of schoolchildren. In R.J. Shephard (Ed.), *Frontiers of Fitness*. Springfield, IL, Charles C. Thomas, pp. 319–45.

1376. Shephard, R.J. (1977). *Endurance Fitness*. Toronto, University of Toronto Press.

1377. Shephard, R.J. (1982). *Physical Activity and Growth*. Chicago, Year Book Medical Publishers.

1378. Shephard, R.J. (1984). Physical activity and "wellness" of the child. In R.A. Boileau (Ed.), *Advances in Pediatric Sport Sciences, Vol. 1, Biological issues*. Champaign, IL, Human Kinetics, pp. 1–28.

1379. Shephard, R.J. (1984). Tests of maximum oxygen intake. A critical review. *Sports Medicine*, **1**, 99–124.

1380. Shephard, R.J. (1986). Fitness of a nation. *Medicine and Sport Science*, **22**, 1–185.

1381. Shephard, R.J. (1986). The Canada fitness survey, some international comparisons. *Journal of Sports Medicine and Physical Fitness*, **26**, 292–300.

1382. Shephard, R.J. (1992). Effectiveness of training programmes for prepubescent children. *Sports Medicine*, **13**, 194–213.

1383. Shephard, R.J. (1994). *Aerobic Fitness and Health*. Champaign, IL, Human Kinetics.

1384. Shephard, R.J. and Bar-Or, O. (1970). Alveolar ventilation in near maximum exercise. Data on pre-adolescent children and young adults. *Medicine and Science in Sports*, **2**, 83–92.

1385. Shephard, R.J. and Godin, G. (1985). Behavioural intentions and activity of children. In J. Rutenfranz, R. Mocellin and F. Klimt (Eds.), *Children and Exercise XII*. Champaign, IL, Human Kinetics, pp. 103–9.

1386. Shephard, R.J., Jequier, J.C., Lavallée, H., La Barre, R. and Rajic, M. (1980). Habitual physical activity: effects of sex, milieu, season and required activity. *Journal of Sports Medicine and Physical Fitness*, **20**, 55–66.

1387. Shephard, R.J., Lavallée H., Jequier, J.C., La Barre, R., Rajic, M. and Beaucage, C. (1978). Seasonal differences in aerobic power. In R.J. Shephard and H. Lavallée (Eds.), *Physical Fitness Assessment – Principles, Practice and Application*. Springfield, IL, Charles C. Thomas, pp. 194–210.

1388. Shephard, R.J., Volle, M., Lavallée H., La Barre, R., Jequier, J.C. and Rajic, M. (1984). Required physical activity and academic grades: a controlled study. In J. Ilmarinen and I. Valimaki (Eds.), *Children and Sport*. Berlin, Springer, pp. 58–63.

1389. Shepherd, J. (1992). Lipoprotein metabolism: an overview. *Annals of the Academy of Medicine*, **21**, 106–13.

1390. Shuleva, K.M., Hunter, G.R., Hester, D.J. and Dunaway, D.L. (1990). Exercise oxygen uptake in 3 through 6 year old children. *Pediatric Exercise Science*, **2**, 130–9.

1391. Siegel, J.A., Camaione, D.N. and Manfredi, T.G. (1989). The effects of upper body resistance training on prepubertal children. *Pediatric Exercise Science*, **1**, 145–54.

1392. Silber, T.J. and Mayer, N.S. (1995). Eating disorders. In B. Goldberg (Ed.), *Sports and Exercise for Children with Chronic Health Conditions*. Champaign, IL, Human Kinetics, pp. 323–34.

1393. Sime, W.E. (1990). Discussion: exercise, fitness and mental health. In C. Bouchard, R.J. Shephard, T. Stephens, J.R. Sutton and B.D. McPherson (Eds.), *Exercise, Fitness, and Health*. Champaign, IL, Human Kinetics, pp. 627–33.

1394. Simon, G., Berg, A., Dickhuth, H.H., Simon-Alt, A. and Keul, J. (1981). Bestimmung der anaeroben Schwelle in Abhängigkeit von Alter und von der Leistungsfähigkeit. (Determination of the anaerobic threshold depending on age and performance potential). *Deutsche Zeitschrift für Sportsmedizin*, **32**, 7–14.

1395. Simon J., Young, J.L., Blood, D.K., Segal, K.R., Case, R.B. and Gutin, B. (1986). Plasma lactate and ventilation threshold in trained and untrained cyclists. *Journal of Applied Physiology*, **60**, 777–81.

1396. Simon, J., Young, J.L., Gutin, B., Blood, D.K. and Case, R.B. (1983). Lactate accumulation relative to the anaerobic and respiratory compensation thresholds. *Journal of Applied Physiology*, **54**, 13–17.

1397. Simons, J., Beunen, G.P., Renson, R., Claessens, A.L.M., Vanreusel, B. and Lefevre, J.A.V. (1990). *Growth and Fitness of Flemish Girls*. Champaign, IL, Human Kinetics.

1398. Simons-Morton, B.G., O'Hara, N.M., Parcel, G.S., Huand, I.W., Baranowski, T. and Wilson, B. (1990). Children's frequency of participation in moderate to vigorous physical activities. *Research Quarterly for Exercise and Sport*, **61**, 307–14.

1399. Simons-Morton, B.G., O'Hara, N.M., Simons-Morton, D.G. and Parcel, G.S. (1987). Children and fitness: a public health perspective. *Research Quarterly for Exercise and Sport*, **58**, 295–302.

1400. Simons-Morton, B.G., Parcel, G.S., O'Hara, N.M., Blair, S.N. and Pate, R.R. (1988). Health-related physical fitness in childhood. *Annual Reviews of Public Health*, **9**, 403–25.

1401. Simons-Morton, B.G., Taylor, W.C. and Huang, I.W. (1994). Validity of the physical activity interview and caltrac with pre-adolescent children. *Research Quarterly for Exercise and Sport*, **65**, 84–8.

1402. Simons-Morton, B.G., Taylor, W.C., Snider, S.A., Huang, I.W. and Fulton, J.E. (1994). Observed level of elementary and middle school children's physical activity during physical education classes. *Preventive Medicine*, **23**, 437–41.

1403. Sinclair, D. (1975). *Human Growth After Birth*. Oxford University Press.

1404. Singh, K.B. (1981). Menstrual disorders in college students. *American Journal of Obstetrics and Gynecology*, **140**, 299–302.

1405. Sinzinger, H. and Virgolini, I. (1988). Effects of exercise on parameters of blood coagulation, platelet function and the prostaglandin system. *Sports Medicine*, **6**, 238–45.

1406. Siri, W.E. (1961). Body composition from fluid spaces and density: analysis of methods. In J. Brozek and A. Henschel (Eds.), *Techniques for Measuring Body Composition*. Washington, DC, National Academy of Sciences, pp. 223–4.

1407. Sjodin, B. (1982). The relationship between running economy, aerobic power, muscle power, and onset of blood lactate accumulation in young boys (11–15 years). In P.V. Komi (Ed.), *Exercise and Sport Biology*. Champaign, IL, Human Kinetics, pp. 57–60.

1408. Sjodin, B. and Jacobs, I. (1981). Onset of blood lactate accumulation and marathon running performance. *International Journal of Sports Medicine*, **2**, 23–6.

1409. Sjodin, B., Jacobs, I. and Karlsson, J. (1981). Onset of blood lactate accumulation and enzyme activities in m. vastus lateralis in man. *International Journal of Sports Medicine*, **2**, 166–70.

1410. Sjodin, B., Schele, R., Karlsson, J., Linnarsson, D. and Wallensten, R. (1982). The physiological background of onset of blood lactate accumulation. In P.V. Komi (Ed.), *Exercise and Sport Biology*. Champaign, IL, Human Kinetics, pp. 43–55.

1411. Sjodin, B. and Svedenhag, J. (1992). Oxygen uptake during running as related to body mass in circumpubertal boys: a longitudinal study. *European Journal of Applied Physiology*, **65**, 150–7.

1412. Sjostrom, L. and Kvist, H. (1988). Regional body fat measures with CT-scan and evaluation of anthropometric predictions. *Acta Medica Scandinavica*, **723** (Suppl.), 169–77.

1413. Skinner, J.S., Bar-Or, O., Bergsteinova, V., Bell, C.W., Royer, D. and Buskirk, E.R. (1971). Comparison of continuous and intermittent tests for determining maximal oxygen intake in children. *Acta Paediatrica Scandinavica*, **217**, 24–8.

1414. Slaughter, M.H., Lohman, T.G., Boileau, R.A., Horswill, C.A., Stillman, R.J., VanLoan, M.D. *et al.* (1988). Skinfold equations for examination of body fatness in children and youth. *Human Biology*, **60**, 709–23.

1415. Sleap, M. (1990). Promoting health in primary school physical education. In N. Armstrong (Ed.), *New Directions in Physical Education, Vol. 1*. Champaign, IL, Human Kinetics, pp. 17–36.

1416. Sleap, M. and Warburton, P. (1992). Physical activity levels of 5–11-year-old children in England determined by continuous observation. *Research Quarterly for Exercise and Sport*, **63**, 238–45.

1417. Sleap, M. and Warburton, P. (1994). Physical activity levels of preadolescent children in England. *British Journal of Physical Education Research Supplement*, **14**, 2–6.

1418. Slemenda, C.W., Christian, J.C., Williams, C.J., Norton, J.A. and Johnston, C.C. (1991). Genetic determinants of bone mass in adult women: a reevaluation of the twin model and the potential importance of gene interaction on heritability estimates. *Journal of Bone Mineral Research*, **6**, 561–7.

1419. Slemenda, C.W., Hui, S.L., Longcope, C. and Johnston, C.C. (1989). Cigarette smoking, obesity and bone mass. *Journal of Bone Mineral Research*, **4**, 737–41.

1420. Slemenda, C.W., Miller, J.Z., Hui, S.L., Reister, T.K. and Johnston, C.C. (1991). Role of physical activity in the development of skeletal mass in children. *Journal of Bone and Mineral Research*, **6**, 1227–33.

1421. Slemenda, C.W., Reister, T.K., Hui, S.L., Miller, J.Z., Christian, J.C. and Johnston, C.C. (1994). Influences on skeletal mineralization in children and adolescents: evidence for varying effects of sexual maturation and physical activity. *Journal of Pediatrics*, **125**, 201–7.

1422. Slemenda, C.W., Reister, T.K., Peacock, M. and Johnson, C.C. (1993). Bone growth in children following the cessation of calcium supplementation. *Journal of Bone Mineral Research*, **8** (Suppl.), S154.

1423. Smith, B.W., Methrey, W.P. and Sparrow, A.W. (1986). Serum lipid and lipoprotein profiles in elite age group runners. In M.R. Weiss and D. Gould (Eds.), *Sport for Children and Youths*. (1984 Olympic Scientific Congress Proceedings, Vol. 10). Champaign, IL, Human Kinetics, pp. 269–73.

1424. Smith, D.M., Nance, W.E., Kang, K.W., Christian, J.C. and Johnston, C.C. (1973). Genetic factors in determining bone mass. *Journal of Clinical Investigations*, **52**, 2800–8.

1425. Smith, E.L., Smith, K.A. and Gilligan, C. (1990). Exercise, fitness, osteoarthritis and osteoporosis. In C. Bouchard, R.J. Shephard, T. Stephens, J.R. Sutton and B.D. McPherson (Eds.), *Exercise, Fitness and Health*. Champaign, IL, Human Kinetics, pp. 607–26.

1426. Smith, J.C. and Hill, D.W. (1991). Contribution of energy systems during a Wingate power test. *British Journal of Sports Medicine*, **25**, 196–9.

1427. Smith, M.L. and Mitchell, J.H. (1993). Cardiorespiratory adaptations to exercise training. In J.L. Durstine, A.C. King, P.L. Painter, J.L. Roitman, L.D. Zwiren and W.L. Kenney (Eds.), *ACSM's Resource Manual for Guidelines for Exercise Testing and Prescription*. Philadelphia, PA, Lea and Febiger, pp. 75–81.

1428. Smith, T.K. (1984). Preadolescent strength training, some considerations. *Journal of Physical Education, Recreation and Dance*, **15**, 91–102.

1429. Smoll, F.L. and Schutz, R.W. (1980). Children's attitudes toward physical activity: a longitudinal analysis. *Journal of Sport Psychology*, **2**, 137–47.

1430. Snedecor, G.W. and Cochran, W.G. (1980). *Statistical Methods, 7th edition*. Ames, IA, Iowa Press.

1431. Snook, G.A. (1979). Injuries in women's gymnastics. *American Journal of Sports Medicine*, **7**, 241–4.

1432. Snow-Harter, C. and Marcus, R. (1991). Exercise, bone mineral density, and osteoporosis. *Exercise and Sport Sciences Reviews*, **19**, 351–88.

1433. Sofranko, A.J. and Nolan, M.F. (1972). Early life experiences and adult sports participation. *Journal of Leisure Research*, **4**, 6–18.

1434. Sonstroem, R.J. (1984). Exercise and self-esteem. *Exercise and Sport Sciences Reviews*, **12**, 123–55.

1435. Sonstroem, R.J. and Morgan, W.P. (1989). Exercise and self-esteem: rationale and model. *Medicine and Science in Sports and Exercise*, **21**, 329–37.

1436. Sorensen, T.I.A. and Sonne-Holm, S. (1977). Mortality in extremely overweight young men. *Journal of Chronic Disease*, **30**, 359–67.

1437. Soto, K.I., Zauner, C.W. and Otis, A.B. (1983). Cardiac output in pre-adolescent competitive swimmers and in untrained normal children. *Journal of Sports Medicine and Physical Fitness*, **23**, 291–300.

1438. South Western Council for Sport and Recreation (1984). *From School to Community*. Crewekerne, Sports Council.

1439. Soutter, W.P., Sharp, F. and Clark, D.M. (1978). Bedside estimation of whole blood lactate. *British Journal of Anaesthesia*, **50**, 445–50.

1440. Spady, D.W. (1980). Total daily energy expenditure of healthy, free ranging schoolchildren. *American Journal of Clinical Nutrition*, **33**, 755–66.

1441. Speakman, J.R., Nair, K.S. and Goran, M.I. (1993). Revised equations for calculating CO_2 production from doubly labelled water in humans. *American Journal of Physiology*, **264**, E912–E917.

1442. Sports Council (1993). *Women and Sport*. London, Sports Council.

1443. Sports Council (1993). *Young People and Sport*. London, Sports Council.

1444. Sports Council (1995). *Young People and Sport: National Survey Selected Findings*. London, Sports Council.

1445. Sports Council for Wales (1995). *Why Boys and Girls Come Out to Play*. Cardiff, Sports Council for Wales.

1446. Sprynarová, S. (1987). The influence of training on physical and functional growth before, during and after puberty. *European Journal of Applied Physiology*, **56**, 719–24.

1447. Sprynarová, S., Párizková, J. and Bunc, V. (1987). Relationships between body dimensions and resting and working oxygen consumption in boys aged 11 to 18 years. *European Journal of Applied Physiology*, **56**, 725–36.

1448. Sprynarová, S., Párizková, J. and Irinová, I. (1978). Development of the functional capacity and body composition of boy and girl swimmers aged 12–15 years. In J. Borms and M. Hebbelinck (Eds.), *Pediatric Work Physiology*. Basel, Karger, pp. 32–8.

1449. Spurr, G.B. and Reina, J.C. (1990). Daily pattern of % $\dot{V}O_2$ max and heart rate in normal and undernourished schoolchildren. *Medicine and Science in Sports and Exercise*, **22**, 643–52.

1450. Stager, J.M., Robertshaw, D. and Miescher, E. (1984). Delayed menarche in swimmers in relation to age at onset of training and athletic performance. *Medicine and Science in Sports and Exercise*, **16**, 550–5.

1451. Stamler, J. (1978). Lifestyles, major risk factors, proof and public policy. *Circulation*, **58**, 3–19.

1452. Stamler, J., Berkson, D.M., Lindberg, H.A., Hall, Y., Miller, W., Mojonnier, L. *et al.* (1966). Coronary risk factors. *Medical Clinics of North America*, **50**, 230–54.

1453. Stanitski, C.L. (1989). Common injuries in preadolescent and adolescent athletes. Recommendations for prevention. *Sports Medicine*, **7**, 32–41.

1454. Stary, H.C. (1983). Macrophages in coronary artery and aortic intima and in atherosclerotic lesions of children and young adults up to age 29. In G. Schettler, A.M. Gotto, G. Middelhoff, A.J.R. Habenicht and K.R. Jurutka (Eds.), *Atherosclerosis VI*. Berlin, Springer, pp. 462–6.

1455. Stary, H.C. (1983). Structure and ultrastructure of the coronary artery intima in children and young adults up to age 29. In G. Schettler, A.M. Gotto, G. Middelhoff, A.J.R. Habenicht and K.R. Jurutka (Eds.), *Atherosclerosis VI*. Berlin, Springer, pp. 82–6.

1456. Staten, M.A., Totty, W.G. and Kohrt, W.M. (1989). Measurement of fat distribution by magnetic resonance imaging. *Investigating Radiology*, **24**, 345–9.

1457. Steen, S.N. and Brownell, K.D. (1986). Nutrition assessment of college wrestlers. *The Physician and Sports Medicine*, **14**, 100–16.

1458. Stefanick, M.L. (1993). Exercise and diabetes mellitus. *Exercise and Sport Sciences Reviews*, **21**, 363–96.

1459. Stefanik, P.A., Heald, F.P. and Mayer, J. (1959). Caloric intake in relation to energy output of obese and non-obese adolescent boys. *American Journal of Clinical Nutrition*, **7**, 55–62.

1460. Stegmann, H. and Kindermann, W. (1982). Comparison of prolonged exercise tests at the individual anaerobic threshold and the fixed anaerobic threshold of 4 mmol.l^{-1}. *International Journal of Sports Medicine*, **3**, 105–10.

1461. Stephens, K.E., Van Huss, W.D., Olson, H.W. and Montoye, H.J. (1984). The longevity, morbidity and physical fitness of former athletes – an update. In H.M. Eckert and H.J. Montoye (Eds.), American Academy of Physical Education, *Exercise and Health*. Champaign, IL, Human Kinetics, pp. 101–9.

1462. Steplock, D.A., Veicsteinas, A. and Mariani, M. (1971). Maximal aerobic and anaerobic power and stoke volume of the heart in a subalpine population. *Internationale Zeitschift für Angewandte Physiologie*, **29**, 203–14.

1463. Stevens, G.H.J., Wilson, B.W. and Raven, P.B. (1986). Aerobic contribution to the Wingate test. *Medicine and Science in Sports and Exercise*, **18** (Suppl.), S2.

1464. Stewart, K.J. and Goldberg, A.P. (1992). Exercise, lipids and obesity in adolescents with parental history of coronary disease. *American Journal of Health Promotion*, **6**, 430–6.

1465. Stewart, K.J. and Gutin, B. (1976). Effects of physical training on cardiorespiratory fitness in children. *Research Quarterly*, **47**, 110–20.

1466. Stolz, H.R. and Stolz, L.M. (1951). *Somatic Development of Adolescent Boys*. New York, MacMillan.

1467. Stone, M.H. and Obryant, H.S. (1987). *Weight Training: A Scientific Approach*. Minneapolis, MN, Bellwether Press.

1468. Stone, M.H., Fry, A.C., Ritchie, M., Stoessel-Ross, L. and Marsit, J.L. (1994). Injury potential and safety aspects of weightlifting movements. *National Strength and Conditioning Association Journal*, **16**, 15–21.

1469. Strand, B. and Reeder, S. (1993). Using heart rate monitors in research of fitness levels of children in physical education. *Journal of Teaching in Physical Education*, **12**, 215–20.

1470. Stransky, A.W., Mickelson, R.J., Van Fleet, C. and Davis, R. (1979). Effects of a swimming training regimen on hematological, cardiorespiratory and body composition changes in young females. *Journal of Sports Medicine and Physical Fitness*, **19**, 347-54.

1471. Stratton, G. and Armstrong, N. (1990). Children's physical activity in physical education lessons as assessed by heart rate telemetry and observational techniques. *Journal of Sport Sciences*, **8**, 299.

1472. Stratton, G. and Armstrong, N. (1991). Children's heart rate responses to indoor games lessons. *Journal of Sport Sciences*, **9**, 432.

1473. Stratton, R., Wilson, D.P., Endres, R.K. and Goldstein, D.E. (1987). Improved glycemic control in insulin-dependent diabetic adolescents. *Diabetes Care*, **10**, 589–93.

1474. Strauss, R.H. (1989). Anabolic steroid use by young athletes. In N.J. Smith (Ed.), *Common Problems in Pediatric Sports Medicine*. Chicago, Year Book Medical Publishers, pp. 125–30.

1475. Strazzullo, P., Cappuccio, F.P., Trevisan, M., De Lea, L., Krogh, V., Giorgione, N. *et al.* (1988). Leisure time physical activity and blood pressure in schoolchildren. *American Journal of Epidemiology*, **127**, 726–33.

1476. Strobino, L.J., French, G.O. and Colonna, P.C. (1952). The effect of increasing tensions on the growth of epiphyseal bone. *Surgery, Gynecology and Obstetrics*, **95**, 694–700.

1477. Strong, J.P. and McGill, H.C. (1969). The pediatric aspects of atherosclerosis. *Journal of Atherosclerosis Research*, **9**, 251–65.

1478. Strong, J.P., Newman, W.P., Freedman, D.S., Gard, P.D., Tracy, R.E. and Solberg, L.A. (1986). Atherosclerotic disease in children and young adults: relationship to cardiovascular risk factors. In G.S. Berenson (Ed.), *Causation of Cardiovascular Risk Factors in Children*. New York, Raven Press, pp. 27–41.

1479. Strong, W.B. (1978). *Atherosclerosis: Its Pediatric Aspects*. New York, Grune and Stratton.

1480. Strong, W.B. (1990). Physical activity and children. *Circulation*, **81**, 1697–701.

1481. Strong, W.B., Miller, M.D., Striplin, M. and Salehbhai, M. (1978). Blood pressure response to isometric and dynamic exercise in healthy black children. *American Journal of Diseases of Children*, **132**, 587–91.

1482. Stucky-Ropp, R.C. and Di Lorenzo, T.M. (1993). Determinants of exercise in children. *Preventive Medicine*, **22**, 880–9.

1483. Stunkard, A.J. and Burt, V. (1967). Obesity and the body image: II. Age at onset of disturbances in the body. *American Journal of Psychiatry*, **123**, 1443.

1484. Stunkard, A.J. and Pestka, J. (1962). The physical activity of obese girls. *American Journal of Diseases of Children*, **103**, 116–21.

1485. Sundberg, S. and Elovainio, R. (1982). Cardiorespiratory function in competitive endurance runners aged 12–16 years compared with ordinary boys. *Acta Paediatrica Scandanavica*, **71**, 987–92.

1486. Sundgot-Borgen, J. (1992). *Eating disorders in female elite athletes*. Department of Biology and Sports Medicine, Norwegian University of Sport and Physical Education, Oslo.

1487. Sundgot-Borgen, J. (1993). Prevalence of eating disorders in female elite athletes. *International Journal of Sport Nutrition*, **3**, 29–40.

1488. Sundgot-Borgen, J. (1994). Eating disorders in female athletes. *Sports Medicine*, **17**, 176–88.

1489. Sundgot-Borgen, J. (1994). Risk and trigger factors for the development of eating disorders in female elite athletes. *Medicine and Science in Sports and Exercise*, **26**, 414–19.

1490. Sundgot-Borgen, J. and Corbin, C.B. (1987). Eating disorders among female athletes. *The Physician and Sports Medicine*, **15**, 89–95.

1491. Sundgot-Borgen, J. and Larsen, S. (1993). Pathogenic weight-control methods and self-reported eating disorders in female elite athletes and controls. *Scandinavian Journal of Medicine and Science in Sports*, **3**, 150–5.

1492. Sundgot-Borgen, J. and Larsen, S. (1993). Preoccupation with weight and menstrual function in female elite athletes. *Scandinavian Journal of Medicine and Science in Sports*, **3**, 156–63.

1493. Sunnegardh, J. and Bratteby, L.E. (1987). Maximal oxygen uptake, anthropometry and physical activity in a randomly selected sample of 8 and 13 year old children in Sweden. *European Journal of Applied Physiology*, **56**, 266–72.

1494. Sunnegardh, J., Batteby, L.E., Sjölin, S., Hagman, U. and Hoffstedt, A. (1985). The relation between physical activity and energy intake of 8 and 13 year old children in Sweden. In R.A. Binkhorst, H.C.G. Kemper and W.H.M. Saris (Eds.), *Children and Exercise XI*. Champaign, IL, Human Kinetics, pp. 183–93.

1495. Superko, R.H. (1991). Exercise training, serum lipids, and lipoprotein particles: is there a change threshold? *Medicine and Science in Sports and Exercise*, **23**, 677–85.

1496. Suter, E. and Hawes, M.R. (1993). Relationship of physical activity, body fat, diet and blood lipid profile in youths 10–15 yr. *Medicine and Science in Sports and Exercise*, **25**, 748–54.

1497. Szmukler, G.I., Eisler, I., Gillis, I. and Hayward, M.E. (1985). The implications of anorexia nervosa in a ballet school. *Journal of Psychiatric Research*, **19**, 177–81.

1498. Tall, A.R. (1990). Plasma high density lipoproteins: metabolism and relationship to atherogenesis. *Journal of Clinical Investigation*, **86**, 379–84.

1499. Talmage, R.U. and Anderson, J.J.B. (1984). Bone density loss in women: effects of childhood activity, exercise, calcium intake and estrogen therapy. *Calcified Tissue International*, **36**, 552.

1500. Tamir, I., Heiss, G., Glueck, C.J., Christensen, B., Kwiterovich, P. and Rifkind, B.M. (1981). Lipid and lipoprotein distribution in white children ages 6–19 yr. The Lipid Research Clinics Program Prevalence Study. *Journal of Chronic Disease*, **34**, 27–39.

1501. Tanaka, H. and Shindo, M. (1985). Running velocity at blood lactate threshold of boys aged 6–15 years compared with untrained and trained young males. *International Journal of Sports Medicine*, **6**, 90–4.

1502. Tanner, J.M. (1949). Fallacy of per-weight and per-surface area standards and their relation to spurious correlation. *Journal of Applied Physiology*, **2**, 1–15.

1503. Tanner, J.M. (1962). *Growth at Adolescence, 2nd edition*. Oxford, Blackwell Scientific Publications.

1504. Tanner, J.M. (1975). *Foetus into Man*. London, Open Books.

1505. Tanner, J.M., Whitehouse, R.H., Marshall, W.A., Healy, M.J.R. and Goldstein, H. (1983). *Assessment of Skeletal Maturity and Prediction of Adult Height (TW2 Method), 2nd edition*. London, Academic Press.

1506. Tanner, J.M., Whitehouse, R.J. and Takaishi, M. (1966). Standards from birth to maturity for height, weight, height velocity and weight velocity: British children, 1965 – I. *Archives of Disease in Childhood*, **41**, 454–71.

1507. Tappe, M.K., Duda, J.L. and Ehrnwald, P.M. (1989). Perceived barriers to exercise among adolescents. *Journal of School Health*, **59**, 153–5.

1508. Taras, H.L., Sallis, J.F., Patterson, T.L., Nader, P.R. and Nelson, J.A. (1989). Television's influence on children's diet and physical activity. *Developmental and Behavioral Pediatrics*, **10**, 176–80.

1509. Taylor, C.B., Sallis, J.F. and Needle, R. (1985). The relations of physical activity and exercise to mental health. *Public Health Reports*, **100**, 195–200.

1510. Taylor, H.L., Buskirk, E.R. and Henschel, A. (1955). Maximal oxygen intake as an objective measure of cardiorespiratory performance. *Journal of Applied Physiology*, **8**, 73–80.

1511. Tejada, C., Strong, J.P., Montenegro, M.R., Restrepo, C. and Solberg, L. (1968). Distribution of coronary and aortic atherosclerosis by geographic location, race and sex. *Laboratory Investigations*, **18**, 509–26.

1512. Telema, R. and Laakso, L. (1983). Habitual physical activity. *Publications of the National Board of Health, Series Original Reports, Helsinki*, **4**, 49–69. Cited by R. Telema, J. Viikari, I. Valimaki, H. Siren-Tiusanen, H.K. Akerblom, M. Uhari *et al.* (1985). Atherosclerosis precursors in Finnish children and adolescents. X. Leisure-time physical activity. *Acta Paediatrica Scandinavica*, **318**, 169–80.

1513. Telema, R. and Silvennoinen, M. (1979). Structure and development of 11- to 19-year-olds' motivation for physical activity. *Scandinavian Journal of Sports Science*, **1**, 23–31.

1514. Telema, R., Viikari, J., Valimaki, I., Siren-Tiusanen, H., Akerblom, H.K., Uhari, M. *et al.* (1985). Atherosclerosis precursors in Finnish children's and adolescents' leisure time physical activity. *Acta Paediatrica Scandinavica*, **318**, 169–80.

1515. Tell, G.S. (1985). Cardiovascular disease risk factors related to sexual maturation: the Oslo Youth Study. *Journal of Chronic Disease*, **38**, 633–42.

1516. Tell, G.S. and Vellar, O.D. (1988). Physical fitness, physical activity and cardiovascular disease risk factors in adolescence. The Oslo Youth Study. *Preventive Medicine*, **17**, 12–24.

1517. Tell, G.S., Vellar, O.D. and Monrad-Hansen, H.P. (1981). Risk factors for chronic diseases in Norwegian schoolchildren. *Preventive Medicine*, **10**, 211–25.

1518. Terney, R. and McClain, L.G. (1990). The use of anabolic steroids in high school students. *American Journal of Diseases of Children*, **144**, 99–103.

1519. Tharp, G.D., Newhouse, R.K., Uffelman, L., Thorland, W.G. and Johnson, G.O. (1985). Comparison of sprint and run times with performance on the Wingate anaerobic test. *Research Quarterly for Exercise and Sport*, **56**, 73–6.

1520. Theintz, G.E. (1994). Endocrine adaptation to intensive physical training during growth. *Clinical Endocrinology*, **41**, 267–72.

1521. Theintz, G., Buchs, B., Rizolli, R., Slosman, D., Clavien, H., Sizonenko, P.E. *et al.* (1992). Longitudinal monitoring of bone mass accumulation in healthy adolescents: evidence for a marked reduction after 16 years of age at the levels of lumbar spine and femoral neck in female subjects. *Journal of Clinical Endocrinology and Metabolism*, **75**, 1060–6.

1522. Thirlaway, K. and Benton, D. (1993). Physical activity in primary- and secondary-school children in West Glamorgan. *Health Education Journal*, **52**, 37–41.

1523. Thoden, J.S. (1991). Testing aerobic power. In J.D. MacDougall, H.A. Wenger and H.J. Green (Eds.), *Physiological Testing of the High-Performance Athlete*. Champaign, IL, Human Kinetics, pp. 107–74.

1524. Thomas, J.R. and French, K.E. (1985). Gender differences across age in motor performance: a meta-analysis. *Psychological Bulletin*, **98**, 260–82.

1525. Thomas, J.R. and French, K.E. (1986). The use of meta-analysis in exercise and sport: a tutorial. *Research Quarterly for Exercise and Sport*, **57**, 196–204.

1526. Thomas, J.R. and Thomas, K.T. (1988). Development of gender differences in physical activity. *Quest*, **40**, 219–29.

1527. Thomasset, A. (1962). Bio-electrical impedance measurements. *Lyon Medical*, **207**, 107–18.

1528. Thomasset, A. (1963). Bio-electrical properties of tissues. *Lyon Medical*, **209**, 1325–52.

1529. Thompson, J.K., Jarvie, G.J., Lahey, B.B. and Cureton, K.J. (1982). Exercise and obesity: etiology, physiology and intervention. *Psychological Bulletin*, **91**, 55–9.

1530. Thorland, W.G. and Gilliam, T.B. (1981). Comparison of serum lipids between habitually high and low active pre-adolescent males. *Medicine and Science in Sports and Exercise*, **13**, 316–21.

1531. Tietz, N.W. (1986). *Textbook of Clinical Chemistry*. Philadelphia, PA, W.B. Saunders.

1532. Tipton, C.M. (1984). Exercise, training and hypertension. *Exercise and Sport Sciences Reviews*, **12**, 245–306.

1533. Tipton, C.M. (1991). Exercise, training and hypertension: an update. *Exercise and Sport Sciences Reviews*, **15**, 447–505.

1534. Tolfrey, K. and Armstrong, N. (1992). The relationship between blood lactate responses to incremental exercise and age. *Journal of Sports Sciences*, **10**, 563–4.

1535. Torg, J.S., Pavlov, H., Cooley, L.H., Bryant, M.H. and Arnoczky, S.P. (1982). Stress fractures of the tarsal navicular: a retrospective study of twenty-one cases. *Journal of Bone and Joint Surgery*, **64A**, 700–12.

1536. Torun, B. (1983). Inaccuracy of applying energy expenditure rates of adults to children. *American Journal of Clinical Nutrition*, **38**, 813–14.

1537. Toth, M.J., Goran, M.I., Ades, P.A., Howard, D.B. and Poehlman, E.T. (1993). Examination of data normalization procedures for expressing peak $\dot{V}O_2$ data. *Journal of Applied Physiology*, **75**, 2288–92.

1538. Toten, L. (1986). Practical considerations in strengthening the prepubescent athlete. *National Strength and Conditioning Association Journal*, **8**, 38–40.

1539. Townsend, J., Wilkes, H., Haines, A. and Jarvis, M. (1991). Adolescent smokers seen in general practice: health, lifestyle, physical measurements, and response to antismoking advice. *British Medical Journal*, **303**, 947–50.

1540. Tran, Z.V., Weltman, A., Glass, G.V. and Mood, D.P. (1983). The effects of exercise on blood lipids and lipoproteins: a meta-analysis of studies. *Medicine and Science in Sports and Exercise*, **15**, 393–402.

1541. Treiber, F.A., Musante, L., Hartdagan, S., Davis, H., Levy, J. and Strong, W.B. (1989). Validation of a heart rate monitor for children in laboratory and field settings. *Medicine and Science in Sports and Exercise*, **21**, 338–42.

1542. Treloar, A.E., Boynton, R.E., Behn, B.G. and Brown, B.W. (1967). Variation of human menstrual cycle through reproductive life. *International Journal of Fertility*, **12**, 77–126.

1543. Trevisan, L., Bents, R., Bosworth, E. and Elliot, D. (1989). A sequential study of anabolic steroid use and availability among high school football athletes. *Medicine and Science in Sport and Exercise*, **21** (Suppl.), S25.

1544. Tsanakas, J.N., Bannister, O.M., Boon, A.W. and Milner, R.D.G. (1986). The "Sport Tester" a device for monitoring the free running test. *Archives of Disease in Childhood*, **61**, 912–14.

1545. Tucker, L.A. (1986). The relationship of television watching to physical fitness and obesity. *Adolescence*, **21**, 797–806.

1546. Tullos, H.S. and King, J.W. (1972). Lesions of the pitching arm in adolescents. *Journal of the American Medical Association*, **220**, 264–71.

1547. Turner, J.G., Gilchrist, N.L., Ayling, E.M., Hassall, A.J., Hooke, E.A. and Sadler, W.A. (1992). Factors affecting bone mineral density in high school girls. *New Zealand Medical Journal*, **105**, 95–6.

1548. Tursz, A. and Crost, M. (1986). Sports-related injuries in children: a study of their characteristics, frequency and severity with comparison to other types of accidental injuries. *American Journal of Sports Medicine*, **14**, 294–9.

1549. Tylavsky, F.A., Anderson, J.J.B., Talmage, R.V. and Taft, T.N. (1992). Are calcium intakes and physical activity patterns during adolescence related to radial bone mass of white college-age females? *Osteoporosis International*, **2**, 232–40.

1550. Uhari, M. (1985). Evaluation of the measurement of children's blood pressure in an epidemiological multicentre study. *Acta Paediatrica Scandinavica*, **318**, 79–88.

1551. Updyke, W.F. and Willett, M.S. (1989). *Physical Fitness Trends in American Youth, 1980–1989*. Bloomington, IN, Indiana University.

1552. Vaccaro, P. and Clarke, D.H. (1978). Cardiorespiratory alterations in 9 to 11 year old children following a season of competitive swimming. *Medicine and Science in Sports*, **10**, 204–7.

1553. Vaccaro, P., Clarke, D.H. and Morris, A.F. (1980). Physiological characteristics of young well-trained swimmers. *European Journal of Applied Physiology*, **44**, 61–6.

1554. Vaccaro, P. and Mahon, A. (1987). Cardiorespiratory responses to endurance training in children. *Sports Medicine*, **4**, 352–63.

1555. Vaccaro, P. and Mahon, A.D. (1989). The effects of exercise on coronary heart disease risk factors in children. *Sports Medicine*, **8**, 139–53.

1556. Vaccaro, P., Zauner, C.W. and Updyke, W.F. (1977). Resting and exercise respiratory function in well-trained child swimmers. *Journal of Sports Medicine and Physical Fitness*, **17**, 297–306.

1557. Valimaki, I., Hursti, M.L., Pihlakoski, L. and Viikari, J. (1980). Exercise performance and serum lipids in relation to physical activity. *International Journal of Sports Medicine*, **1**, 132–6.

1558. van der Walt, L.A., Wilmsen, E.N. and Jenkins, T. (1978). Unusual sex hormone patterns among desert dwelling gatherers. *Journal of Clinical Endocrinology and Metabolism*, **46**, 658–63.

1559. Van Loan, M.D. (1990). Bioelectrical impedance analysis to determine fat-free mass, total body water and body fat. *Sports Medicine*, **10**, 205–17.

1560. Van Praagh, E., Bedu, M., Falgairette, G., Fellmann, N. and Coudert, J. (1991). Oxygen uptake during a 30s supramaximal exercise in 7 to 15 year old boys. In R. Frenkl and I. Szmodis (Eds.), *Children and Exercise, Pediatric Work Physiology XV*. Budapest, National Institute for Health Promotion, pp. 281–7.

1561. Van Praagh, E., Falgairette, G., Bedu, M., Fellmann, N. and Coudert, J. (1989). Laboratory and field tests in 7-year-old boys. In S. Oseid and K.H. Carlsen (Eds.), *Children and Exercise XIII*. Champaign, IL, Human Kinetics, pp. 11–17.

1562. Van Praagh, E., Fellmann, N., Bedu, M., Falgairette, G. and Coudert, J. (1990). Gender difference in the relationship of anaerobic power output to body composition in children. *Pediatric Exercise Science*, **2**, 336–48.

1563. VandenBergh, M.F.Q., DeMan, S.A., Witteman, C.M., Hofman, A., Trouerbach, W.T. and Grobbee, D.E. (1995). Physical activity, calcium intake, and bone mineral content in children in the Netherlands. *Journal of Epidemiology and Community Health*, **49**, 299–304.

1564. Vanderburgh, P.M., Mahar, M.T. and Chou, C.H. (1995). Allometric scaling of grip strength of body mass in college-age men and women. *Research Quarterly for Exercise and Sport*, **66**, 80–4.

1565. Vanderschueren-Lodeweyckx, M. (1990). Endocrinological control of growth. In G. Beunen, J. Ghesquiére, T. Reybrouck and A.L. Claessens (Eds.), *Children and Exercise*. Stuttgart, Enke, p. 64–76.

1566. Vandewalle, H., Peres, G. and Monod, H. (1987). Standard anaerobic exercise tests. *Sports Medicine*, **4**, 268–89.

1567. Vanreusel, B., Renson, R., Beunen, G., Claessens, A., Lefevre, J., Lysens, R. et al. (1993). Adherence to sport from youth to adulthood: a longitudinal study on socialization. In W. Duquet, P. de Knop and L. Ballaert (Eds.), *Youth Sport*. Brussels, Belgium, VUB Press, pp. 99–109.

1568. Vartiainen, E., Puska, P. and Salonen, J.T. (1982). Serum total cholesterol, HDL-cholesterol and blood pressure levels in 13-year-old children in Eastern Finland. The North Karelia Youth Project. *Acta Medica Scandinavica*, **211**, 95–103.

1569. Vartiainen, E., Puska, P. and Tossavainen, K. (1987). Serum total cholesterol, HDL-cholesterol and blood pressure levels in 15-year-old adolescents in Eastern Finland. *Acta Paediatrica Scandinavica*, **76**, 332–7.

1570. Vartiainen, E., Tuomilehto, J. and Nissen, A. (1986). Blood pressure in puberty. *Acta Paediatrica Scandinavica*, **75**, 626–31.

1571. Vered, Z., Battler, A., Segal, P., Liberman, D., Yerushalmi, Y., Berezin, M. et al. (1984). Exercise induced left ventricular dysfunction in young men with asymptomatic diabetes mellitus (diabetic cardiomyopathy). *American Journal of Cardiology*, **54**, 633–7.

1572. Verschuur, R. and Kemper, H.C.G. (1985). Habitual physical activity. *Medicine and Sport Science*, **20**, 56–65.

1573. Verschuur, R. and Kemper, H.C.G. (1985). Habitual physical activity in Dutch teenagers measured by heart rate. In R.A. Binkhorst, H.C.G. Kemper and W.H.M. Saris (Eds.), *Children and Exercise XI*. Champaign, IL, Human Kinetics, pp. 194–202.

1574. Verschuur, R. and Kemper, H.C.G. (1985). The pattern of daily physical activity. *Medicine and Sport Science*, **20**, 169–86.

1575. Verschuur, R., Kemper, H.C.G. and Besseling, C.W.M. (1984). Habitual physical activity and health in 13- and 14-year-old teenagers. In J. Ilmarinen and I. Valimaki (Eds.), *Children and Sport*. New York, Springer, pp. 255–61.

1576. Vignos, P.J. and Watkins, M.P. (1966). The effect of exercise in muscular dystrophy. *Journal of the American Medical Association*, **197**, 843–8.

1577. Viikari, J., Akerblom, H.K. and Uhari, H. (1985). Atherosclerosis precursors in children and adolescents. *Acta Paediatrica Scandinavica*, **74** (Suppl. 318), 1–237.

1578. Viikari, J., Akerblom, H.K. and Uhari, M. (1987). Atherosclerosis precursors in Finnish children and adolescents. In B.S. Hetzel and G.S. Berenson (Eds.), *Cardiovascular Risk Factors in Childhood: Epidemiology and Prevention*. Amsterdam, Elsevier, pp. 21–42.

1579. Vikan, A. (1985). Psychiatric epidemiology in a sample of 1510 ten-year-old children: 1. prevalence. *Journal of Child Psychology and Psychiatry*, **26**, 55–75.

1580. Vincent, L.M. (1979). *Competing with the sylph: dancers and the pursuit of the ideal body form*. New York, Andrews and McMeel.

1581. Vitug, A., Schneider, S.H. and Rudermman, N.B. (1988). Exercise and type I diabetes mellitus. *Exercise and Sport Sciences Reviews*, **16**, 285–304.

1582. Vokac, Z., Bell, H., Bautz-Holter, H. and Rodahl, K. (1975). Oxygen uptake/heart rate relationship in leg and arm exercise, sitting and standing. *Journal of Applied Physiology*, **39**, 54–9.

1583. Voller, R.D. and Strong, W.B. (1981). Pediatric aspects of atherosclerosis. *American Heart Journal*, **101**, 815–36.

1584. von Dobeln, W. (1956). Maximal oxygen intake, body size and total hemoglobin in normal man. *Acta Physiologica Scandinavica*, **38**, 193–9.

1585. Von Noorden, C. (1907). *Obesity, Metabolism and Practical Medicine, Vol. 3.* Chicago, IL, Kenner.

1586. Vrijens, J. (1978). Muscle strength development in the pre- and post-pubescent age. *Medicine and Sport*, **11**, 152–8.

1587. Wagner, J.A., Robinson, S., Tzankoff, S.P. and Marino, R.P. (1972). Heat tolerance and acclimatization to work in the heat in relation to age. *Journal of Applied Physiology*, **33**, 616–22.

1588. Wallace, J.P., McKenzie, T.L. and Nader, P.R. (1985). Observed vs recalled exercise behaviour, a validation of a 7-day exercise recall for boys 11–13 years old. *Research Quarterly for Exercise and Sport*, **56**, 161–5.

1589. Wallberg-Henriksson, H. (1992). Exercise and diabetes mellitus. *Exercise and Sport Sciences Reviews*, **20**, 339–68.

1590. Walsh, M.L. and Bannister, E.W. (1988). Possible mechanisms of the anaerobic threshold: a review. *Sports Medicine*, **5**, 269–302.

1591. Wanne, O., Viikari, J. and Valimaki, I. (1984). Physical performance and serum lipids in 14–16 year old trained, normally active and inactive children. In J. Ilmarinen and I. Valimaki (Eds.), *Children and Sport*. New York, Springer, pp. 241–6.

1592. Wardle, J. and Beales, S. (1986). Restraint, body image and food attitudes in children from 12 to 18 years. *Appetite*, **7**, 209–17.

1593. Warren, M.P. (1980). The effects of exercise on pubertal progression and reproductive function in girls. *Journal of Clinical Endocrinology and Metabolism*, **51**, 1150–6.

1594. Warren, M.P. (1983). Effects of undernutrition on reproductive function in the human. *Endocrinology Reviews*, **4**, 363–77.

1595. Warren, M.P., Brooks-Gunn, J., Hamilton, L.H., Warren, L.F. and Hamilton, W.G. (1986). Scoliosis and fractures in young ballet dancers: relation to delayed menarche and secondary amenorrhea. *New England Journal of Medicine*, **314**, 1348–53.

1596. Washburn, R.A. and Montoye, H.J. (1986). The assessment of physical activity by questionnaire. *American Journal of Epidemiology*, **123**, 563–76.

1597. Washington, R.L. (1989). Anaerobic threshold in children. *Pediatric Exercise Science*, **1**, 244–56.

1598. Washington, R.L. (1993). Anaerobic threshold. In T.W. Rowland (Ed.), *Pediatric Laboratory Exercise Testing*. Champaign, IL, Human Kinetics, pp. 115–30.

1599. Washington, R.L., VanGundy, J.C., Cohen, C., Sondheimer, H. and Wolfe, R. (1988). Normal aerobic and anaerobic exercise data for North American school-age children. *Journal of Pediatrics*, **112**, 223–33.

1600. Wasserman, K. (1984). The anaerobic threshold measurement to evaluate exercise performance. *American Review of Respiratory Disease*, **129** (Suppl.), S35–S40.

1601. Wasserman, K., Whipp, B.J., Koyal, S.N. and Beaver, W.L. (1973). Anaerobic threshold and respiratory gas exchange during exercise. *Journal of Applied Physiology*, **35**, 236–43.

1602. Watkins, L.O. and Strong, W.B. (1984). The child: when to begin preventative cardiology. *Current Problems in Pediatrics*, **14**, 1–71.

1603. Watson, A.W.S. and O'Donovan, D.J. (1977). Influences of level of habitual activity on physical work capacity and body composition of postpubertal school boys. *Quarterly Journal of Experimental Physiology*, **62**, 325–32.

1604. Watson, R. (1974). Bone growth and physical activity in young males. In R. Mazess (Ed.), *International Conference on Bone Mineral Measurements*. Washington, DC, US Government Printing Office, pp. 380–5.

1605. Weaver, M.R. and Vadgama, P.M. (1986). An O_2 based enzyme electrode for whole blood lactate measurement under continuous flow conditions. *Clinica Chimica Acta*, **155**, 295–308.

1606. Webb, D.R. (1990). Strength training in children and adolescents. *Pediatric Clinics of North America*, **37**, 1187–210.

1607. Webber, L.S., Baugh, J.G., Cresanta, J.L. and Berenson, G.S. (1983). Transition of cardiovascular risk factors from adolescence to young adulthood: the Bogalusa post high school study. *Circulation*, **74** (Suppl.), 111–60.

1608. Webber, L.S., Cresanta, J.L., Voors, A.W. and Berenson, G.S. (1983). Tracking of cardiovascular disease risk factor variables in school age children. *Journal of Chronic Diseases*, **36**, 647–60.

1609. Webber, L.S., Srinivasen, S.R., Wattigney, W.A. and Berenson, G.S. (1991). Tracking of serum lipids and lipoproteins from childhood to adulthood. *American Journal of Epidemiology*, **133**, 884–99.

1610. Weber, G., Kartodihardjo, W. and Klissouras, V. (1976). Growth and physical training with reference to heredity. *Journal of Applied Physiology*, **40**, 211–15.

1611. Weil, M.H., Leavy, J.A., Rackow, E.C. and Halfman, C.J. (1986). Validation of a semi-automated technique for measuring lactate in whole blood. *Clinical Chemistry*, **32**, 2175–7.

1612. Weiner, J.S. and Lourie, J.A. (Eds.) (1981). *Practical Human Biology*. London, Academic Press.

1613. Weirman, M.E. and Crowley, W.F. (1986). Neuroendocrine control of the onset of puberty. In F. Falkner and J.M. Tanner (Eds.), *Human Growth, Vol. 2, Postnatal Growth*. London, Plenum Press, pp. 225–41.

1614. Weissinger, E., Housh, T.J., Johnson, G.O. and Evans, S.A. (1991). Weight loss behaviour in high school wrestling: wrestler and parent perceptions. *Pediatric Exercise Science*, **3**, 64–73.

1615. Welch, M.J. and Priest, R.F. (1989). Anabolic steroid use among high school athletes. *Medicine and Science in Sports and Exercise*, **21** (Suppl.), S25.

1616. Welk, G.J. and Corbin, C.B. (1995). The validity of the Tritrac-R3D activity monitor for the assessment of physical activity in children. *Research Quarterly for Exercise and Sport*, **66**, 202–9.

1617. Wells, C.L. (1985). *Women, Sport and Performance: a Physiological Perspective*. Champaign, IL, Human Kinetics.

1618. Wells, C.L. (1986). The effects of physical activity on cardiorespiratory fitness in children. In American Academy of Physical Education, *Effects of Physical Activity on Children*. Champaign, IL, Human Kinetics, pp. 114–26.

1619. Wells, C.L. and Plowman, S.A. (1988). Relationship between training, menarche and amenorrhea. In E.W. Brown and C.F. Branta (Eds.), *Competitive Sports for Children and Youth*. Champaign, IL, Human Kinetics, pp. 195–211.

1620. Welsman, J. and Armstrong, N. (1992). Daily physical activity and blood lactate indices of aerobic fitness. *British Journal of Sports Medicine*, **26**, 228–32.

1621. Welsman, J. and Armstrong, N. (1995). The interpretation of peak volume oxygen ($\dot{V}O_2$) in prepubertal children. In F.J. Ring (Ed.), *Children in Sport*. Bath, Centre for Continuing Education, pp. 64–9.

1622. Welsman, J.R. and Armstrong, N. (1996). Post-exercise lactates in children and adolescents. In E. Van Praagh (Ed.), *Anaerobic Power and Capacity During Childhood and Adolescence*. Champaign, IL, Human Kinetics, (in press).

1623. Welsman, J., Armstrong, N. and Kirby, B. (1994). Serum testosterone is not related to peak $\dot{V}O_2$ and submaximal blood lactate responses in 12–16 year old males. *Pediatric Exercise Science*, **6**, 120–7.

1624. Welsman, J.R., Armstrong, N., Nevill, A.M., Winter, E.M. and Kirby, B.J. (1996). Scaling peak $\dot{V}O_2$ for differences in body size. *Medicine and Science in Sports and Exercise*, **28**, 259–65.

1625. Welsman, J.R., Armstrong, N. and Winsley, R.J. (1996). Scaling the relationship between thigh volume, thigh muscle volume and peak $\dot{V}O_2$ in prepubertal girls. *Pediatric Exercise Science*, **8**, 177–8.

1626. Welten, D.C., Kemper, H.C.G., Post, G.B., Van Mechelen, W., Twisk, J., Lips, P. *et al.* (1994). Weight-bearing activity during youth is a more important factor for peak bone mass than calcium intake. *Journal of Bone and Mineral Research*, **9**, 1089–96.

1627. Welten, D.C., Post, G.B. and Kemper, H.C.G. (1995). Bone mineral density and dietary calcium intake. In H.C.G. Kemper (Ed.), *The Amsterdam Growth Study*. Champaign, IL, Human Kinetics, pp. 236–46.

1628. Weltman, A. (1989). Weight training in prepubertal children: physiologic benefit and potential damage. In O. Bar-Or (Ed.), *Advances in Pediatric Sport Sciences, Vol. 3*. Champaign, IL, Human Kinetics, pp. 101–30.

1629. Weltman, A., Janney, C., Rians, C.B., Strand, K., Berg, B., Tippitt, S. *et al.* (1986). The effects of hydraulic resistance strength training in pre-pubertal males. *Medicine and Science in Sports and Exercise*, **18**, 629–38.

1630. Weltman, A., Janney, C., Rians, C.B., Strand, K. and Katch, F.I. (1987). The effects of hydraulic-resistance strength training on serum lipid levels in prepubescent boys. *American Journal of Diseases of Children*, **141**, 777–80.

1631. Weltman, A., Snead, D., Seip, R., Schurrer, R., Levine, S., Rutt, R. *et al.* (1987). Prediction of lactate threshold and fixed blood lactate concentrations from 3200m running performance in male runners. *International Journal of Sports Medicine*, **8**, 401–6.

1632. Weltman, A., Tippett, S., Janney, C., Strand, K., Rians, C., Cahill, B.R. *et al.* (1988). Measurement of isokinetic strength in prepubertal males. *Journal of Orthopaedic and Sports Physical Therapy*, **9**, 345–51.

1633. Weltman, J., Seip, R., Levine, S., Snead, D., Rogol, A. and Weltman, A. (1989). Prediction of lactate threshold and fixed blood lactate concentrations from

3200m time trial running performance in untrained females. *International Journal of Sports Medicine*, **10**, 207–11.

1634. Wenger, H.A. and Bell, G.J. (1986). The interactions of intensity, frequency and duration of exercise training in altering cardiorespiratory fitness. *Sports Medicine*, **3**, 346–56.

1635. Wessel, J.A., Montoye, H.J. and Mitchell, H. (1965). Physical activity assessment by recall method. *American Journal of Public Health*, **55**, 1430–6.

1636. Westcott, W.L. (1979). Female responses to weight training. *Journal of Physical Education*, **77**, 31–3.

1637. Westcott, W.L. (1980). Effects of teacher modelling on children's peer encouragement behavior. *Research Quarterly for Exercise and Sport*, **51**, 585–7.

1638. Westerp, K.R., Brouns, F., Saris, W.H.M. and Hoor, F.T. (1988). Comparison of doubly labelled water method with respirometry at low and high-activity levels. *Journal of Applied Physiology*, **65**, 53–6.

1639. Westgard, J.O., Lahmeyer, B.L. and Birnbaum, M.L. (1972). Use of the DuPont "Automatic Clinical Analyser" in direct determination of lactic acid in plasma stabilised with sodium fluoride. *Clinical Chemistry*, **18**, 1334–8.

1640. Weymans, M., Reybrouck, T., Stijns, H. and Knops, J. (1985). Influence of age and sex on the ventilatory anaerobic threshold in children. In R.A. Binkhorst, H.C.G. Kemper and W.H.M. Saris (Eds.), *Children and Exercise XI*. Champaign, IL, Human Kinetics, pp. 114–18.

1641. Weymans, M.L., Reybrouck, T.M., Stijns, H.J. and Knops, J. (1986). Influence of habitual levels of physical activity on the cardiorespiratory endurance capacity of children. In J. Rutenfranz, R. Mocellin and F. Klimt (Eds.), *Children and Exercise XII*. Champaign, IL, Human Kinetics, pp. 149–56.

1642. Wheeler, G.D., Wall, S.R., Belcastro, A.N. and Cumming, D.C. (1984). Reduced serum testosterone and prolactin levels in male distance runners. *Journal of the American Medical Association*, **252**, 514–16.

1643. Whipp, B.J. and Wasserman, K. (1972). Oxygen uptake kinetics for various intensities of constant load work. *Journal of Applied Physiology*, **33**, 351–6.

1644. White, C.M., Hergenroeder, A.C. and Klish, W.J. (1992). Bone mineral density in 15- to 21-year-old eumenorrheic and amenorrheic subjects. *American Journal of Diseases of Children*, **146**, 31–5.

1645. Widdowson, E.M. (1947). A study of individual children's diets. *Medical Research Council Special Series No. 257*. London, His Majesty's Stationery Office.

1646. Wieliczko, M.C., Gobert, M. and Mallet, E. (1991). La practique du sport chez l'enfant diabetique. Enquete dans la region Rouennaise. *Annals of Pediatrics (Paris)*, **38**, 84–8.

1647. Wilkins, K.E. (1980). The uniqueness of the young athlete: musculoskeletal injuries. *American Journal of Sports Medicine*, **5**, 377–82.

1648. Willerman, L. (1973). Activity level and hyperactivity in twins. *Child Development*, **44**, 288–93.

1649. Willerman, L. and Plomin, R. (1973). Activity level in children and their parents. *Child Development*, **44**, 854–8.

1650. Williams, A. (1979). Physical education in the junior school: a study of the teachers involved. *Bulletin of Physical Education*, **15**, 5–13.

1651. Williams, A. (1988). Physical activity patterns among adolescents – some curriculum implications. *Physical Education Review*, **11**, 28–39.

1652. Williams, A. (1996). Physical education at key stage 2. In N. Armstrong (Ed.), *New Directions in Physical Education, Vol. 3, Change and Innovation*. London, Cassell, pp. 62–72.

1653. Williams, C. and Armstrong, N. (1995). Optimised peak power output of adolescent children during maximal sprint pedalling. In F.J. Ring (Ed.), *Children in Sport*. Bath, Centre for Continuing Education, pp. 40–4.

1654. Williams, C.A., Armstrong, N. and Powell, J. (1995). The effects of continuous and interval training programmes on the anaerobic and aerobic performance of prepubertal boys. *Paper presented to the XVIII International Seminar on Pediatric Work Physiology*, Faaborg, Denmark,.

1655. Williams, C.L., Carter, B.J. and Wynder, E.L. (1981). Prevalence of selected cadiovascular and cancer risk factors in a pediatric population: the "Know Your Body" Project, New York. *Preventive Medicine*, **10**, 235–50.

1656. Williams, J.R. and Armstrong, N. (1991). Relationship of maximal lactate steady state to performance at fixed blood lactate reference values in children. *Pediatric Exercise Science*, **3**, 333–41.

1657. Williams, J.R. and Armstrong, N. (1991). The influence of age and sexual maturation on children's blood lactate responses to exercise. *Pediatric Exercise Science*, **3**, 111–20.

1658. Williams, J.R., Armstrong, N. and Kirby, B. (1990). The 4 mmol·L^{-1} blood lactate level as an index of exercise performance in 11–13 year old children. *Journal of Sports Sciences*, **8**, 139–47.

1659. Williams, J.R., Armstrong, N. and Kirby, B. (1992). The influence of the site of sampling and assay medium upon the measurement and interpretation of blood lactate responses to exercise. *Journal of Sports Sciences*, **10**, 95–107.

1660. Williams, J.R., Armstrong, N., Winter, E.M. and Crichton, N. (1992). Changes in peak oxygen uptake with age and sexual maturation in boys: physiological fact or statistical anomaly? In J. Coudert and E. Van Praagh (Eds.), *Children and Exercise XVI*. Paris, Masson, pp. 35–7.

1661. Williams, P.T., Krauss, R.M., Vranizan, K.M. and Wood, P.D. (1990). Changes in lipoprotein subfractions during diet-induced and exercise-induced weight loss in moderately overweight men. *Circulation*, **81**, 1293–1304.

1662. Williams, T.M. and Handford, A.G. (1986). Television and other leisure activities. In T.M. Williams (Ed.), *The Impact of Television: A Natural Experiment in Three Communities*. Orlando, FL, Academic Press, pp. 143–213.

1663. Wilmore, J.H. (1983). Body composition in sport and exercise: direction for future research. *Medicine and Science in Sports and Exercise*, **15**, 21–31.

1664. Wilmore, J.H. (1991). Eating and weight disorders in female athletes. *International Journal of Sport Nutrition*, **1**, 104–17.

1665. Wilmore, J.H. (1995). Disordered eating in the young athlete. In C.J.R. Blimkie and O. Bar-Or (Eds.), *New Horizons in Pediatric Exercise Science*. Champaign, IL, Human Kinetics, pp. 161–78.

1666. Wilmore, J.H. and Costill, D.L. (1994). *Physiology of Sport and Exercise.* Champaign, IL, Human Kinetics.

1667. Wilmore, J.H. and McNamara, J.J. (1974). Prevalence of coronary heart disease risk factors in boys, 8 to 12 years of age. *Journal of Pediatrics*, **84**, 527–33.

1668. Wilmore, J.H., Constable, S.H., Stanforth, P.R., Tsao, W.Y., Rotkis, T.C., Paicius, R.M. *et al.* (1982). Prevalence of coronary heart disease risk factors in 13- to 15-year-old boys. *Journal of Cardiac Rehabilitation*, **2**, 223–33.

1669. Wilmore, J.H., Wambsgans, K.C., Bremner, M., Broeder, C.E., Paijmans, I., Volpe, J.A. *et al.* (1992). Is there energy conservation in amenorrheic compared with eumenorrheic distance runners? *Journal of Applied Physiology*, **72**, 15–22.

1670. Windsor, R. and Dumitru, D. (1989). Prevalence of anabolic steroid use by male and female adolescents. *Medicine and Science in Sports and Exercise*, **21**, 494–7.

1671. Winsley, R., Armstrong, N. and Welsman, J. (1995). Leg volume is not related to peak oxygen uptake in 9-year-old boys. In F.J. Ring (Ed.), *Children in Sport*. Bath, Centre for Continuing Education, pp. 70–6.

1672. Winter, E.M. (1991). Cycle ergometry and maximal intensity exercise. *Sports Medicine*, **11**, 351–7.

1673. Winter, E.M. (1992). Scaling: partitioning out differences in size. *Pediatric Exercise Science*, **4**, 296–301.

1674. Winter, E.M., Brooks, F.B.C. and Hamley, E.J. (1991). Maximal exercise performance and lean leg volume in men and women. *Journal of Sports Sciences*, **9**, 3–13.

1675. Winter, J.S.D. (1978). Prepubertal and pubertal endocrinology. In F. Falkner and J.M. Tanner (Eds.), *Human Growth, Vol. 2, Postnatal Growth*. New York, Plenum Press, pp. 183–213.

1676. Wirth, A., Trager, E., Scheele, K., Mayer, D., Diehm, K., Reisch, K. *et al.* (1978). Cardiopulmonary adjustment and metabolic response to maximal and submaximal physical exercise of boys and girls at different stages of maturity. *European Journal of Applied Physiology*, **39**, 229–40.

1677. Wood, P.D. (1987). Exercise, plasma lipids, weight regulation. In Coronary Prevention Group, *Exercise Heart Health*. London, Coronary Prevention Group, pp. 35–46.

1678. Wood, P.D. and Stefanick, M. (1990). Exercise, fitness and atherosclerosis. In C. Bouchard, R.J. Shephard, T. Stephens, J.R. Sutton and B.D. McPherson (Eds.), *Exercise, Fitness and Health*. Champaign, IL, Human Kinetics, pp. 409–24.

1679. Wood, P.D., Stefanick, M.L., Dreon, D.M., Fray-Hewitt, B., Garay, S.C., Williams, P.T. *et al.* (1988). Changes in plasma lipids and lipoproteins in overweight men during weight loss through dieting as compared with exercise. *New England Journal of Medicine*, **319**, 1173–9.

1680. Wood, P.D., Stefanick, M.L., Williams, P.T. and Haskell, W.L. (1991). The effects on plasma lipoproteins of a prudent weight-reducing diet, with or without exercise, in overweight men and women. *New England Journal of Medicine*, **325**, 461–6.

1681. Woods, E.R., Wilson, C.D. and Masland, R.P. (1988). Weight control methods in high school wrestlers. *Journal of Adolescent Health Care*, **9**, 394–7.

1682. Working Group on Arteriosclerosis of the National Heart, Lung and Blood Institute (1981). Report of the Working Group on Arteriosclerosis of the National Heart, Lung and Blood Institute, Vol. 2. *National Institute of Health Publication No. 81-2035*, Washington, USA.

1683. Working Party on Ethics of Research in Children (1980). Guidelines to aid ethical committees considering research involving children. *British Medical Journal*, **280**, 229–31.

1684. Working Part on Research in Children (1991). *The Ethical Conduct of Research in Children*. London, Medical Research Council.

1685. World Health Organization (1947). Constitution of the World Health Organization. *Chronicle of the World Health Organization*, **1**, 1–2.

1686. World Health Organization (1982). *Prevention of Coronary Heart Disease*. (Technical Report Series 678). Geneva, World Health Organization.

1687. World Health Organization (1985). *Blood Pressure Studies in Children*. (Technical Report 715). Geneva, World Health Organization.

1688. World Health Organization (1994). Report of WHO study group: assessment of fracture risk and its application to screening for post-menopausal osteoporosis. *WHO Technical Series*, 843. Geneva, World Health Organization.

1689. Woynarowska, B. (1980). The validity of different estimations of maximal oxygen uptake in children 11–12 years of age. *European Journal of Applied Physiology*, **43**, 19–23.

1690. Wright, D. (1993). Treating and managing injuries in children. In M. Lee (Ed.), *Coaching Children in Sport*. London, Spon, pp. 225–35.

1691. Wynder, E.L., Williams, C.L., Laakso, K. and Levenstein, M. (1981). Screening for risk factors for chronic disease in children from fifteen countries. *Preventive Medicine*, **10**, 121–32.

1692. Yates, A. (1991). *Compulsive exercise and eating disorders*. New York, Brunner-Mazel.

1693. Yates, C. and Grana, W.A. (1981). Adaptations of prepubertal children to exercise. *Journal of Oklahoma State Medical Association*, **74**, 173–7.

1694. Ylitalo, V.M. (1984). Exercise performance and serum lipids in obese schoolchildren before and after a reconditioning program. In J. Ilmarinen and I. Valimaki (Eds.), *Children and Sport*. Berlin, Springer, pp. 247–54.

1695. Yoesting, D.R. and Burkhead, D.L. (1973). Significance of childhood recreation experience on adult leisure behaviour. An explanatory analysis. *Journal of Leisure Research*, **5**, 25–36.

1696. Yoshida, T. (1984). Effect of exercise duration during incremental exercise on the determination of anaerobic threshold and the onset of blood lactate accumulation. *European Journal of Applied Physiology*, **53**, 196–9.

1697. Yoshida, T. (1987). Current topics and concepts of lactate and gas exchange thresholds. *Journal of Human Ergology*, **16**, 103–21.

1698. Yoshida, T., Chida, M., Khioka, M. and Suda, Y. (1987). Blood lactate parameters related to aerobic capacity and endurance performance. *European Journal of Applied Physiology*, **56**, 7–11.

1699. Yoshida, T., Suda, Y. and Takeuchi, N. (1982). Endurance training regimen based upon arterial blood lactate: effects on anaerobic threshold. *European Journal of Applied Physiology*, **49**, 223–30.

1700. Yoshizawa, S. (1972). A comparative study of aerobic work capacity in urban and rural adolescents. *Journal of Human Ergology*, **1**, 45–65.

1701. Yoshizawa, S., Honda, H., Urushibara, M. and Nakamura, N. (1989). Aerobic-anaerobic energy supply and daily physical activity level in young children. In S. Oseid and K.-H. Carlsen (Eds.), *Children and Exercise XIII*. Champaign, IL, Human Kinetics, pp. 47–56.

1702. Yoshizawa, S., Ishizake, T. and Honda, H. (1977). Physical fitness of children aged 5 and 6 years. *Journal of Human Ergology*, **6**, 41–51.

1703. Yost, L.J., Zauner, C.W. and Jaeger, M.J. (1981). Pulmonary diffusing capacity and physical working capacity in swimmers and non-swimmers during growth. *Respiration*, **42**, 8–14.

1704. Young, C.M. and DiGiacomo, M.M. (1965). Protein utilization and changes in body composition during weight reduction. *Metabolism*, **14**, 1084–94.

1705. Young, T.L. and Rogers, T.L. (1986). School performance characteristics preceding onset of smoking in high school students. *American Journal of Diseases of Children*, **140**, 257–9.

1706. Zakus, G., Lee Chin, M., Cooper, H. Jr., Makovsky, E. and Merrill, C. (1981). Treating adolescent obesity: a pilot project in a school. *Journal of School Health*, December, 663–6.

1707. Zanconato, S., Buchthal, S., Barstow, T.J. and Cooper, D.M. (1993). $_{31}$P-magnetic resonance spectroscopy of leg muscle metabolism during exercise in children and adults. *Journal of Applied Physiology*, **74**, 2214–18.

1708. Zanconato, S., Cooper, D.M. and Armon, Y. (1991). Oxygen cost and oxygen uptake dynamics and recovery with 1 min of exercise in children and adults. *Journal of Applied Physiology*, **71**, 993–8.

1709. Zapletal, A., Misur, M. and Samanek, M. (1971). Static recoil pressure of the lungs in children. *Bulletin de Physiopathologie Respiratoire*, **7**, 139–43.

1710. Zauner, C.W. and Benson, N.Y. (1981). Physiological alterations in young swimmers during three years of intensive training. *Journal of Sports Medicine and Physical Fitness*, **21**, 179–85.

1711. Zauner, C.W., Maksud, M.G. and Melichna, J. (1989). Physiological considerations in training young athletes. *Sports Medicine*, **8**, 15–31.

1712. Zeek, P. (1930). Juvenile arteriosclerosis. *Archives of Pathology*, **10**, 417–46.

1713. Zimmerman, D.R. (1987). Maturation and strenuous training in young female athletes. *The Physician and Sports Medicine*, **15**, 219–22.

1714. Zinman, B., Murray, F.T., Vranic, M., Albiser, A.M., Leiobel, S., McClean, P.A. *et al.* (1977). Glucoregulation during moderate exercise in insulin treated diabetics. *Journal of Clinical Endocrinology and Metabolism*, **45**, 641–52.

Index